FIGHTING GOLIATH

Exposing the flawed science and statistics behind the COVID-19 event

First Edition

Prof. (Emeritus) Norman Fenton PhD

Prof. Martin Neil PhD

With foreword by Nick Hudson

Sovereign Rights Publishing

DISCLAIMER

The content of this book is intended for informational and educational purposes only and is not a substitute for professional medical advice, diagnosis, or treatment. Readers are advised that the information contained herein should not be used to make any health-related decisions without consulting a qualified healthcare professional. The authors and publisher of this book make no representations or warranties with respect to the accuracy, applicability, fitness, or completeness of the contents of this book. They shall not be liable for any direct, indirect, consequential, or exemplary damages arising from the use or misuse of any information provided. Always seek the advice of your physician or other qualified health provider with any questions you may have regarding a medical condition.

This book contains information obtained from authentic and highly regarded sources. Reasonable efforts have been made to publish reliable data and information, but the authors and publisher cannot assume responsibility for the validity of all materials or the consequences of their use. The authors and publishers have attempted to trace the copyright holders of all materials reproduced in this publication and apologize to copyright holders if permission to publish in this form has not been obtained. If any copyright material has not been acknowledged, please write and tell us how we may rectify in any future reprint.

Sovereign Rights Publishing

Printed in the United Kingdom

Available from Amazon.com

First Printing Edition, 2024

ISBN: 978-1-0687498-2-7

"Fenton & Neil were pioneers in exposing the extent to which flawed and easily manipulated data were used to mislead the public about Covid-19 vaccine safety. This book catalogues their findings."

— **Robert F. Kennedy Jnr**

"So much of the official narrative regarding Covid science was based on faulty methods and faulty ideas. In this book, Norman Fenton & Martin Neil detail the work and thinking they did to untangle the mess and make sense of the data. The next time there is a pandemic declared, the world would do well to embrace incisive voices and thinkers like Norman and Martin so that the policy responses imposed do not create more suffering than they prevent."

— **Professor Jay Bhattacharya PhD**, Director of Stanford University's Center for Demography and Economics of Health and Aging

"This book chronicles Norman & Martin's fight against lockdowns and the narrative of a miraculous vaccine that saved us from a deadly virus"

— **Toby Young**, Associate Editor of The Spectator magazine and creator of the Daily Sceptic blog

"This book documents how the medical community, public health officials, and government agencies misled an unsuspecting public into taking what appears to be the most unsafe vaccine in human history. This book is a two-edged sword. On the one hand, it explains to the public how the authorities manipulated the data to fool the public. On the other hand, it also serves as a guidebook to people in power on how to mislead the public without getting caught."

— **Steve Kirsch**, entrepreneur and founder of the Vaccine Safety Research Foundation

"This is an important book because it reveals the extent to which Governments used flawed studies to deceive most of the population into unnecessarily taking a vaccine which is now known to have caused harm to many".

— **Dr Aseem Malhotra**, cardiologist & writer

"When confronted with a new challenge scientific knowledge and critical analysis should be applied objectively, without bias and groupthink and free of manipulation by external vested interests. This book exposes how the public health and scientific establishments failed these critical tests during Covid-19 leading to a catastrophe for humanity."

— **John Campbell PhD**, retired nurse teacher and former clinical nurse

"Instead of debate, science was censored. Norman & Martin compile the questions that were not allowed to be asked."

— **Dr Clare Craig**, diagnostic pathologist and co-founder of HART (Health Advisory and Recovery Team)

"Fenton and Neil's brilliant substack 'Where are the numbers?' was the authoritative 'go to' for Covid-19 sceptics and dissenters, over the period of Lockdown and its contrived novel 'vaccine' exit. The scrupulous analyses they produced of the official statistics and other significant research data provided a vital resource during that period for all those questioning the official narrative. Its chronological compilation in book form now supplies a critical historic record of the statistical deceit and manipulation practised by Government and media to prop up their narrative."

— **Kathy Gyngell**, editor of The Conservative Woman

"A compelling chronicle of Fenton & Neil's intellectually honest, scientifically rigorous, and relentless pursuit of truth during a time of government-directed data distortion and pandemic propaganda."

— **Jessica Hockett PhD**, independent Covid-19 researcher

"If telling the truth in a time of deceit is a revolutionary act, then Professors Fenton and Neil are honest-to-goodness revolutionaries. Beginning in the early days of the Covid-19 scare, this book traces their valiant struggle against the deluge of falsehoods, armed only with bar charts, unassailable logic and the courage to face the facts no matter the personal or professional cost. You don't need a PhD to understand their work - all you need is an open mind."

— **Josh Guetzkow PhD**, Senior Lecturer, Hebrew University

"Professors Neil and Fenton have consistently and courageously applied rigorous critical thinking to their analyses of the events of the covid era, always eschewing popularity in favour of the pursuit of truth. Their invaluable insights span the entirety of the period since early 2020. Taken as a whole, one is left wondering whether - without the insane response - anything unusual would have been noticed at all and, therefore, whether the 'pandemic' was a totally policy-induced phenomenon rather than a biological event."

— **Dr. Jonathan Engler**, healthcare entrepreneur, co-founder of HART (Health Advisory and Recovery Team)

"With millions of us now aware of the truth behind the Covid-19 'measures' I am grateful to the authors of this book for their persistent efforts to expose this truth."

— **Jessica Rose PhD**, independent Covid-19 researcher

"Epidemiological statistics is hard. But it's practically impossible when the world is bouncing as one about a 'once-in-a-century pandemic'. Norman & Martin kept their cool, and their sober takes throughout put in proportion the real risks of Covid-19, and the massive harms of the interventions."

— **Mark Changizi PhD**, theoretical cognitive scientist and independent Covid-19 researcher

"In the beginning there were two types of people; those who went along, and those who spoke out. However, unlike many who felt something wasn't right but couldn't explain why, Fenton and Neil were uniquely positioned to find the evidence, do the analysis, *and* present the results in easily understood bite-sized pieces. This book brings together their work and, like cleansing water that creates a sinkhole, erodes the foundation on which Goliath stood."

— **Scott McLachlan PhD**, Lecturer in Digital Technologies for Health, Kings College London

"During the Covid-19 pandemic, Fenton & Neil were very rare amongst academics and journalists, in persistently searching for the truth. Despite facing relentless propaganda and attempts to discredit them, they produced an honest chronicle of the real pandemic - iatrogenesis. Their work has exposed the globalist cabal's efforts to control the narrative and revealed the harms caused by pandemic measures. It is a valuable resource."

— **Joel Smalley**, independent Covid-19 researcher

"A wonderful book, by two brave and brilliant scientists who were prepared to stand against the government narrative due to their own findings. from lock downs to masks to vaccines, these men show us the major flaws in what we were told was 'the science'"

— **Leilani Dowding**, media personality, conservative commentator and former Miss Great Britain

"Fenton and Neil are a modern-day Holmes and Watson. A rare example of thinking that is not only independent, but also both meticulous and expansive."

— **Danny Emmett**, independent Covid-19 researcher

"This volume captures the authors' evolving understanding of what has happened to the scientific method, clinical trial ethics, medical and other freedoms, honesty in public discourse and governance since 2020. Careful reading of the book reveals that what has happened is much more frightening than anything an alleged novel pathogen might have done to the way we live our lives."

— **Mike Yeadon, PhD**, ex Chief Scientist and VP, Pfizer Inc.

Table of Contents

Foreword ix

Preface xi

Acknowledgements xv

Online xvii

Authors xix

List of contributing co-authors xxi

Chapter 1. The beginning 1

1.1. In the UK football is the tipping point for Coronavirus lockdown 1

1.2. Coronavirus country comparisons 1

1.3. Problems with studies into Covid-19 risk factors 3

1.4. Covid-19 Infection and fatality rates 4

1.5. UK Covid-19 death rates by religion 6

1.6. A privacy-preserving Bayesian network model 7

1.7. People and Pandemics – A Better World? 7

Chapter 2. The scam starts to be revealed 9

2.1. What is the evidence of a big second wave? 9

2.2. Critical flaw in the Covid-19 'hospital admissions' data 10

2.3. The impact of false positives in Covid testing 12

2.4. Hospital admissions data: evidence of exponential increase? 15

2.5. Why we know so little about Covid-19 from testing data 16

2.6. Covid-19 is Not a High Consequence Infectious Disease 18

2.7. Why the continued Covid-19 lockdowns and restrictions? 19

2.8. Our evidence submitted to UK Parliament 21

2.9. An increasing proportion of people testing positive? 26

Chapter 3. Faking the data to prepare for new lockdown and vaccine rollout 29

3.1. Latest UK Covid-19 statistics roundup 29

3.2. UK Covid Testing data: tests and positivity rate by regions 31

3.3. London goes into Tier 4 lockdown - but the data are flawed 33

3.4. The curious pooled Covid-19 testing ... 34
3.5. How many people 'with Covid' are actually ill? ... 37
3.6. On false positives in Covid-19 testing again ... 38
3.7. The "1 in 3 people with Covid 19 have no symptoms" claim ... 41
Chapter 4. More data shenanigans and censorship as the vaccine is rolled out ... 45
4.1. The Tiffany Dover (collapsing nurse) cover-up ... 45
4.2. Major problem with UK lighthouse laboratories testing ... 46
4.3. The Times attacks our vaccine scepticism ... 48
4.4. The barriers to academic publication ... 50
4.5. NFL Covid-19 protocols ... 51
4.6. The problem with ALL studies into the risks/benefits of Covid-19 vaccines ... 52
4.7. Simpson's paradox and vaccine effectiveness ... 53
4.8. Analysis of COVID-19 vaccine death reports from VAERS ... 54
Chapter 5. The Lancet and the Pfizer study ... 57
5.1. Is the Pfizer vaccine as effective as claimed? ... 57
5.2. The curious case of Dr Sharon Alroy-Preis ... 61
5.3. The Lancet has become a laughing stock ... 63
5.4. The Lancet heavily redact response to our subject access request ... 67
Chapter 6. The 'safe and effective' vaccine narrative crumbles ... 71
6.1. Comparing vaccinated and unvaccinated mortality rates ... 71
6.2. Is vaccine efficacy a statistical illusion? ... 73
6.3. Impact of miscategorising deaths when evaluating vaccine safety ... 77
6.4. Further concerns about systematic miscategorisation ... 78
6.5. New ONS report on deaths by vaccination ... 79
6.6. Covid-19: Definitions matter - and these are real ... 81
6.7. Undercounting of deaths in first two weeks of vaccination ... 83
6.8. Why are UKHSA obfuscating data on stillbirths by vaccine status ... 84
6.9. The Bangladesh Mask Study ... 86
6.10. Why did Frontiers publish a flawed study? ... 87
Chapter 7. How the BBC and ONS pushed a false narrative about the unvaccinated ... 89

7.1. The BBC claim of "8% unvaccinated against Covid" 89
7.2. BBC's biased 'vaccine experts' 90
7.3. Critique of BBC2 documentary 'Unvaccinated' 91
7.4. BBC response to our complaint about 'Unvaccinated' 95
7.5. More updates on BBC2 documentary 'Unvaccinated' 96
7.6. BBC response to our follow-up complaint 96
7.7. Did the documentary breach regulations? 98
7.8. About that ONS estimate of only 8% adults unvaccinated 100
7.9. BBC's final response 101
Chapter 8. More Lies, cover-up and censorship over vaccine safety 103
8.1. Is the vaccine safe for pregnant and breastfeeding women? 103
8.2. Does ONS have data for accurate assessment of vaccine safety? 104
8.3. Are vaccinees especially healthy or especially unhealthy? 105
8.4. ONS data on vaccine mortality not fit for purpose 107
8.5. About those estimates of '20 million lives saved' by the vaccine 109
8.6. A Study in Stupidity 111
8.7. Scientific paper preprint sites censor submissions 111
8.8. How many lives did the Covid-19 vaccines really save? 112
8.9. The CDC's data on covid vaccine safety signals 115
Chapter 9. The Iatrogenesis Hypothesis 119
9.1. The deadly spring 2020 Covid-19 wave 119
9.2. Covid-19 deaths exaggerated by re-attribution. 122
9.3. What really caused the surge in Covid-19 deaths in early 2020? 122
9.4. In defence of alternative explanations for excess deaths 125
Chapter 10. A regulatory win, but bad news and bad data continue 133
10.1. Scottish cardiac ambulance data 133
10.2. UK Statistics Regulator agrees with us 134
10.3. How to create the illusion your vaccine is 90% effective 135
10.4. The latest ONS data on deaths by covid vaccination status 139
10.5. Postmodern science delivers immortality benefits 143

10.6. Summary remarks on new ONS data release 144
Chapter 11. The vanishing flu 145
11.1. Playing hide and seek with the flu 145
11.2. Peek-a-Boo Flu 146
Chapter 12. The vanishing flu detection system 157
12.1. Sensors set to off 157
12.2. Finding the Flu is easy, just Google it! 163
12.3. Do Not Seek and Ye Shall Not Find 165
Chapter 13. The fightback against vaccine hesitancy relied on dodgy data 175
13.1. Claims the unvaccinated were at higher risk were wrong 175
13.2. The 'fact checkers' can't find the target never mind hit it 180
Chapter 14. Censored by academia and the media 183
14.1. Retrospective censorship 183
14.2. Misinformation from the Times and other media sources 185
14.3. The scandal of the AstraZeneca vaccine 186
14.4. How many deaths were caused by the covid vaccines? 188
Chapter 15. The cheap trick, exaggerated mortality and FDA lies 195
15.1. The Cheap Trick 195
15.2. When lack of safety means safety 198
15.3. The UK Government's flawed Covid-19 death numbers 200
15.4. The Very Best of Cheap Trick 202
Chapter 16. Blasphemer's begone! Censorship, secrets and it gets personal 213
16.1. Blasphemers begone: cancelled by the NHS! 213
16.2. Censored by the academic preprint servers 221
16.3. Why is the MHRA hiding critical vaccine safety data? 223
16.4. AstraZeneca's second most lethal batch 228
Chapter 17. Were Covid-19 respiratory symptoms caused by bacterial pneumonia? 231
17.1. Why this hypothesis? 231
17.2. Mens rea: "the act is not culpable unless the mind is guilty". 231
17.3. Whodunnit opening scene – the first victim 232

17.4. Scene two: Panic! 233
17.5. Which was first on the crime scene: SARS-CoV-2 or pneumonia? 234
17.6. But the pneumonia coinfection rates were low! 236
17.7. Pneumonia has 'previous' 239
17.8. Evidence from the crime scene 240
17.9. A pinpoint pandemic? 241
17.10. The EPIC and other studies 241
17.11. Discussion 242
Chapter 18. Why more ventilation and opioids but fewer antibiotics? 243
18.1. How did antibiotics use change? 243
18.2. Policy for the treatment Covid-19 243
18.3. Changes in antibiotic prescribing patterns 245
18.4. Physicians defying public health authorities 245
18.5. Was ventilation an accomplice? 248
18.6. Increased Fentanyl and Midazolam use in NYC hospitals 253
18.7. But they were given antibiotics in ICU! 254
18.8. DNRs and official recognition of higher mortality 255
18.9. Covid-19 ventilation: A policy made in America 256
Chapter 19. Celebrating the NHS, informed consent, and eye-opening discussions 261
19.1. I helped protect the NHS 261
19.2. The scandal of the EU/Pfizer contract is even worse than reported 264
19.3. Informed consent statement on covid policies 265
19.4. An explosive discussion with ex-CDC scientist 268
Chapter 20. Was Covid-19 novel and deadly? 273
20.1. 'Spikeopathy' does not explain Covid-19's 'novel' symptoms 273
20.2. The debate – dissecting Dr Kory's response 286
20.3. Differential diagnosis 291
Chapter 21. From horror fiction to cross reactivity in PCR testing 293
21.1. A New Years Eve Horror Story 293
21.2. Unacceptably high cross reactivity in PCR testing 294

21.3. The Australian respiratory season puzzle ... 304
21.4. PCR positives using single genes as the rule ... 308
Chapter 22. Virus origins and gain (claim) of function research ... 311
22.1. There is nothing novel about a novel virus ... 311
22.2. MERS-CoV and SARS and the fallacy of a single cause ... 312
22.3. Would we recognise a novel virus when we see it? ... 314
22.4. Are spike proteins, inserts and furin cleavage sites dangerous or novel? ... 317
22.5. Novelty of the SARS-CoV-2 furin cleavage site ... 319
22.6. Is engineering of more lethal viruses possible? ... 320
22.7. Gain (or loss) of function experiments ... 323
22.8. Contradictory evidence on zoonotic origins ... 325
22.9. GoF research is routine and involves creating (infectious?) clones ... 327
22.10. If not lab leak or wet market, then how did 'it' arise? ... 329
22.11. Discussion ... 331
Chapter 23. Dodgy epidemiology and the ONS admit the cheap trick ... 335
23.1. Exaggerated estimates from epidemiological modelling ... 335
23.2. We were right! ... 344
Chapter 24. Conclusions and Recommendations ... 347
24.1. Virus origins ... 348
24.2. Covid-19 lethality ... 348
24.3. PCR testing ... 349
24.4. Lockdowns and other non-pharmaceutical interventions ... 351
24.5. Vanishing flu ... 351
24.6. Vanishing flu detection system ... 352
24.7. The illusion of a pandemic and Covid-19 waves ... 353
24.8. Virus symptom novelty, spread and risk ... 353
24.9. Swabs and the 'nasal filter' ... 354
24.10. Bacterial pneumonia ... 355
24.11. Iatrogenesis ... 355
24.12. Censorship ... 356

24.13. Vaccine safety and efficacy 356
24.14. Recommendations 358
References 359
Index 393

Foreword

The covid phenomenon has been one of the strangest events in history. From very early on it was clear that official representations regarding the purported pandemic were consistently false. Clear to whom? Not many. To pierce through the ginned-up hysteria of the time, you needed to be willing and able to disregard the headlines, to ferret out and analyze emergent data, and to critique the disconnect between fact and media fiction. It turned out that only a minority of people were able to do that, and the few among that minority who had the courage to speak out were systematically and relentlessly censored and attacked via multiple avenues.

Keeping your head while all about you were losing theirs turned out to be the preserve of a few fortunately independent or very brave souls. Norman Fenton and Martin Neil were two of those. Although the ranks of the covid sceptic community swell inexorably, late joiners are late for a reason, having been let down for some while by a mix of cowardice and uncritical thought processes. Several of these have vaulted into relative media stardom, with meek criticisms of discrete elements of the covid narratives — the "vaccines" or suppression of 'early treatment' being topics seemingly within the new Overton Window, augmented by dubious propositions that add to the burden faced by credible sceptics in their effort to replace a tangled fabrication with an account of things that conforms with reality.

But to master the complexity of the covid phenomenon, to perceive the enormity of the lie, one must stay focused on what the early voices said and how they navigated the elaborate, prodigiously funded and wholly false official narrative. For such purposes, this anthology of articles is a treasure trove. Throughout we mark the signs of clear thought—never saying more than needs to be said, spotting inconsistencies and spelling out the questions they provoke, and originating hypotheses that might account for them.

What is the official narrative? According to it, a "novel deadly virus" sprang into existence in Wuhan in late 2019, either from a zoonotic event or from a lab leak. Hospitals were overwhelmed. Millions were saved by lockdowns, social distancing, contact tracing and mask mandates. The right treatment for the sick involved ventilators or high flow oxygen, and on-label pharmaceuticals such as Remdesivir and Paxlovid. It was useless to use antibiotics or steroids. We had to keep deploying these measures until vaccines arrived. When they did arrive, they were fortunately safe and effective, making you into a dead-end for the virus.

These articles deal a devastating blow to this official narrative. The whole story could be invalidated by one or two refutations, but Norman and Martin leave nothing standing. Can we begin to describe an alternative narrative that bears closer correspondence with reality? I think we can, and it goes something like this:

Inconsequential variants of a virus that was already endemic and of no particular clinical significance were increasingly detected by the spread of inappropriately designed and applied PCR tests. Media, politicians, regulators and officials, thoroughly captured by the pharmaceutical industry, were suddenly all over the false notion that something dangerous was spreading. Pharmaceutical companies faked the development of a vaccine, using studies riddled with scientific fraud. None of the policy measures prevented mortality or morbidity. Instead, serious alterations to standards of care for influenza-like illness killed many. Much of the data used to prop up various elements of the narrative was manipulated or conjured out of thin air. Many of the salient media events were staged. Censorship saw to it that solid refutations of the official narrative never saw the light of day, as far as the general public were concerned. Millions were killed by this, with millions more deaths to come. Unprecedented transfers of wealth to the wealthiest at the expense of all others added insult to injury. Worse still, the intention to recapitulate this catastrophic hoax is clear.

It is unclear whether this alternative narrative will replace the false official one in the minds of a sufficient mass of people to prevent further deterioration in the prospects of mankind. But if we are successful in achieving such a 'coming to Jesus' moment, it will in no small part be due to the assiduous and courageous efforts of Norman and Martin, and the many plucky individuals they influenced along the way.

Nick Hudson

Preface

This book is about how the official Covid-19 narrative was based on flawed and manipulated data and science. This narrative claimed that a deadly virus emerged from China, creating a 'pandemic' and that humanity was eventually saved by unprecedented interventions: lockdowns, and the deployment of a safe and effective miracle vaccine. We question these official claims and show how statistics and science were manipulated to create the hysteria needed to convince people to fear 'the virus' and in response adopt extraordinary changes in their behaviour.

We describe our fight against the establishment 'Goliath', exposing the fact that the data and science underlying the Covid-19 event, in both its origins and response, did not 'add up'. This includes battles against the UK government, regulators, the Orwellian manipulation of the BBC, and academic censorship. We describe our attempts to reveal the flawed and dangerous scientific ideas and wrongheaded assumptions that resulted in the unnecessary collapse of economies and global decline in health.

We expose the flawed and manipulative thinking that underlies modern virology, epidemiology and respiratory medicine and how these latent scientific vulnerabilities were exploited to spin a narrative used to manipulate medical decision making, public health and personal behaviour.

Based on our substack blog, 'Where Are the Numbers?' it asks questions about the data and numbers behind the Covid-19 event. The number of covid cases. The number of dead. The number of positive PCR tests. The number of people vaccinated or unvaccinated. The numbers behind the vaccine clinical trials and observational studies. Our questions are not a shrill request for data, but a challenge to authority to justify and explain the established narrative and its analyses and assumptions.

Unlike most scientific books ours is (mostly) arranged chronologically to provide an honest account of how our analyses, models, hypotheses, and conclusions changed as the 'pandemic' evolved. Hence, the reader can clearly see how our prior views and assumptions were updated over time based on our reactions to new information, in the form of official statistics, scientific studies, data and propaganda. Likewise, the reader will also see how our perspectives radically changed as we engaged with the established media, online trolls, the security services, regulators, government, and big Pharma. For instance, one example of this is how we moved from calling both the virus and the disease Covid-19* (or COVID-19 to use the official nomenclature) to drawing the distinction between the virus (SARS-CoV-2) and the disease (Covid-19). Hence earlier chapters fail to draw this distinction whilst later chapters are much more careful to do so, reflecting our altered views.

We are not claiming that we had the answers from the outset of the 'pandemic' in March 2020 and neither are we claiming that we reached a fully formed unassailable conclusion of the event by the end of it. By organising the book chronologically the reader will see, with the benefit of hindsight, where we took wrong turns or where we made naive assumptions early on, either because we took elements of the official narrative on faith or assumed aspects of the science were sufficiently settled that they could be relied upon.

Why is it important to present the story in this way? Most scientific texts present their contents as fait accompli, as finished fully formed works, with a linear narrative. But that can create the false impression of coherence and certainty. It also fails to place the ideas in a historical, potentially turbulent, and contested context, within which the ideas must be understood. As well as presenting a historical chronology of events as we saw them, much of it is written from a journalistic perspective even though we are not trained journalists; our background is in mathematics, statistics, and computer science. Our justification for writing as journalists, as well as scientists, was simply that so few journalists were brave and independent enough to fulfil this crucial societal function. Someone had to do it, so it fell on us and others.

* Note that throughout this book we will refer to Covid-19, or sometimes Covid, rather than COVID-19, not because there is any semantic distinction between them but simply because it is easier on the eye when repeated many times in a body of text.

Dedicated to

Elma

&

Naomi

Acknowledgements

We are indebted to many people who were co-authors, collaborators and/or colleagues who in their personal or professional capacity, commented on, supported or promoted our work during the last four years, even when it so fiercely challenged the prevailing narrative.

These include (in alphabetical order)*:

Frank Ahmet, Tim Anderson, Glynis Barber, Lorraine Barrat, Amber-Rose Bate St Cliere, Randy Bock, Bryan Bishko, Paul Brennan, Andrew Bridgen, Del Bigtree, Rachel Butcher, John Campbell, Mark Changizi, Jennifer Clark, Rachel Collins, Philip Davies, David Dickson, Laura Dodsworth, Alberto Donzelli, Peter Doshi, Leilani Dowding, Lee and Yvonne Drury, Sonia Elijah, Danny Emmett, Debi Evans, Mike Farris, Mitch Feierstein, Sean Flanagan, Nizza Fluss, Laurence Fox, James Freeman, Shahar Gavish, Maryann Gebauer, Jekka Geffre, Mark Girardo, Cheryl Grainger, Joshua Guetzkow, Tore Gulbrandson, Leslie Katon, Stacey Kauder, Linda Keen, Flor Kent, Pierre Kory, Kathy Gyngell, Karen Harradine, Phil Harper, Tedd Hilbert, Francis Hoar, Renée Hoenderkamp, Seth Holehouse, Arabella Howell, Nick Hudson, Ros Jones, Will Jones, Robert F Kennedy Jnr., Steve Kirsch, Helen Lasn, Matt Le Tissier, Retsef Levi, Kat Lindley, Aseem Malhotra, Robert Malone, Rachel Marcus, David Wiseman, Alexandra Marshall, Peter McCullough, Michael McConville, Peter McIlvenna, Alan Miller, Maajid Nawaz, David Paton, Georgina Prodhan, Neil Oliver, Magda Osman, Claire Pain, Norman Picniazek, Sonia Poulton, Gerry Quinn, RemnantMD, Robbie Robertson, Mike Ryan, Jessica Rose, Ralph Schoelhammer, David Scott, Adrian Shaw, Mark Skidmore, Yaffa Shir Az, Joel Smalley, Mark Steyn, June Slater, Nazarin Veronica, Kate Wand, Howard Stupak, Bret Weinstein, Alex Williams, Mike Yeadon and Toby Young.

We would like to give special thanks to Clare Craig, Jonathan Engler, Scott McLachlan and Jessica Hockett for their contributions to the book, conversations, reviews, comments, humour and insights.

We also acknowledge the vaccine injured who gave their time speaking with us: Alex Mitchell, Jules Serkin and John Watt.

* Note that by listing the named individuals above we are making no implicit or explicit claim that they endorse the contents of this book. The views contained herein, along with any errors or omissions, are entirely the responsibility of the authors and should not be interpreted as representing the opinions, partially or wholly, of any of the above.

Online

Much of our material can be accessed here on our substack 'Where Are the Numbers?' (WATN), by subscription:

wherearethenumbers.substack.com

Note that many of the articles that appear here are abridged versions of the original articles that appear on WATN.

For corrections and updates the book landing page is:

wherearethenumbers.substack.com/fighting-goliath

Other blogs and websites contain additional material:

probabilityandlaw.blogspot.com

www.normanfenton.com

On X / Twitter we are @MartinNeil9 and @profnfenton

On YouTube: https://www.youtube.com/@normanfenton81

On Rumble: rumble.com/user/normanfenton

On Bitchute: bitchute.com/channel/zUwHexBX1ZJH/

On Odysee: odysee.com/@NormanFenton

Authors

Norman E. Fenton is a British mathematician and computer scientist. He is the Professor (Emeritus) of Risk in the School of Electronic Engineering and Computer Science at Queen Mary University of London. Norman has published 7 books and over 400 peer reviewed articles. His research works covers multiple domains including especially Bayesian probability, statistics and its relationship to the law and forensics (he has been an expert witness in major criminal and civil cases), software engineering, and medical health. Since 2020 has been active in analysing data related to the Covid-19 event. Norman has written for the Daily Sceptic, The Conservative Woman, Epoch Times, UK Column, appeared on the BBC, Fox News, GBNews, NDT News, Spectator TV, TNT Radio and multiple podcasts.

Martin Neil is a British statistician and computer scientist. He is a Professor of Computer Science and Statistics in the School of Electronic Engineering and Computer Science at Queen Mary University of London. Martin has published two books and over 100 peer reviewed articles. His research works covers the application of statistics and Bayesian probabilistic reasoning to systems engineering, AI, finance, medical expert systems, computer programming and cyber risk. Since 2020 has been active in analysing data and the science related to the Covid-19 event. Martin has written for The Conservative Woman, Daily Sceptic and Open Guardian.

List of contributing co-authors

Chapter 9 with Nick Hudson and Dr Jonathan Engler

Chapter 11 with Jessica Hockett PhD and Dr Jonathan Engler

Chapter 12 with Jessica Hockett PhD and Dr Jonathan Engler

Chapter 15 with Scott McLachlan PhD

Chapter 17 with Jessica Hockett PhD and Dr Jonathan Engler

Chapter 18 with Jessica Hockett PhD and Dr Jonathan Engler

Chapter 19 with Jessica Hockett PhD and Dr Jonathan Engler

Chapter 20 with Jessica Hockett PhD and Dr Jonathan Engler

Chapter 21 with Dr Jonathan Engler

Chapter 22 with Dr Jonathan Engler

Chapter 23 with Scott McLachlan PhD

Chapter 1. The beginning

1.1. In the UK football is the tipping point for Coronavirus lockdown

13 March 2020

Yesterday the UK Prime Minister, Boris Johnson announced the importance of not cancelling major sporting events; and the Premier League announced there would certainly be no cancellations of this weekend's matches. But anybody with any football knowledge knew that - whatever the Government's risk mitigation plans were for Coronavirus - they would become irrelevant if a single high profile Premiership player or manager became infected. As soon as it was confirmed that Arsenal manager Mikel Arteta had the virus last night, it was inevitable that a total shutdown of all professional football would start and that is precisely what has happened.

Again, anybody with any UK football knowledge knows that this is also a game-changer as far as the whole UK economy is concerned. Millions who were previously unmoved to make any changes will voluntarily go into lock-down after panic buying (Norman noted that the shelves in his supermarket immediately emptied). Note that nothing much changed when it was announced that the Government's own Health Minister got the virus a few days ago. But one key football person getting it was the single trigger for mass change.

We can only assume that the Government risk experts/advisors did not include a single person with football knowledge.

1.2. Coronavirus country comparisons

They are pointless unless we account for these biases in testing (2 April 2020)

Suppose we wanted to estimate how many car owners there are in the UK and how many of those own a Ford Fiesta, but we only have data on those people who visited Ford car showrooms in the last year. If 10% of the showroom visitors owned a Fiesta, then, because of the bias in the sample, this would certainly overestimate the proportion of Ford Fiesta owners in the country.

Estimating death rates for people with Covid-19 is currently undertaken largely along the same lines. In the UK, for example, almost all testing of Covid-19 is performed on people already hospitalised with Covid-19 symptoms. At the time of writing, there are 29,474 confirmed Covid-19 cases (analogous to car owners visiting a showroom) of whom 2,352 have died (Ford Fiesta owners who visited a showroom). But it misses out all the people with mild or no symptoms.

Concluding that the death rate from Covid-19 is on average 8% (2,352 out of 29,474) ignores the many people with Covid-19 who are not hospitalised and have not died (analogous to car owners who did not visit a Ford showroom and who do not own a Ford Fiesta). It is therefore equivalent to making the mistake of concluding that 10% of all car owners own a Fiesta.

There are many prominent examples of this sort of conclusion. The Oxford Covid-19 Evidence Service have undertaken a thorough statistical analysis [1]. They acknowledge potential selection bias and add confidence intervals showing how big the error may be for the (potentially highly misleading) proportion of deaths among confirmed Covid-19 patients.

They note various factors that can result in wide national differences – for example the UK's 8% (mean) "death rate" is very high compared to Germany's 0.74%. These factors include different demographics, for example the number of elderly in a population, as well as how deaths are reported. For example, in some countries everybody who dies after having been diagnosed with Covid-19 is recorded as a Covid-19 death, even if the disease was not the actual cause, while other people may die from the virus without actually having been diagnosed [2] with Covid-19.

However, the models fail to incorporate explicit causal explanations in their modelling that might enable us to make more meaningful inferences from the available data, including data on virus testing.

In the full version of this article [3], which was also published here [4] we produced an initial prototype "causal model" which shows that the Covid-19 death rate is as much a function of sampling methods, testing and reporting, as it is determined by the underlying rate of infection in a vulnerable population. The links between the named variables in the model show how they are dependent on each other. These links, along with other unknown variables, are captured as probabilities. As data are entered for specific, known variables, all of the unknown variable probabilities are updated using a method called Bayesian inference.

Therefore, different countries may appear to have different death rates, but only because they have applied different sampling and reporting policies. It is not necessarily because they are managing the virus any better or that the virus has infected fewer or more people.

With a causal model [5] that explains the process by which the data is generated, we can better account for these differences between countries. We can also more accurately learn the underlying true population infection and death rates from the observed data. Such a model could be extended to include demographic factors, as well as social distancing and other prevention policies. We have developed such models for many similar problems [6] and are currently gathering data required for populating our causal model.

In the absence of community-wide testing, only random testing applied throughout the population will enable us to learn about the number of people with Covid-19 who are asymptomatic or have already recovered. Only when we know how many people don't show symptoms, will we know the underlying infection and death rate. It will also enable us to learn about the accuracy of the tests (false positive and false negative rates).

Random testing therefore remains the most effective strategy to avoid selection bias and reduce the distortions in reported statistics. Ideally, this should be combined with a causal model.

Currently it seems there are no state-wide protocols in place in any country for randomised community testing of citizens for Covid-19. Spain did attempt it. But that involved purchasing large volumes of rapid Covid-19 tests, and they soon discovered that some Chinese-sourced tests had poor validity [7] and reliability delivering only 30% accuracy – resulting in high numbers of false positives.

Countries like Norway have proposed introducing such tests [8], but there is uncertainty around how to legislatively compel citizens to test – and what might constitute an appropriate randomisation protocol. In Iceland, they have voluntary sampling [9] which has covered 3% of the population, but this isn't random. Some countries with large scale testing, like South Korea, might get closer to being random.

The reason it is so hard to achieve random testing is that you have to account for several practical and psychological factors. How does one collect samples randomly? Gathering samples from volunteers may not be sufficient as it does not prevent self-selection bias.

During the H1N1 influenza pandemic of 2009–2010, there was a lot of anxiety about the disease that created "mass psychogenic illness" [10]. This is when hypersensitivity to particular symptoms leads to healthy people self-diagnosing as having a virus – meaning they would be highly incentivised to get tested. This could, in part, further contribute to false positive rates if the sensitivity and specificity of the tests are not fully understood.

While self-selection bias is not going to be eliminated, it could be reduced by running field tests. This could involve asking the public to volunteer samples in locations where, even in a lockdown state, they might be expected to attend and also from those in self-imposed isolation or quarantine.

In any event, when statistics are communicated at press conferences or in the media, it is very important that their limitations are explained and any relevance to the individual or population are properly delineated. It is this which we contend is lacking in the current crisis.

On 9 April 2020 (as an update to the above) in a detailed report [11] we explained the importance of causal modelling in understanding the results of different types of Covid-19 testing in order to expose what is lacking and what is needed to reduce the uncertainty in classifying an individual as infected with Covid-19.

1.3. Problems with studies into Covid-19 risk factors

Why most studies may be producing flawed conclusions - and how to fix the problem (15 May 2020)

In a new paper [12] we extend the recent work by Griffith et al [13] which highlights how 'collider bias' in studies of Covid-19 undermines our understanding of the disease risk and severity. This is typically caused by the data being restricted to people who have undergone Covid-19 testing, among whom healthcare workers are over-represented. For example, collider bias caused by smokers being under-represented in the dataset may (at least partly) explain recent empirical results that suggest smoking reduces the risk of Covid-19.

The new paper makes more explicit use of graphical causal models to interpret observed data. We show that the Griffith et al smoking example can be clarified and improved using

Bayesian network models with realistic data and assumptions. We show that there is an even more fundamental problem for risk factors like 'stress' which, unlike smoking, is more rather than less prevalent among healthcare workers; in this case, because of a combination of collider bias from the biased dataset and the fact that 'healthcare worker' is a confounding variable, it is likely that studies will wrongly conclude that stress reduces rather than increases the risk of Covid-19. Indeed, exactly this has been claimed for hypertension [14] and the same data could even - bizarrely - find factors like 'being in close contact with Covid-19 patients' reducing the risk of Covid-19. To avoid such erroneous conclusions, any analysis of observational data must take account of the underlying causal structure including colliders and confounders. If analysts fail to do this explicitly then any conclusions, they make about the effect of specific risk factors on Covid-19 are likely to be flawed.

1.4. Covid-19 Infection and fatality rates

Infection rates are higher, fatality rates lower than widely reported (26 May 2020)

In a new study [14] we used a Bayesian Network (BN) analysis of Covid-19 data to reveal higher infection prevalence rates and lower fatality rates than have been widely reported:

> "Widely reported statistics on Covid-19 across the globe fail to take account of both the uncertainty of the data and possible explanations for this uncertainty. This study uses a Bayesian Network (BN) model to estimate the Covid-19 infection prevalence rate (IPR) and infection fatality rate (IFR) for different countries and regions, where relevant data are available. This combines multiple sources of data in a single model."

The results show that Chelsea Mass. USA and Gangelt Germany have relatively higher infection prevalence rates (IPR) than Santa Clara USA, Kobe, Japan and England and Wales. In all cases the infection prevalence is significantly higher than what has been widely reported, with much higher community infection rates in all locations. For Santa Clara and Chelsea, both in the USA, the most likely IFR values are 0.3-0.4%. Kobe, Japan is very unusual in comparison with the others with values an order of magnitude less than the others at, 0.001%. The IFR for Spain is centred around 1%. England and Wales lie between Spain and the USA/German values with an IFR around 0.8%.

Our first estimate was of the proportion of people infected as detected from seroprevalence testing, infection prevalence rate (IPR) (note that the rate here is measured on a scale of 0 to 1 rather than as a percentage 0 to 100), as shown in Figure 1.

There remains some uncertainty around these estimates but an IFR greater than 1% looks remote for all regions/countries. We said:

> "We use a Bayesian technique called 'virtual evidence' to test the sensitivity of the IFR to two significant sources of uncertainty: survey quality and uncertainty about Covid-19 death counts. In response the adjusted estimates for IFR are most likely to be in the range 0.3%-0.5%."

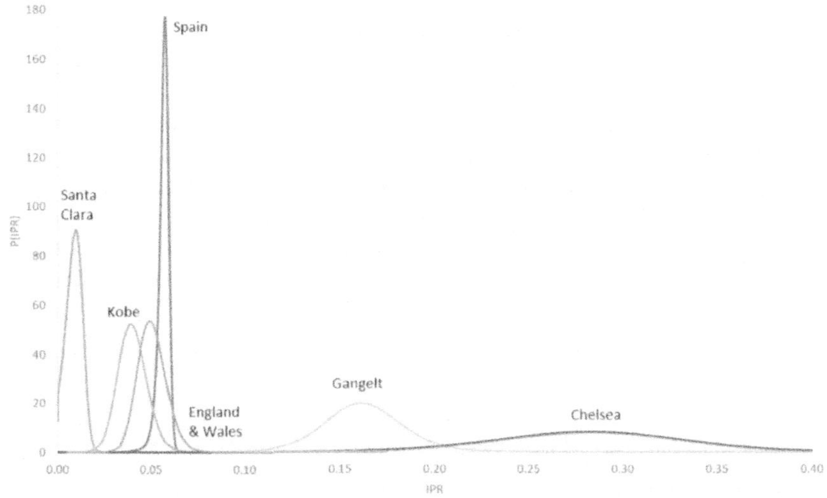

Figure 1 Distribution of Infection prevalence rate for countries/regions

Our second estimate was of the infection fatality rate. Before making any adjustment for the mortality data Figure 2 shows what we estimated for each country/region.

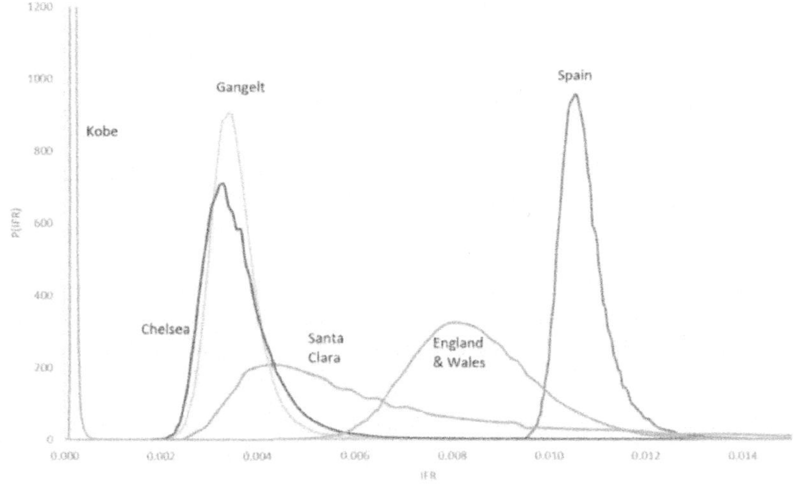

Figure 2 Distribution of Infection fatality rate for countries/regions

This can be contrasted with the study by Feguson et al, [17] which calculated a 1.38% case fatality ratio and the initial reports, by the World Health Organization (WHO) [18] that China had experienced a 3.4% fatality rate.

1.5. UK Covid-19 death rates by religion

15 July 2020

The most recent UK Office of National Statistics (ONS report on Covid-19 deaths by religion [19] (covering the period 2 March - 15 May) provides the overall number of fatalities for each religious group but, curiously, provides no simple overall fatality rate by religious group. So, we have done it ourselves. Using Table 2 of the report (which provides the total deaths per religious group) and Table 1 of the report (which provides the population proportion per religion) and assuming the UK population size is 65 million, we get the results shown in Table 1.

So, looking only at these population totals, Jews (by far) and then Christians have the highest death rate with atheists (no religion) by far the lowest (it is fair to assume these are atheists because these are people who declared "no religion" as opposed to those who did not declare any religion, i.e. those who fall into the category "not stated or required").

Now, while there are many Black Christians who come under the "BAME" (Black And Minority Ethnic) classification, there are very few Black Jews in the UK. So the results here seem to contradict the widely accepted narrative about BAME being 'by far' the highest risk group [21].

Table 1 Deaths per 100K by religion

Religion	*Deaths per 100,000*
Jewish	139
Christian	76
Hindu	61
Sikh	50
Muslim	41
Buddhist	38
Other religion	38
No religion	21
Not stated or required	59

The question is whether an obvious confounding factor like age is causing a Simpson's paradox [22] effect here whereby - although the overall rate is highest for a particular class of people - it may be possible that a different class is highest in each age sub-category. For example, as Dana Mackenzie shows for US statistics [23]:

> "although in every age category (except ages 0-4), whites have a lower case fatality rate than non-whites, when we aggregate all of the ages, whites have a higher fatality rate. The reason is simple: whites are older."

So, is that what we have here also, i.e. is it all explained by the fact that Jews and Christians are older? Well, according to the statistical analysis in the ONS report it ***may be to a certain extent***. The report uses 'age standardised mortality rates' to take account of the age distribution differences and concludes that Muslims, rather than Jews, have the highest fatality risk (something which seems very surprising given the above table).

However, the report does not define how the 'age standardised mortality rates' are calculated and it does not provide the raw data to check the results either (just as this Barts study [24] failed to provide the necessary raw data to check if its bold claims about higher risk for BAME people were valid). Another concerning aspect of the report is that a lot of it focuses on the under 65s. Yet, the total number of fatalities in the under 65s is dwarfed by the number of fatalities in the over 65s.

Our approach to this problem is to construct causal (probabilistic) models (this is, of course, also the approach recommended by Pearl and Mackenzie in their excellent "Book of Why", reviewed here [25]).

Note that there are many factors other than just age that must be incorporated into any analysis of the observed data before making definitive conclusions about risk based on religion/ethnicity. Moreover, if we discount unknown genetic factors, then religion and ethnicity have NO impact at all on a person's Covid-19 death risk once we know their age, underlying medical conditions, work/living conditions, and extent of social distancing.

A detailed version of this article, which includes the causal model can be found here [26].

1.6. A privacy-preserving Bayesian network model

For personalised Covid-19 risk assessment and contact tracing (May 2020)

Concerns about the practicality and effectiveness of using Contact Tracing Apps (CTA) to reduce the spread of Covid-19 have been well documented and, in the UK, led to the abandonment of the NHS CTA shortly after its release in May 2020.

One of the key non-technical obstacles to widespread adoption of CTA has been concerns about privacy. In this new paper [27], [28] our group presented a causal probabilistic model (a Bayesian network) that provides the basis for a practical CTA solution that does not compromise privacy. Users of the model can provide as much or little personal information as they wish about relevant risk factors, symptoms, and recent social interactions. The model then provides them feedback about the likelihood of the presence of asymptotic, mild or severe Covid-19 (past, present and projected). When the model is embedded in a smartphone app, it can be used to detect new outbreaks in a monitored population and identify outbreak locations as early as possible. For this purpose, the only data needed to be centrally collected is the probability the user has Covid-19 and the GPS location.

1.7. People and Pandemics – A Better World?

22 July 2020

Norman was one of four Queen Mary University of London academics to take part in this panel [28] session today. It was a disturbing experience as it revealed just how politicised the pandemic had become and, indeed, how it seemed to be part of a grander scheme for more worldwide authoritarian control - as the title of the panel suggested. Four months into the ridiculous lockdowns and these other academics were talking about the "opportunity for a Great Reset using the exact same terminology as Klaus Schwab of the World Economic Forum and other world leaders. Not just here, but also talking to other academic colleagues it was clear that many were salivating over lockdowns - openly praising them for their effect on "reducing carbon emissions" and demanding that such lockdowns continue even if Covid-19 was defeated. It seems that Covid-19 lockdowns are going to be the precursor for climate lockdowns Yet there has still been no cost and risk benefit analysis for the lockdowns.

Academics (almost exclusively on the extreme Left politically) have played a lead role in pushing the Government into the extreme restrictions and lockdowns. These academics and other leftist commentators and politicians have traditionally claimed to be most protective of our civil liberties, and yet are now leading the attack on these civil liberties. In future years people will look back on this time as one of total shame for academia. The very people who should have been leading the charge to question what Governments are telling us and pursuing the truth are now the ones most prominent in censoring any attempts to pursue the truth. Often these academics are not even qualified in the relevant areas, and they provide no rigorous evidence for the recommendations they make. They include psychologists who are prominent in promoting the psyops propaganda campaign of fear to force people to comply with increasingly harsh restrictions These academics are completely unaffected by the negative consequences of their recommendations. They have no skin in the game. In contrast to the independent workers and small business owners who lose their whole livelihoods, not one of these academics or politicians has lost a single day's work or pay. In fact, for most, their lives are made easier by being able to work from home because these are a generally privileged elite who have nice homes with gardens. Meanwhile it is the poorest in society, the ones they still expect to stack shelves and deliver stuff to their homes, who suffer the most from the restrictions and lockdowns.

Chapter 2. The scam starts to be revealed

2.1. What is the evidence of a big second wave?

14 September 2020

The UK now enters a new period of 'semi lockdown' with private gatherings restricted to groups of 6 people. This seems to be in response to an 'increase in confirmed cases'; but such an increase is inevitable as more people are being tested (especially young people, many of whom will not suffer any major symptoms), and with the false positive problem [29]. It seems that the most relevant Covid-19 trend plot should be number of deaths per 100K people tested. We've not seen such a plot - so we just downloaded the relevant raw data [30] and produced the plot for the UK from 1 April 2020 shown in Figure 3.

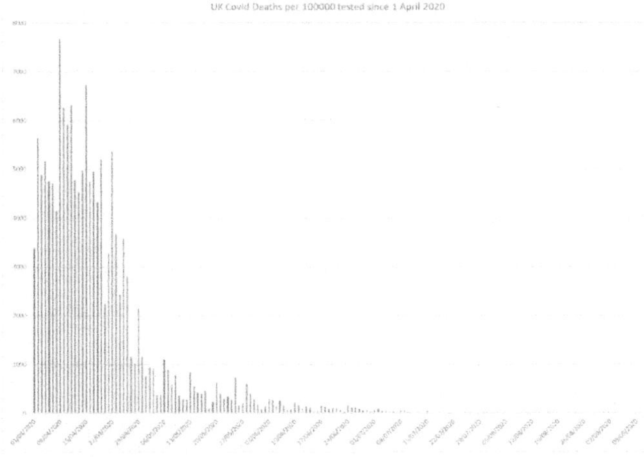

Figure 3 Covid deaths per 100k tested

It does seem that the introduction now of the new UK rules is a very strange move.....

17 September 2020

Following on from the previous article (and using the same dataset), Figure 4 is a plot of the number of new cases per 1000 people tested (for each day since 8 April - the first date for which there is a record of number of people tested.). Contrary to what is being shown by the media, this plot is the one that should be used to base decisions on if and when new social distancing or lockdown rules are needed.

When we consider that a higher proportion of new cases now (compared to the first 2 months) are minor or totally asymptomatic (as evidenced by the continued very low death rates shown in the previous piece). It is rather incredible that the Government and almost all media outlets are not showing this graph, but instead only showing the graph of new cases per day (that indicate a 'second wave'). Such a graph does not take account of the increase in number of people tested. Neither does it take account of the decrease in proportion of deaths per cases, nor the false positive test rate [29] (and so further exaggerates the scale of the problem).

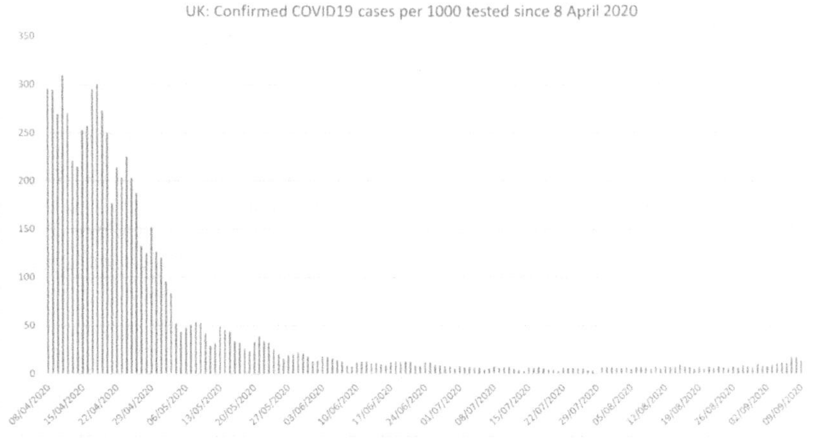

Figure 4 New cases per 1000 tested

Of course, evidence of a 'second wave' is something which better fits the narrative of a lot of influential people. But the Government's own latest data (as of 18 Sept 2020) on hospitalisations and deaths (as opposed to 'cases') provides no evidence of a second wave (screenshots of the plots can be found in the full version [31] of this article).

24 September 2020

Our short paper[33] uses Bayesian analysis to examine the latest (up to 22 Sept) Covid-19 data to determine whether there is evidence to support the Government claim of an exponential 'second wave'. As Figure 5 shows there remains insufficiently solid evidence, despite the number of tests done, to support any such claim. There is no reason to panic.

2.2. Critical flaw in the Covid-19 'hospital admissions' data

27 September 2020

We discovered today that the data on hospital admissions are not only flawed but also reveal a systematic problem with any data based on "suspected" Covid-19 cases. The website says:

> "Wales include suspected Covid-19 patients while the other nations include only confirmed cases"

The raw data in Table 2 (which includes the most recent complete data for all 4 nations) shows Wales is massively overestimating the number of Covid-19 hospital admissions.

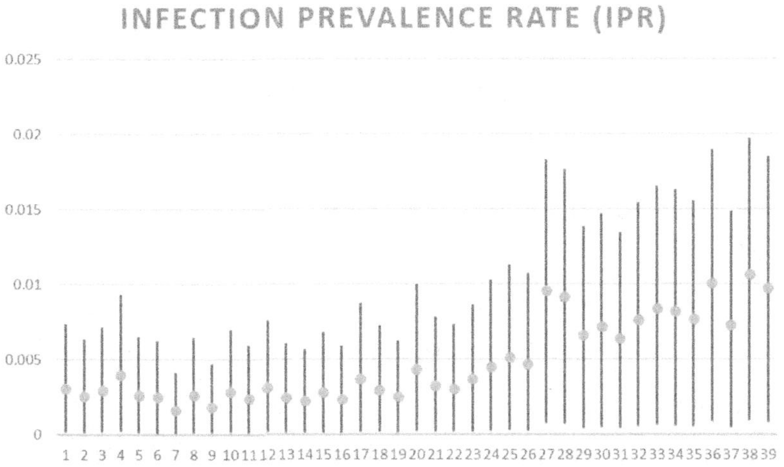

Figure 5 Infection prevalence rates by week with uncertainty bounds

Note that Scotland consistently has about twice the number of new confirmed case as Wales, yet Wales typically has about TWENTY times the number of admissions than Scotland. In fact, based on the above data, whereas in England, Scotland and NI on average around 4% of Covid-19 cases are admitted to hospital, for Wales the figure is 61%.

Table 2 Raw data on hospital admissions and cases

	Hospital admissions				Confirmed cases			
	England	NI	Scotland	Wales	England	NI	Scotland	Wales
15/09/2020	194	2	7	53	3,031	110	238	164
14/09/2020	172	7	9	59	2,882	125	186	191
13/09/2020	153	2	4	55	1,704	93	178	165
12/09/2020	143	4	6	55	2,202	109	214	140
11/09/2020	135	4	8	70	2,847	74	216	145
10/09/2020	143	5	8	49	3,101	82	231	186
09/09/2020	136	1	2	56	2,849	100	223	158
08/09/2020	99	10	5	65	2,995	56	103	143
07/09/2020	84	1	5	46	3,461	73	166	159
06/09/2020	85	4	2	42	2,053	107	154	131
05/09/2020	94	1	3	27	2,183	91	137	128
04/09/2020	67	1	8	69	2,582	131	170	149
03/09/2020	69	1	1	70	2,663	108	201	125
02/09/2020	79	0	5	59	2,614	92	191	95
01/09/2020	58	4	1	69	1,915	66	199	57
31/08/2020	52	5	3	29	1,255	54	143	44
30/08/2020	38	3	2	33	968	35	102	46
29/08/2020	52	3	2	52	1,037	44	94	44
28/08/2020	44	5	4	83	1,379	89	105	52
27/08/2020	69	3	3	70	1,335	81	97	50

Indeed, in July (not shown above but you can find it all on the website) when there were almost zero hospital admissions in the rest of the UK (and very few new cases) Wales was typically reporting 50-100 new Covid-19 hospital admissions every day.

Unless Wales is routinely admitting people who should not be hospitalised, we can conclude that at least 90% of the Wales 'Covid-19' admissions were not Covid-19 at all and that 'suspected' Covid-19 cases are generally not Covid-19. With UK admissions currently being recorded as around 250 per day including around 60 in Wales this means the real UK admissions number should be reduced to less than 200.

There are two lessons to be drawn from this:

- Any graphs/analysis of hospital admissions should exclude Wales.
- Any data about ***suspected*** Covid-19 cases (whether with respect to hospital admissions, deaths, or anything else) should be completely ignored or treated as massively exaggerated.

2.3. The impact of false positives in Covid testing

30 September 2020

There has been much recent debate - and controversy - about the impact of false positives in Covid testing. As Norman showed in this video [29], if the current rate of infection is 1 in 200 (i.e. 1 in every 200 people is currently infected with the virus) and if a person is selected ***at random*** to be tested then, if that person tests positive, there is actually only about a 1 in 6 chance (less than 17%) the person actually has the virus. This assumes the test has a 2% false probability rate (i.e. 2 out of every 100 people who don't have the virus will wrongly be tested positive) and a 20% false negative rate (i.e. 20 out of every 100 people with the virus will wrongly be tested negative).

Obviously the 1 in 200 pre-test (i.e. 'prior') probability assumption is critical. A person who is tested ***because*** they have been in contact with somebody confirmed as having the virus will have a much higher pre-test probability of having the virus. If we assumed it was 50% then, if that person tests positive, there is a 97% chance they have the virus.

The BMJ have produced an excellent infographic [35], which allows you to adjust all of the key parameters (namely the pre-test probability, false positive rate, and false negative rate). However, there is a severe limitation. The graphic does not allow you to enter pre-test probabilities of less than 1% (as I found out when I tried to enter the value 0.5% that I had used in my video - it automatically rounded it up to 1%). This is a curious limitation, given that the current infection rate is widely believed to be much lower than 1%; if it was 1% this would mean 680,000 people in the UK were infected right now, i.e. not including those who were previously infected (if it was that high this would confirm the belief of many that the virus goes unnoticed in most people).

Moreover, it also very curious that the default setting in the BMJ infographic has the pre-test probability set at a ludicrously high 80%. Even for a person with symptoms and having been in contact with a person with Covid this is actually too high. With that prior assumption somebody testing positive is, of course, almost certain to have the virus.

By focusing on the notion that people getting tested have a relatively high pre-test probability of having the virus, an article [37] in the Huffington Post, uses the BMJ infographic to hammer those claiming that most people testing positive do not have the virus. For example, they suggest a scenario where the pre-test probability is 20% and the false positive rate is 1%. With these assumptions, somebody testing positive has a 94% chance of having the virus.

In reality there is massive uncertainty about all of the three parameters as explained in this article [33]. Very early on during this crisis we argued that a more intelligent approach to data collection and analysis was needed to learn these parameters; in particular, there was a need to consider causal models to explain observed data. A basic causal model showed that it was critical to distinguish between people who had no, mild and severe symptoms, both when recording those being tested and when recording those testing positive. Yet there are no publicly available data on those being tested which makes these distinctions (we just have 'total tested' per day) and neither do we have it for those testing positive; all we can do is make some crude inferences based on the number hospitalised, but even then, this published daily number includes all patients hospitalised **with** Covid not **because** of Covid. And, even worse, as we shared in the previous article there are fundamental errors in some of the UK data on hospital admissions.

Contrary to what has been assumed, there is no 'gold standard' test for Covid and hence there is no way to determine the accuracy of the PCR and other tests. On the issue of what is known about test accuracy, our colleague Dr Scott McLachlan says:

> "During the last five months we have collected every preprint and journal publication that we could locate on Covid-19 testing with rt-PCR and antibodies. The issues of false positives (FP) and false negatives (FN) are more complicated than test product developers, some academic authors, and the mass and social media have presented.
>
> First, discussion of a single FP or FN rate completely misses the fact that there are multiple tests from different vendors being used at the moment. The NHS alone are using at least five different primary rt-PCR tests. Each has a different manufacturer or seeks a different RNA target and therefore has a different sensitivity and specificity profile. What we do not have as yet is independent laboratory verification of the manufacturer's claimed sensitivity and specificity. As well as those five there are a range of perhaps three or four, including the DNANudge cartridge test that comes from the UCL company that also market DNA NFC identity wristband in malls such as White City Westfield. Their test documentation focuses predominately on their claims of near zero FNs - because FNs have been the leading subject of much media and academic literature in recent weeks, and brushes over the fact that by their own numbers they make around 3% FP.
>
> Second, we have very little in the way of credible independent 3rd party verification for any of the Covid-19 tests. Everything we get at the moment either consists of self-validation by the manufacturer lab (which should not be accepted wholesale without independent verification but sadly has been during Covid-19 times), or of poorly constructed literature from well-meaning medics who, in one example, used an unvalidated PCR test as the standard by which to assess the accuracy of chest CT/CXR for diagnosing Covid-19 (for the record, the CT did far better than the

PCR test they used as *cough gold-standard… and they ended up acknowledging the PCR test resulted in FNs and FPs at far higher levels than expected).

As best as we have been able to identify from the literature collected that has assessed the rt-PCR and lab-based antibody tests:

FNs are occurring at a rate of between 3-30% for rt-PCR Covid-19 tests - depending on the test type, manufacturer, and the lab that ran the tests.

FPs are occurring at a rate of between 0.8% (lowest value accepted in the literature) and 7.9% (in a recent EU-based preprint) for rt-PCR Covid-19 tests.

Sens/Spec for rt-PCR Covid-19 tests ranges from 87%-100% depending on which manufacturers test and whether they performed their own testing or wrote their own academic report.

The antibody tests have an accuracy of somewhere between 30 and 93%, again depending on whose antibody test you review, whether it was IgG or IgM, and whether they averaged the score of all antibodies the test assayed for, or reported them individually. Antibody tests tended to be really good at identifying one antibody (often IgG), and less accurate or specific for the other (most often IgM)."

There is plenty of anecdotal evidence that most people testing positive either really don't have the virus or will be totally unaffected by it. For example, as part of the standard testing of professional footballers earlier this week 18 out of 25 of Leyton Orient's players - and many of their staff - tested positive. None of these people had - or will have - any symptoms at all. The same is true of the many other footballers and staff (including many older managers/trainers) who have tested positive and the hundreds of Scottish University students who tested positive this week. See also this important article "Waiting for Zero" [40] by Dr Clare Craig.

That is why we have been posting on twitter updates of our *cases (i.e. positive tests) per 1000 tested* graph as a contrast to the naive cases only graph which all the media post (obviously cases have been rising as number of tests have been rising). It is curious that the website produces all kinds of plots but not this most obvious and informative one. As we explained in earlier articles this shows that, contrary to the Government claims made this week, there is no real evidence of exponential growth in the virus.

People have been responding by saying 'ah but in April we were only testing those hospitalised with severe symptoms'; this is generally true (in fact the testing 'strategy' - i.e. who primarily gets tested has changed several times, which is why we argued long ago it needs to factored into a causal model [39]); so the proportion of positives among those tested in April was obviously a lot higher than now. However, it is also the case that the proportion of people now testing positive who will be totally unaffected by the virus (whether they have it or not) is ***also*** much higher. That is why we need to distinguish between mild, severe and asymptomatic cases. We really need to see the plot of severe cases, and as I mentioned above, hospitalisations is the best approximation we have for that. However, that is also compromised for reasons explained above and the fact that we are now entering the normal flu season when hospital admission inevitably rise significantly.

2.4. Hospital admissions data: evidence of exponential increase?

2 October 2020

We have been arguing that using the simple plot of daily 'number of cases' (which just means 'number testing positive') is an inappropriate way to monitor the Covid-19 trend. This is because much of the increase in 'cases' is explained by an increase in the number of people tested, and that many of the 'positives' are either false positives or people who are asymptomatic (or who will only ever have mild symptoms). Hence, we argued that a better, but still simple alternative plot, is daily 'cases per 1000 people tested'.

Many have responded by saying that it is daily Covid-19 hospital admissions which is the key plot to focus on. It is certainly a better indicator of the Covid-19 trend than just 'cases' and it is all plotted daily [29].Today's data (note: screenshots can be seen in the full article [42]) shows a small recent increase – averaging 300 daily for the past week compared to the summer lows of 80, but well below the 3,000 average in late March to early April.

However, even if we ignore the major problem with the data for Wales (which artificially inflates the admissions data as explained in Section 2.2), there is still a problem in using this plot to monitor the progress of Covid-19. To see why, here is what the website says about the England data:

> "data include people admitted to hospital who tested positive for Covid-19 in the 14 days prior to admission, and those who tested positive in hospital after admission. Inpatients diagnosed with Covid-19 after admission are reported as being admitted on the day prior to their diagnosis"

In other words, we have no idea how many of the 'Covid-19 hospital admissions' were people admitted ***because*** of Covid-19. A person entering hospital for, say, cancer treatment who recently tested positive for Covid-19 will be officially classified as a Covid-19 case. The same is true of those entering hospital for any treatment who have not previously been tested positive for Covid-19 but 'test positive' at some time during their stay. We must therefore assume that - as in the public generally - a proportion of the 'Covid-19 hospital admissions' are people who either a) don't have Covid-19; or b) are asymptomatic (or who will only ever have mild symptoms).

It also means that, as with 'Covid-19 cases', much of the recent increase in 'Covid-19 hospital admissions' may be explained by the general increase in number of people being tested. Unfortunately, we do not have the daily data for number of people being tested before and during UK hospital admissions. But it is not unreasonable to assume the number is roughly proportional to the total number of people being tested in the UK. So, it makes sense to plot the daily hospital 'Covid-19 admissions per 1000 people tested' in preference to simply the Covid-19 admissions. This plot shows a much lower recent increase – averaging 0.9 per 1000 tested daily for the past week compared to the summer lows of 0.4, but massively below the spring peak. In fact, data for number of people tested are only provided from 22 April (when the number of hospital admissions had already fallen well below the earlier peak). On 22 April the number of admissions per 1000 tested was 68.

This suggests that, indeed some (but not all) of the recent increase is explained by the increase in testing. And - before anybody suggests that it's "Covid-19 deaths" not hospital admissions we should be looking at - everything we said above is also relevant to those classified as Covid-19 deaths.

2.5. Why we know so little about Covid-19 from testing data

11 Oct 2020

This article provides some context for a short article (with Scott McLachlan and Magda Osman) [43] that was published in Lockdown Sceptics and which has received quite a bit of attention.

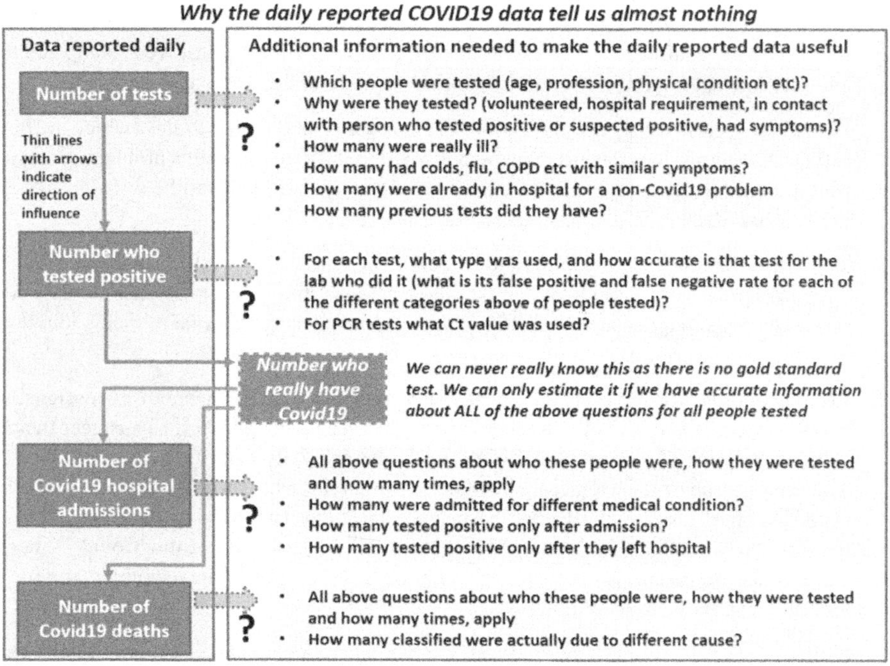

Figure 6 Why the daily reported covid data tells us almost nothing

The daily monitoring of Covid-19 cases are intended ultimately to determine what the 'current' population infection rate really is and how it is changing. However, in the absence of a gold-standard test for Covid-19, it is always uncertain whether a person has the virus (let alone whether a person can infect someone else). This is explained in Figure 6.

Obviously, this means that the population infection rate (sometimes referred to as the community infection prevalence rate) on a given day is also unobservable. The best we can do is estimate it from data that are observable. To get a feel for how complex this really is to do properly - and why current estimates are unreliable, a schematic showing the *minimum* regular information we need to get these estimates is provided in the full version of this article.

There are 31 separate boxes in the schematic representing different necessary pieces of information we need to 'know' for accurate estimation. Of these, 21 are ***unobservable,*** including some related to people currently with Covid (such as the proportion of people with symptoms, and the test false negative rate) and some related to people who do not have covid (such as the proportion of people with covid-like symptoms and the test false positive rate). Hence, we are totally reliant on 10 other pieces of information which ***are*** observable. Fortunately, using Bayesian causal inference, we know how to provide good estimates of the unobservable variables if we had the data for the observable variables.

But the BIG problem is that the only accessible daily data [29] we have are for 2 of the 10 observable variables: number of tests processed and number of people testing positive. Others, such as number of people with (and without) symptoms tested are not available. This means that any estimates of the things we really want to know are poor and highly uncertain (including the regular updates we have been providing based on this data). Yet, in principle, we should easily be able to get daily data for all the observable variables and, if we did, our estimates would be far more accurate. Given the critical need to know these things more accurately, it is a great shame that these data are not available.

As complex as our schematic is, there are still several simplified assumptions, notably:

- We make a crucial distinction between people who *do* and *do not* have Covid-19 symptoms - for the important reason that a) the former are more likely to be tested than the latter, and b) the testing accuracy rates will be different in each case. However, we don't (but really should) also distinguish between people who *have* and *have not* been in recent contact with a person tested positive, because again a) the former are more likely to be tested; and b) the testing accuracy rates will be different in each case. It could also be reasonably argued that we should also distinguish between different age categories.
- We are making the massively simplified assumption that the testing process is somehow 'constant'. Not only are there many different types of tests, but for the most common - PCR testing - there are massive variations depending on what 'Ct value' is used [51] (i.e. the number of cycles) and small changes can lead to radically different false positive rates. If there are government changes to the ct value guidelines then this can cause apparent (but non-real) massive changes in the 'population infection rate' from one day to the next.
- While we have allowed for the fact that some people are tested multiple times (hence the observable, but never reported, variable number of people tested more than once) this massively over-simplifies a very complex problem. If a person tests positive where the Ct value was above 40, then (because it is known that ct values even above 30 lead to many false positives) the recommendation is to retest, but we do not know if and when this happens and how many retests are performed. Similarly, some people may receive multiple negative tests before a single positive test and such people would count only as one of the people testing positive.

The schematic is a representation of what is called a Bayesian network; the direction of the arrows is important because every variable (box) that has arrows going into it is calculated as an arithmetic or statistical function of the variable which are its 'parents'.

As all unobserved variables like population infection rate are never known for certain they will always be represented as a probability distribution (which could be summarised, for example as "a 95% chance of being between 0.1% and 20%" or something like that). As we enter observed data (such as number of people testing positive) we can calculate the updated probability of each unobserved variable; so, for example, the population infection rate might change to "a 95% chance of being between 0.1 and 10%". The more data we enter for the observable variables the more accurate the estimates for the unobserved variables will be. Unlike traditional statistical methods, Bayesian inference works 'backwards' (in the reverse direction of the arrows) as well as forwards. So, for example, if we know the proportion of people with symptoms who are tested, we can revise our estimates of the proportion of people with covid and symptoms who are tested and the proportion of people not with covid (but with similar symptoms) who are tested.

2.6. Covid-19 is Not a High Consequence Infectious Disease

So Why Lockdown? (27th October 2020)

Lockdown Sceptics have published our article [44] based on a twitter thread [45] pointing out that Covid-19 was not classified as a high consequence infectious disease by the UK authorities.

1. On 19th March the UK 4 nation's public health "High Consequence Infectious Disease" (HCID) group made a decision that Covid-19 is NOT a HCID. This was published on a government website for public access.
2. The statement also said: "The Advisory Committee on Dangerous Pathogens (ACDP) is also of the opinion that Covid-19 should no longer be classified as an HCID."
3. In the UK an HCID is defined as an acute infectious disease, with high case-fatality rate requires an enhanced individual, population and system response.
4. Professor Neil Ferguson is a member of The Advisory Committee on Dangerous Pathogens (ACDP), as listed here[46].
5. We understand the committee reached the UNANIMOUS view, that Covid-19 is NOT a HCID, at a meeting on 13th March 2020.
6. Despite this the UK SAGE group, Whitty and Vallance published a document [47] recommending enhanced individual, population and system responses to Covid-19 on 14th March. This was the day after the ACDP committee decision and five days before the HCID group's decision.
7. They therefore made this decision despite, and in contradiction to, official scientific advice.

8. What happened between 13th and 14th March? Why did Ferguson, Vallance and Whitty change direction before the 4 nations HCID group made their decision on 19th March?
9. Professor Neil Ferguson is a member of SAGE and a member of the ACDP. How can he make a decision one day and then contradict it the next?

We also came into possession of a copy of a letter (dated 13 March 2020) from Professor Tom Evans, chair of the ACDP (a screenshot of the letter is in the full article [44]) saying:

> "Dear DHSA.
>
> Classification of Covid-19 as a HCD
>
> I am writing as Chair of the Advisory Committee on Dangerous Pathogens (ACDP). The committee discussed today the classification of Covid-19 as a high consequence disease. The unanimous view of the committee was that this infection should NOT be classified as a HCD.
>
> Best wishes
>
> Yours sincerely
>
> Professor Tom Evans"

In this YouTube clip [45] from the Downing Street Corona Briefing on May 11th 2020, Prof. Chris Whitty - the UK's Chief Medical Officer - says that, to most people, the coronavirus is entirely harmless. He said:

> "Most people will never get it. Most of the people who get it won't ever experience symptoms. Most of the people who experience symptoms won't need medical care. Most of the people who need medical care won't be need emergency or critical care. And even the tiny percentage of people who need who DO need critical care will survive, regardless of risk factors or medical history."

This message was no aberration, for two-weeks before, on 30th April 2020, he had made clear his views [48] in similar terms. Note that both of these messages went out AFTER the HCID committee made its decision, yet the country was locked down against a 'pandemic'.

2.7. Why the continued Covid-19 lockdowns and restrictions?

Time to demand the evidence to support them (25th October 2020)

In this article we presented the latest (as of 24 Oct 2020) plot of daily UK Covid-19 deaths per 1000 cases with a 28-day delay (the reason for the delay is because of the delay between confirmed cases and death). The 28-day delay simply means we divide the number of deaths reported on day N by the number of cases reported on day N minus 28. Contrary to the current hysteria created by the increasing number of 'covid deaths', this plot has remained more or less steady at about 25 deaths per 1000 cases for the last month, and well below the 220 per 100 cases in early May.

Obviously, as we have explained in previous articles, there is a causal explanation for the higher numbers in May: 28 days prior to that it was mainly hospitalised people being tested and recorded as 'cases'. And there are lots of other causal explanations to consider, along with the general weakness of the data provided as was explained in Section 2.5 Moreover, as Clare Craig has shown Covid-19 deaths are clearly being over-counted **[52]**.

Figure 7 provides an interesting comparison between the UK and Sweden (where there has been no lockdowns) which suggests lockdowns do not reduce cases or deaths.

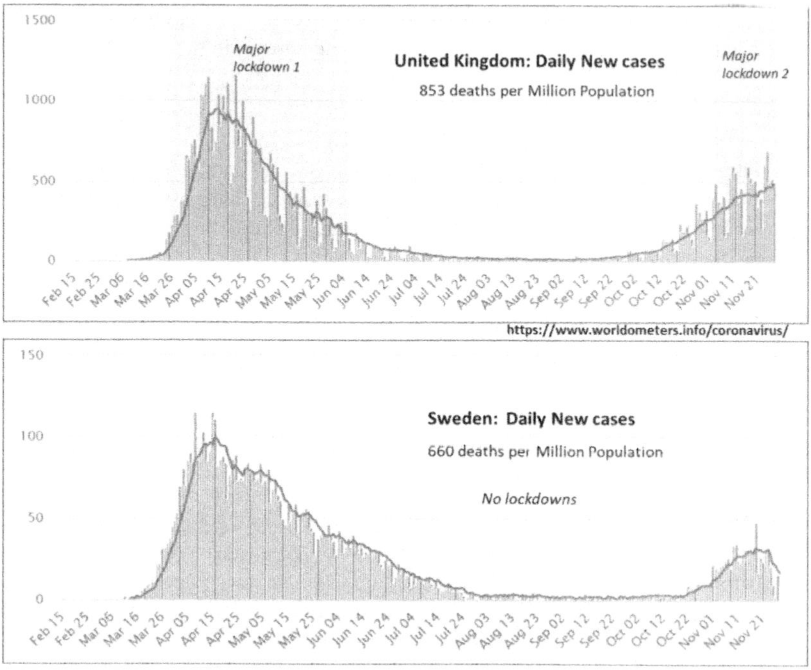

Figure 7 UK v Sweden comparison

Increasingly it is clear that the continued response to the virus is not in proportion to its deadliness. It is time for the Government and SAGE to provide real evidence to support the continued lockdowns and infringements of civil liberties and they can start by putting some numbers on the various related factors that we displayed in the schematic here [49]. This separated the 'Costs' from the 'Benefits'.

The costs included all the factors leading to increases in cancer and other diseases through reduced access to non-covid health services; all the factors leading to reduced long term health and employment prospects of children, all the factors leading to increased unemployment (including devastation of swathes of the economy, tourism, arts, culture and sports), increased government spending and debt (leading to future increased taxes and devastation of pensions); and all the factors leading to increases in divorces, violence and suicides. Since we have no evidence at all that fewer people die from covid as a result of the lockdowns, the only demonstrable benefits were reduced NHS costs resulting from restriction of most non-covid services, and fewer injuries and deaths resulting from 'unnecessary' car journeys.

A full analysis should also factor in the personal costs/risks of those people advising and making the lockdown decisions. They are - without exception - those whose own jobs are not threatened as a consequence of their decisions to lockdown and (interestingly) those least likely to be denied or delayed treatment for non-Covid-19 medical conditions.

And note the chart does not include the many billions of pounds already spent or committed on (highly questionable) research, equipment and apps dedicated to 'combatting Covid-19'. Just as there was no cost-benefit analysis for lockdown there has been no cost-benefit analysis for most of that spending, which also comes at the expense of research and equipment needed for other more serious medical conditions that will be with us for much longer.

2.8. Our evidence submitted to UK Parliament

On Covid-19 data transparency and accountability (1 November 2020)

In response to the UK Government "Call for Evidence Regarding Covid-19 Data Transparency and Accountability", Norman, Martin and Scott McLachlan submitted the formal document [56] that can be found here. The full document contains extensive references and figures. Below we present just key text from the document:

1. We are a group of senior researchers in risk assessment, probability, statistics, and public health technologies based at Queen Mary University of London. Since March 2020, we have produced 23 articles/reports (of which 5 have been published in peer reviewed journals) analysing the publicly available Covid-19 statistics and producing risk assessments and models.
2. We believe that the statistics provided to and by the Government during the Covid-19 crisis have been inadequate and have been too easily used by influencers and decision-makers to fit particular narratives that have exaggerated the scale of the crisis.
3. Statistics and data are observed phenomena arising from unobserved processes and their interactions (including causal explanations). The number of observed Covid-19 'cases' clearly depends on how a 'case' is defined and the population infection rate, but it is also influenced by many (normally unreported) causal factors such as how many tests are being performed, who is being tested and why, and the accuracy of the testing. Similarly, while the number of observed Covid-19 'deaths' clearly depends on how a Covid-19 death is defined and reported, it is also influenced by the population demographics, quality of healthcare etc. Hence, contrary to popular conception, data do not 'speak for themselves'.
4. For example, in March and April by focusing only on simple counts of 'cases', 'hospitalisations' and 'deaths', the public was misled into believing that the virus was more deadly than it really was. At that stage testing was essentially limited to those who were either already hospitalised with severe symptoms or were frontline healthcare workers. The reported high death (and hospitalisation) rates of those infected (calculated by simply dividing the number of deaths by the number of 'cases')

were in part explained by the limited testing regime that was essentially only 'finding' the most severe 'cases'.

5. Similarly, the scale of the 'second wave' has been continually exaggerated by focusing on increased 'cases' without considering the simple causal explanation of massively increased testing. When this is done – as shown in the plots of Figure 2 –the trends for cases, hospitalisations and deaths look far less worrying than those presented at https://coronavirus.data.gov.uk using exactly the same data.

6. At the root of the data problem there has been a fundamental misunderstanding about the meaning of terms 'Covid-19 cases' and 'Covid-19 deaths', and what can be interpreted from statistics that use these terms. Even small changes in how these are defined and classified (as has happened several times since March) lead to very different trends and conclusions.

7. The definition of a Covid-19 'case' is especially concerning. In epidemiology, a case definition includes criteria for person (e.g. gender, race, age, or exclusion criteria), place (such as that associated with the outbreak of a disease), time (when illness started) and clinical features. Clinical features are initially normally simple and objective such as 'sudden onset of fever and cough' but should later be characterised by confirmed presence of specific laboratory findings, such as 'ground-glass opacity on Chest CT and positive culture for SARS-CoV-2'. During this crisis, a positive PCR test has improperly become the surrogate replacing all four aspects of case definition. A PCR test may be positive: (i) before clinical features arise; (ii) long after clinical features have abated; or even (iii) when a person has simply come into contact with the disease but without them ever becoming infected. Some argue that reporting cycle threshold (Ct) values may help clinical decision-makers identify at which of these three stages an asymptomatic person may present; however, given that almost all so-called asymptomatic cases never develop active disease, if we leave aside issues with false positives (which increase for high Ct values), we submit that many 'cases' must be type (iii) and therefore did not meet the normal epidemiological standard to be classified or counted as *a case*.

8. Confusion about the definition of a Covid-19 'death' also persist. It is now clear that Government-reported deaths include not just those who died as a direct result of the disease, but also all of those who have died 'with it', thus leading to inflation of the fatality figures. Several studies have also suggested that reported deaths from other pneumonias, influenzas and even lung cancer have dropped well below normal annual levels since March. As such there are questions surrounding whether people who died of these similar conditions were incorrectly classified as Covid-19 deaths.

9. With the massive increase in testing since August, uncertainty about the testing accuracy - especially the false positive rate of PCR tests - means that almost nothing meaningful can be concluded about the increasing cases or fatality rate. The vast majority tested have no symptoms at all, so in the absence of data provided about the proportion of asymptomatic people who were tested and tested positive (as well as the other missing information shown in Figure 3), we do not know what proportion of new 'cases' and reported 'deaths' are people infected with Covid-19 at all. A false positive rate of even just 1% would, together with the massively increased testing, provide a causal explanation for the increase in cases even if the virus has largely subsided. But,

yet again, the narrative presented – and the one on which lockdown decisions are based – is that of a massive 'second wave'.

10. Closed loop thinking means that, once a particular narrative is 'believed', alternative explanations for the observed data are never entertained. Indeed, the lack of data, unscientific closed-shop models, fundamental misunderstandings by decision-makers, manipulation of underlying reporting processes, contradictory goals or the potential for malign intent are all feasible explanations for the observed data and chaotic analysis. The lack of data transparency gives credence to these explanations and leads to a lack of trust in government statistics and decisions made using those statistics.
11. There are many examples of how the crude data, and failure to consider alternative causal explanations, has been used for inappropriate decision-making and even scare-mongering. These include:
    i. Using '100 new cases per 100,000 people' as a threshold beyond which a local borough is required to move to lockdown. With this metric the threshold can be avoided or reached simply by decreasing/increasing the number of tests carried out.
    ii. As explained above the headline figures and graphs – as presented for example, at https://coronavirus.data.gov.uk/ do not factor in the increase in testing. For example, the recent 'exponential' increase in number of cases – which has driven the 'second wave narrative' does not look at all serious when we plot it as number of cases per 1000 tests. The same is true of hospital admissions and deaths; for example, contrary to the frightening 'absolute' increase in hospital cases since September, it turns out that the number of hospital admissions per 1000 cases has remained stable – and may even be decreasing when we factor in the false positives and those admitted for non-COVID reasons who happen to get a positive COVID test after admission.
    iii. The ONS report on Covid-19 deaths by ethnicity is one of many that have produced misleading conclusions without even revealing all relevant data. This particular report exaggerated the increased risk to people from the BAME community by using 'relative risk' to summarise the findings, rather than 'absolute risk' as continually recommended for communicating risk to the public, by Royal Statistical Society Chairman (and member of SAGE) Professor Sir David Spiegelhalter. Moreover, we noted that the claims were almost certainly further exaggerated as they were likely based on out-of-date demographic information (the ONS failed to respond to our request to identify what data were used). Hence the ONS report – which was widely quoted in the media – was likely to create an unjustified level of fear and anxiety among the BAME community. Failure to identify causal explanations for data bias has also led to multiple well-publicised studies with exaggerated - or even flawed - claims that certain communities, or people with certain attributes or habits, are at much higher risk of Covid-19.
    iv. In early October news broke of under-reporting of almost 16,000 positive PCR tests and that, as a result, as many as 48,000 people may not have been informed of their exposure due to close contact with these undisclosed 'cases'. PHE blamed Microsoft's Excel software but this disingenuous

admonition did more to highlight PHE's: (a) reliance on almost 25yr old technology; (b) ignorance of and failure to maintain pace with technology; and (c) lack of any reliable approach to checking and validating data they collect and report. Data security experts describe this as one in a long string of data and information security failings by PHE and the Government and have used it to support eschewing use of the proposed NHSx track and trace apps.

v. Removal or sanitising of flu incidence/death data from 1999 and all previous years from the ONS website making comparisons almost impossible and giving the impression that the 'past is being rewritten or expunged'.

vi. Constant changing of scales and metrics used in data reporting. For example, deaths were recorded as Covid-19 deaths if they occurred within 28 days of a positive test, and this has recently been changed to 60 days if Covid-19 appears on the death certificate. This change was done in reaction to a recommendation that the period should be reduced to 21 days. The change was made with no accompanying explanation of why it was increased rather than decreased.

12. Ultimately the only way to achieve accurate estimates of the critical population infection rate at any given time is to provide the missing – but easy to obtain data shown in [Figure 4].
13. Decisions about lockdown require data to support the evidence shown in [Figure 5]. If these data have been considered in Government decisions, they have certainly not been made public.

In summary, and supported by the arguments above our responses to the eight issues identified in the public call are:

14. In response to Issue 1: *Did the Government have good enough data to make decisions in response to Coronavirus, and how quickly were the Government able to gather new data?*

Data provided by several departments including PHE, NHS and ONS for Government decision-making was observed to be ever-changing, unreliable, and of such poor quality and so inappropriately framed as to be insufficient to support the public health, policy and legislative decisions that resulted.

15. In response to Issue 2: *Was data for decision-making sufficiently joined up across departments?*

Where multiple actors are responsible for collecting and reporting data that will be aggregated and used to direct public policy: definitions, thresholds and processes must observe a consistent standard. The central aggregator, in this case the ONS, should have been responsible for both dictating and enforcing that standard.

As evidenced by anomalies and misrepresentations identified above, the efforts of PHE, NHS and ONS were not sufficiently joined up, fell short of due standards, and severely undermined Government decision-making, independent scrutiny, and ultimately public confidence.

16. In response to Issue 3: *Was relevant data disseminated to key decision-makers in: Central and Local Government; other public services (like schools); businesses; and interested members of the public?*

To be relevant, data must be capable of informing the decision-making process. Relevant data is that which is *accurate, timely, indisputable, optimised* and *fit to inform the known purposes for which it may be used.*

Given that Government was aware most members of the public consume only limited 'views' of such data as are presented in the media, its presentation, accuracy and fitness for purpose should have received greater consideration. While data was made available via the ONS website, for the reasons discussed above the relevance of this data has remained questionable.

17. In response to *Issue 4: Were key decisions (such as 'lockdowns') underpinned by good data and was data-led decision-making timely, clear and transparently presented to the public?*

Government decisions impacting the liberty and freedoms of individuals appear to have been made haphazardly. While each came supported by justifications, it was claimed, that they were 'led by the science', more often it could be argued this was not the case.

Decision making has been presented as being the result of "the science" with the goal of delivering 'consensus'. However, science does not operate as a consensus making mechanism and it is not monolithic. The current crisis has demonstrated that groups like SAGE and the Joint Biosecurity Centre are not following scientific norms of behaviour. Analysis and policy formulation need more stringent oversight in a way that invites and delivers scientific debate from both within and also outside the group.

18. In response to *Issue 5: Was data shared across the devolved administrations and local authorities to enable mutually beneficial decision-making?*

If this were the case it has not been made clear to the public, and in any case, it is likely that the shared data suffered from all of the limitations we have highlighted.

19. In response to *Issue 6: Is the public able to comprehend the data published during the pandemic. Is there sufficient understanding among journalists and parliamentarians to enable them to present and interpret data accurately, and ask informed questions of Government?*

It is difficult to ensure accurate comprehension in circumstances where, as discussed earlier, relevantly framed data has not been provided. Continued reliance on journalists to identify meaning from data has only resulted in sensational headlines that amplified public ignorance and promulgated fear.

What could have been done to improve understanding and who could take responsibility for this?

The current crisis has demonstrated Government must take additional steps to provide context and meaning capable of supporting differing interpretations they wish the public should draw from published data. The public should be trusted to understand nuance and scientific disagreement about what the data might be telling them.

20. In response to *Issue 7: Does the Government have a good enough understanding of data security, and do the public have confidence in the government's data handling?*

The policies and approaches of Government do not seem to have reflected prevailing opinions and wishes of the public. This has never been more obvious than during development and release of both versions of the NHSx Track and Trace smartphone app, and when vision-based population proximity monitoring AI systems were deployed around London suburbs, and once exposed in the media, hastily removed. It seems there is little public confidence in the current approach to securing public and personal data and indeed the potential for increased suspicion of the government's motives in this regard.

21. In response to *Issue 8: How will the change in responsibility for Government data impact future decision-making?*

It is not clear what the change in responsibility is and the motivation for it. Any change in responsibility might simply be akin to 'rearranging the deckchairs on the Titanic'.

2.9. An increasing proportion of people testing positive?

What does this really mean? (6th November 2020)

A few people have argued (see e.g. here [53] and here [54]) that, despite the official Government statistics, real Covid-19 cases are not increasing and that most Covid-19 positive test results are false positives. The obviously strong argument against this is the evidence that the proportion of positive tests is now increasing.

Ignoring the possibility that Covid-19 cases are being redefined, then unless the false positive rate itself is increasing, surely it cannot be possible for the proportion of positive tests to be increasing without a proportional increase in genuine Covid-19 cases? In fact, as we pointed out in Section 2.5, there could be simple causal explanations for an increasing proportion of positive tests being observed even if the underlying Covid-19 infection rate and test accuracy rates are unchanged. The most obvious causal explanation would be a change in the type of people being tested, such as if a lower proportion of people without symptoms were tested, or a higher proportion of older people were tested. In other words, if a higher proportion of people who had the virus were being tested.

However, as Clare Craig pointed out **[55]**, it ***is*** possible for the proportion of people wrongly testing positive (as opposed to the proportion of tests that are wrongly positive) to increase even if there is also no change to the type of people being tested. How? Because if some people are being tested more than once – as is certainly happening for those admitted to hospital – the probability of those people wrongly testing positive at least once does increase. Suppose, for example, the 'constant' false positive rate is 1 in 100 (i.e. 0.01 probability). Then, if you have two tests, the probability you test positive at least once is higher than 0.01. In fact, it is almost double. It is one minus the probability you do NOT test positive both times, i.e.

$$1 - (0.99) \times (0.99) = 1 - 0.9801 = 0.1999$$

which is close to 2%. But we do not even need to use this calculation to show the impact of testing people more than once. Consider the following example:

> Suppose the real Covid-19 infection rate among those being tested is constant at 5% and that 10,000 people in consecutive periods are tested. Suppose the true positive rate for the testing is 80% and the false positive rate is 1%.
>
> In period 1 everybody is tested just once. Then about 500 of these people have Covid-19 and 9500 do not. But then 95 of the 9500 without Covid-19 will wrongly test positive. Hence 495 out of 10000 people test positive – i.e. a proportion of 4.95%
>
> If the rates are unchanged in subsequent periods, then the proportion testing positive remains the same no matter how many more (or less) are tested.
>
> However, suppose that in period 2 some of those – let's say 20% - who test negative are retested and are recorded as a positive case if the second test is positive. Then, if 10,000 are tested in period 2, we know from above that 495 will test positive first time. However, 20% of those who test negative are retested. That means 20 of the 100 who wrongly tested negative and 1881 of those 9405 who correctly tested negative will be retested. Of the 20 with Covid-19, about 16 will test positive. Of the 1881 without Covid-19 about 19 will test positive. Hence, in period 2 – because some get tested twice – the number testing positive is now 529 out of 10,000 – i.e. a proportion of 5.29%.

It follows that if, over a sequence of periods, a steadily increasing proportion of people get retested, then the proportion of people testing positive will also steadily increase even though the true infection rate and false positive rate remain constant and there is no change in the type of people being tested. Moreover, if some people get retested more than twice (as is happening with hospital admissions) then this leads to further increases in the proportion testing positive.

It should be noted that an increase in the true positive rate (i.e. a reduction in the false negative rate) will ***also*** lead to an increase in the proportion of positive tests even if the true infection rate and false positive rate are unchanged, and nobody gets retested. In fact, this is a point which has largely been missed in the discussion about false positives for PCR testing. At the start of the crisis false negatives rates were typically as high as 67% **[57]** and it would be understandable in such cases to both a) do retesting; and b) increase the sensitivity of the tests to reduce the false negative rate. The sensitivity can be increased by increasing the cycle threshold of the PCR test. However, it is this increase which has led to claims of the reduction in specificity (the proportion of true negatives), i.e. an increase in the false positive rate.

It is widely assumed that the false negative rates have been significantly reduced. This would normally lead to an increase in the false positive rate. But if, somehow, the false positive rate remained the same, there would still be an increasing proportion of people testing positive even if there was no change in the infection rate and even if we ignore retesting and just consider proportion of tests that are positive (and not proportion of people who test positive). To see this, consider a similar example as above:

> Period 1 is exactly as above (5% real Covid-19 infection rate among those being tested is constant at 5% a true positive rate of 80% and false positive rate of 1%), so the proportion of positive tests is 4.95%.
>
> Suppose the only thing that changes in period 2 is an increase in the true positive rate to 90%. Then this time 450 (as opposed to 400) of those who have Covid-19 test positive making a total of 545 testing positive, so the proportion of positive tests is now increased to 5.45%.

So, in summary, assuming there are no changes to the way Covid-19 cases are defined, then there are still several different ways in which we could see an increasing proportion of people testing positive even if the underlying Covid-19 infection rate, and the false positive rate, are unchanged, namely:

- Causal explanation such as change in the type of people being tested
- Increasing number of people being retested
- Increasing true positive rate for the testing

Obviously combining any of the above will lead to even greater increases.

Chapter 3. Faking the data to prepare for new lockdown and vaccine rollout

3.1. Latest UK Covid-19 statistics roundup

14 and 15 Dec 2020

We wanted to see some data comparing people with Covid-19 symptoms to the 'case' numbers. The first link we found with relevant data was from Buckinghamshire, whose dashboard provides details of different types of triage numbers [58]. As you can from the screenshots of the day's data in the full version of this article this provides yet more evidence of why counting 'cases' (without considering number of people actually ill with the virus and number tested) is really dumb. Despite the apparently exponentially increasing number of daily 'cases' the daily number of 'cases triaged with suspected Covid-19 symptoms' has completely flatlined to its lowest number in months.

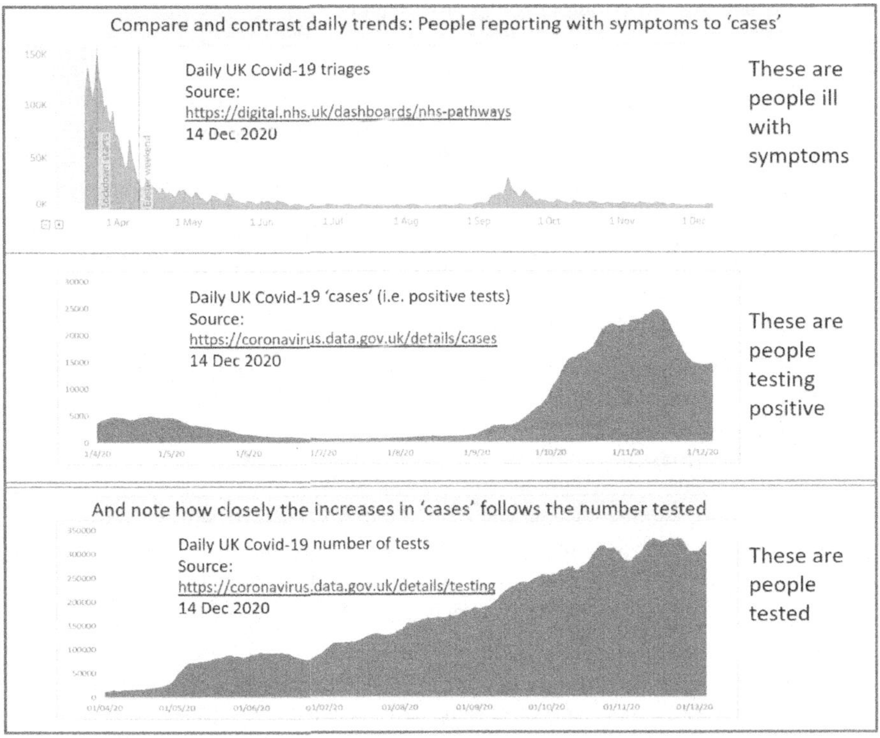

Figure 8 Comparing cases numbers with people ill with symptoms

While we were impressed with the Buckinghamshire dashboard it was surprising that it doesn't have data for numbers tested, which almost certainly have been steadily increasing as elsewhere. After tweeting about that somebody pointed us to a national NHS dashboard for Covid-19 triage [59]. And it turns out that the national figures in Figure 8 also show the stark difference between number of 'cases' (high and increasing) and number of people actually ill with symptoms (consistently low since the usual September blip). So, the 'casedemic' argument grows ever stronger.

It was also interesting to see Tim Spector's analysis of London prevalence rates based on his ZOE css app for monitoring people with symptoms. The average across all the London Boroughs was less than 600 people per 100,000. That is a remarkably low number of people with cold/flu like symptoms for mid-December. This confirms how ludicrous today's Government decision was to move the whole of London to Tier 3 lockdown (caveat: of course, we don't belief there should be **any** lockdowns of any sort **anywhere** for the reasons given below).

Our regular updated plots also destroy the mass pandemic wave narrative. These plots all take account of number of tests (which now includes lateral flow device tests as well as PCR tests). There is a very slight uptick in proportion of positive tests, but as we explained in Chapter 2, there may be multiple explanations for such changes. Similarly, there is a barely perceptible uptick in proportion of 'cases' which lead to hospital admissions (but, as usual, note that any person admitted to hospital who has a positive PCR test within 14 days prior to admission or within 28 days after admission is classified as a Covid-19 admission irrespective of their reason for being in hospital). And we know that many patients now classified as Covid-19 admissions are people who 'contracted' Covid-19 in hospital.

The current case fatality rate (proportion of people currently dying 'with covid' having tested positive any time up to 28 days prior to death) has been steady at around 2% for some time. And the proportion of all people who have died having tested positive any time up to 28 days prior to death continues to drop.

The (Government) decision about whether to move a region into a higher (resp. lower) tier is based on whether the number of "cases" goes above (resp. below) a certain threshold number per 100,000 residents. But, as there are wide variations in the number of people per 100,000 who are ***tested***, this strategy is ludicrous. Because (since July) many (most?) people tested do not have any symptoms and (because of the various reasons why there may be false positives), the more people you test the more "cases" you will find. Hence, a region which has a genuinely low infection rate, but a disproportionately high number of tests, may find itself in Tier 3 lockdown; conversely, a district with a genuinely high infection rate, but a disproportionately low number of tests, may find itself in the relative 'freedom' of Tier 1.

The Government website does provide the national figures for daily number of tests, which means that we can produce plots comparing the daily number of 'cases' (exponentially increasing) with the proportion of tests that are positive (barely changed).

As soon as we produce such plots it becomes clear that the scale of the 'second wave crisis' has been massively exaggerated and that there is merit to the claim that what we have is a 'casedemic'. The people who dispute this say that we are 'wrong' because what matters is that, for example, in London "Covid-19 hospital admissions" and "deaths" are rising. But notwithstanding the fact that overall autumn/winter rises in cases of flu-like illness are inevitable, the problem is that the data on number of hospital admissions and deaths attributed to Covid-19 suffer from the same problems as Covid-19 "case" data: we have no idea at all how many of those are hospitalised or dying because of covid as opposed to simply having had a positive test.

3.2. UK Covid Testing data: tests and positivity rate by regions

Remarkable relationship between them (18th December 2020)

Now even if there was no genuine increase in the population infection rate then, when you massively increase the number of people being tested (as happened in early September), you would expect to see a corresponding increase in number of 'cases' (i.e. positive test results) However, we should not see an increase in the positivity rate (the proportion of those tested who are positive) unless the false positive rate increased (e.g. due to increased human error) as more people were tested.

Since early November there is no obvious correlation between number of tests and positivity rate. Hence, it seems justifiable to conclude that the number of tests performed has no impact on the positivity rate (or vice versa) and hence that the recent (slight) increase in positivity rate since early December represents a genuine increase in spread of the virus that may justify the renewed lockdowns.

However, it turns out the overall UK data is hiding what is happening at the regional level. Figure 9 shows the regional graphs of number of tests versus positivity rate are taken straight from the ONS (the website only has the regional breakdown for England; for Scotland Wales and N Ireland we do not even have the overall number of tests). The trend plots in these main regions are different, with increases and decreases in positivity rates occurring at different times. Yet, in each region since mid-September, the positivity rate very closely correlates with the number of tests irrespective of the direction of movement. But it doesn't stop there. The website also now provides the same data at a lower level of granularity - namely health authorities. And, when you drill down to those, despite some very different trend plots at these local levels, the correlation between number of tests and positivity rates is almost perfect. For example, both the number of tests and the positivity rate for Ashford have recently been steadily increasing while in North Tyneside both the number of tests and the positivity rate have been steadily decreasing.

So, what can we conclude from these remarkable local correlations and why they started in September? (a later article provides some explanation). It suggests some systematic non-natural factor independent of a virus. Otherwise, two possible (causal) hypotheses are:

1. That the testing is highly accurate and since September people have only got tested when they think they might have the virus. As the infection rate increases (resp. decreases) the number of people choosing to get tested increases (resp. decreases).

2. That as the number of people tested increases (resp. decreases) the false positive rate increases (resp. decreases) due to increased (resp. decreased) possibility of human error.

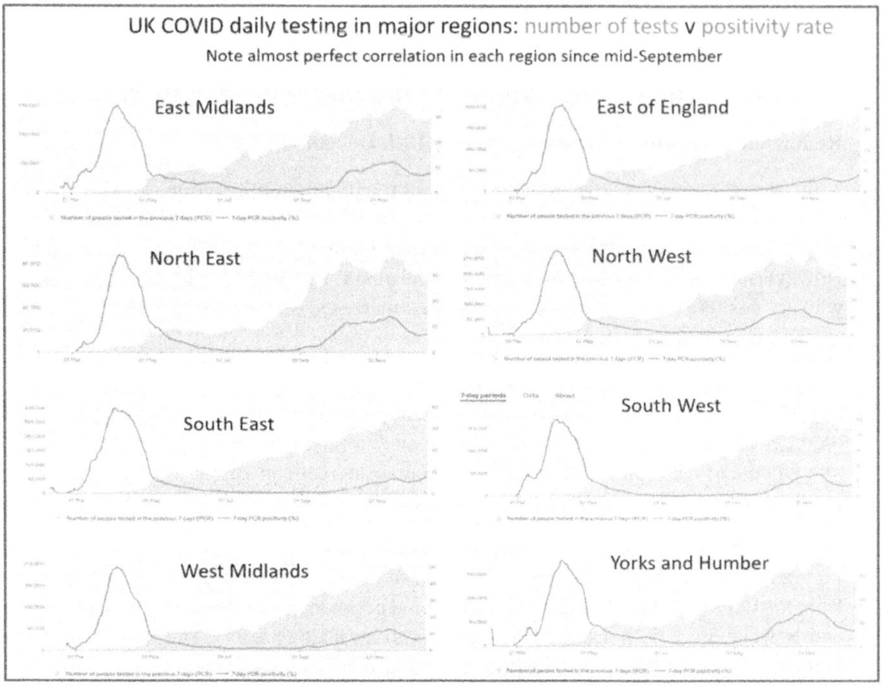

Figure 9 Regional graphs of number of tests versus positivity rates

But if hypothesis 1 were true we would expect to see similarly identical (but delayed) trend plots in hospital admissions and deaths, which does not seem to be the case. Another definite problem with hypothesis 1 is that it relies on the assumption that people only get tested when they either have symptoms or have been in recent contact with a person recently tested positive. But we know this is not the case. A very large proportion of people tested since September (including hundreds of thousands of students) have had neither symptoms nor a recent positive contact.

One possible problem with hypothesis 2 is that it fails to explain what happened between July and September when testing increased but there was no real increase in the positivity rate. Well, on the one hand testing levels were still sufficiently low for there to be plenty of checks in place (including confirmatory tests for positive results); that may not have been possible with such a big increase in testing in the autumn; also nobody doubts that, while the virus was almost gone in the summer there was an increase in cases in the autumn, so it is inevitable that the positivity rate would start rising then. But, in the absence of some systematic non-natural factor independent of a virus, the fact we see remarkable correlations involving rises and falls since September suggest that this must at least in part be explained by hypothesis 2. In other words, if a local authority decides to increase testing, then they would see an increase not just in number of 'cases' but also in the positivity rate. In that case a decision simply to increase testing could lead to a region being moved to a higher lockdown 'tier'.

Of course, because of the massive limitations of what can be concluded from simple data like number of tests and number of positives (as explained in Chapter 2) there is massive uncertainty about any of the above conclusions. The analysis certainly supports the need for the kind of additional data for which we have been arguing for a long time; in particular, we need to know not just number of people being tested but also number of people tested who are asymptomatic and – of those testing positive – the number who subsequently developed real symptoms. Only then might we be able to accurately determine whether the infection rate is really increasing or decreasing.

3.3. London goes into Tier 4 lockdown - but the data are flawed

Proof that the government data for London are flawed (20th December 2020)

With the sudden announcement of the Tier 4 lockdown for London yesterday we decided to look at the London hospital admissions and 'case' data (where, by definition, 'case' = positive test). Using the data here and filtering on London we did a plot of hospital admissions as a percentage of cases (this is a crude measure of 'severity' of the virus at any time).We used 7-day rolling averages for both cases and admissions and assumed a 4-day lag from positive test to admission (none of these assumptions makes a lot of difference to the results). The results are ***very*** interesting for two reasons.

The first reason is that the percentage of 'cases' leading to hospitalisation has been steady at around 7% for over 3 months, so no increase in 'severity'. In fact, as recently as mid-September it was much higher at 12%, and in June it was ***really*** much higher at 120%. Which brings us on the second reason why the results are, to say the least, interesting. It should, of course, be impossible for the number of Covid-19 hospitalisations to be greater than the number of Covid-19 'cases'. Yet it is not our analysis that is in error here. Table 3 shows the raw data, for example, from June.

We have highlighted some examples of admission numbers which do not appear to be feasible given the previous days number of new cases. Now, of course, for any new admission we do not know date of the associated positive specimen. We have assumed on average a hospital admission follows 4-days after a specimen was taken that ended up positive. But we know that a hospital 'admission' is also classified as Covid-19 when there is a (first) positive test ***after*** admission. However, whichever way you look at these data they cannot be correct. The data for Covid-19 hospital admissions (in June at least) must be exaggerated (it cannot be that 'cases' are underestimated because a hospitalisation cannot be classified as Covid-19 without a positive test, i.e. a recorded 'case'). In case anybody thinks the error must be in the way we have extracted the data, the screenshots in the full version of this article for relevant part of June from the government website confirm that that it is not our error.

Table 3 Raw hospitalisation data for London

DATE	New cases by specimen date	New admissions
01/06/2020	49	48
02/06/2020	49	51
03/06/2020	79	68
04/06/2020	57	58
05/06/2020	46	50
06/06/2020	46	46
07/06/2020	45	56
08/06/2020	56	69
09/06/2020	71	35
10/06/2020	52	41
11/06/2020	47	32
12/06/2020	53	30
13/06/2020	39	20
14/06/2020	31	22
15/06/2020	41	49
16/06/2020	46	56
17/06/2020	42	56
18/06/2020	46	50
19/06/2020	37	47
20/06/2020	29	19
21/06/2020	27	25
22/06/2020	51	60
23/06/2020	49	69
24/06/2020	46	51
25/06/2020	57	47
26/06/2020	48	39
27/06/2020	32	29
28/06/2020	22	18
29/06/2020	58	20
30/06/2020	52	28
01/07/2020	42	53

Now, there they may be understandable reasons for errors in the Government data. For example, perhaps only a subset of hospital admissions were recorded in June, or perhaps there are different definitions of what 'London' is defined as for 'cases' compared to 'admissions'. But, whatever, if the Government cannot get such basic data correct, it hardly inspires trust in their Draconian decisions. And how do we know that the number of Covid-19 hospital 'admissions' is still not being exaggerated? The latest London case fatality rate plot confirms there is no need for panic. Not only is the rate steady and very low compared to the spring 2020 numbers (and even compared to as late as June 2020) but the current 1% is ***less*** than the current national average of 1.8%

3.4. The curious pooled Covid-19 testing

Makes the data on 'cases' even more dubious (23 December 2020)

This article [65] by Clare Craig, Jonathan Engler, Mike Yeadon, and Christian McNeill lays out a convincing case why PCR testing for Covid-19 has failed.

While we were aware of many of the issues they raise, until speaking with Clare, Jonathan and also Joel Smalley, Keith Johnson, and Scott McLachlan yesterday we were unaware of another major problem with PCR testing that is not discussed in the article. Specifically, when mass PCR testing for Covid-19 started in the UK in late summer, so too did the idea to implement **pooled testing** as described in this official NHS document. It is not clear how extensively the idea has been implemented, but it could have created more problems.

The motivation for pooled testing for any virus is that you can do much more efficient testing when population infection rates are low. Instead of separately testing each sample you combine, say, 10 samples and test the pooled sample. When prevalence is low then the pooled sample will most likely test negative and so we can conclude that all of the individual samples in it were negative. On the relatively rare occasions when the pooled sample tests positive we conclude that at least one of the individual samples would be positive and so (only when this happens) we retest each of the individual samples to confirm which ones were positive.

A proposed implementation of the NHS Guidelines for pooled testing by McNally and Ball is described here. However, there are the following fundamental problems with using pooled testing for Covid-19.

1. For a start, pooled testing - according to the NHS document - should be used only when the population infection rate is in the range 1% to 2% and when the infection rate among those being tested (the test positivity rate) is around 8%. But many areas currently have much higher test positivity rates (for example, as we can see below, London is now at 15% and the number tested there in the week ending 18 Dec was 410,463 - an increase of over 57% from the 261,075 just one week earlier). So, this should certainly rule out pooled testing. Moreover, the title of the NHS document suggests it should be used only on samples from asymptomatic people, which makes sense since those with symptoms will have a much higher probability of being infected. However, it is not clear if this has been the case. The NHS document says:

   > "It is also expected that as winter approaches the demand for Covid-19-19 testing will increase, putting more pressure on an already stretched system. Sample pooling strategies increase testing capacity when resources are limited."

   If pooled testing was only used on asymptomatics, then testing data that differentiates between symptomatics and asymptomatics would be available, but we are constantly told it is not.

2. As explained here [72], calculating the optimum number of samples (and process) for pooled testing requires prior knowledge of:
   - The current true population infection rate
   - The false positive test rate for asymptomatics (i.e. the probability an asymptomatic person without the virus tests positive)
   - The false negative test rate for asymptomatics (i.e. the probability an asymptomatic person with the virus tests negative)

   Moreover, all these values need to be low for pooled testing to be efficient and accurate. But, as we have made clear many times, NONE of these are known; indeed, one of the main purposes of testing asymptomatics is to find out what these really are.

So, while theoretically the concept of pooled testing (especially if you are testing asymptomatic people) for Covid-19 is sound, practically it seems flawed before we start.

3. Asymptomatics with the virus have low viral load, so even for a single sample it requires high Ct values to detect it. Because pooled samples are mixed from the original samples, even higher Ct values are needed to detect the virus if it is indeed there. But, while high Ct values decrease the false negative rate, they ***increase*** the false positive rate. This is tolerable when the population infection rate is very low because there will be sufficiently few positive samples so that they can all be retested individually. Suppose, for example, that the false positive rate for a pooled sample is 5% and the false positive rate for a single sample is 2%. Then the probability that an individual sample will wrongly test positive is the probability it will wrongly test positive both in a pooled sample and then individually. This is 0.05 times 0.02 which is 0.001, i.e. just 0.1%. Similarly, if there is no pooled testing, but there is confirmatory testing for each individual sample that tests positive, then the probability that a sample will wrongly test positive twice is 0.02 times 0.02 which is 0.0004, i.e. 0.04%.

   This explains why – in the summer when the infection rate was close to zero – the number of 'positives' (and necessarily the number of false positives) was also very low. All those people who have ridiculed the notion of false positive rates above 1% for PCR testing simply do not understand the role of confirmatory testing (whether in pooled or individual testing). But, while the conditions for pooled and/or confirmatory testing were OK for the summer (low population infection rate, lots of testing but mostly asymptomatic people) that changed as soon as the infection rate (as well as illnesses which have similar symptoms) increased in the autumn.

   Even if the population infection rate is stable any big increase in the number of tests conducted is likely to lead to a greater proportion of false positives whether or not pooled testing is used. This is because, as testing increases not only is there greater potential for various types of handling and contamination errors due to limited resources and time, but inevitably it seems **fewer confirmatory tests can be carried out**. If pooled testing is performed without confirmatory testing, then the false positive rate (using the above example figures) increases from 0.1% to 5%. That is a massive increase. If pooled testing is not applied, then the false positive rate rises from 0.04% when confirmatory testing is used to 2% when it is not.

It is difficult to find out just how much pooled testing has been going on and whether and when there has been a drop in confirmatory testing. It is likely that there will have been major differences between labs. But, given the massive increase in testing since September, if for whatever reason it is felt that confirmatory testing cannot be carried out, then this would explain why we are seeing a very close correlation between number of tests and test positivity.

Jonathan Engler raises the following additional relevant points:

"The PCR test has been worked up from bench-top to industrialised scale, in assay development terms, overnight. In particular, there is only quite limited testing of cross-reactivity with other viruses. What testing there was – as outlined in the Drosten paper – revealed some cross-reactivity.

Also, from the Drosten paper they ***do*** report on 4 positive cases out of 310 negative controls containing other viruses: These examples of "weak initial reactivity" are somewhat brushed off, justified by them testing negative 2nd time around, but they do account for >1% of tests. (What if the 306 initial negatives had been tested again – might some of those then have then been positive on their 2nd test?). The point of this in relation to pooling is that there are clearly uncharacterised sources of false positivity, likely including but possibly not limited to unknown or undetected coronaviruses; even a single such instance could contaminate the entire pool, and then testing at high cycle rates could surely magnify such issues greatly."

3.5. How many people 'with Covid' are actually ill?

Divergence between numbers of 'cases' and people reporting symptoms (26-Dec 2020)

On 23 December over half a million people (507,384) - the highest daily total yet - had a COVID-19 test in the UK. That was an increase of 39.2% over the total tested (364,388) just one week earlier on 16 Dec.

Yet, as shown in the screenshot in the full version of this article during exactly the same period there was an average daily total of just 8,500 total NHS triages - **and that number includes all** 999, 111 calls and 111-online reports. The increase from 16 Dec (when it was 8239) to 23 Dec (when it was 9185) was just 11%. The figure also shows how low those numbers are compared to when the virus was at its peak in March; for example, on 19 March there were 152,088 NHS triages.

Four days after those 152,088 people reported symptoms through NHS triages there were, according to the Government website, 1,379 confirmed 'cases' (where, of course, 'cases' simply means a positive test result). On 18 Dec just 7,969 people reported symptoms through NHS triages. Yet, on 22 Dec there were 44,903 'cases'. So, whereas in March less than 1% of the number reporting symptoms through the NHS tested positive, we now have a situation where, for every person reporting symptoms through the NHS we have nearly six testing positive. If that March ratio applied today then the 7,969 people with symptoms would equate to about 72 'cases', not the 44,903 reported.

The remarkably diverging difference between 'cases' and people reporting symptoms provides yet more evidence that the vast majority of those currently testing positive do not have the virus.

There are causal explanations for part of the divergence: in March - unlike now - it was primarily patients hospitalised with the virus who were being tested, so people who may have had the virus but had minor (or no symptoms) may not have been recorded as 'cases'. It is also possible that more people with symptoms now are choosing to go straight for a test and not report their symptoms through the NHS. However, these causal explanations go nowhere near to explaining the scale of the divergence observed (625 times as many cases per people reporting symptoms since March).

It is also important to note that those who point to the Government-backed ZOE COVID symptom app tracker for estimates of number of cases are also being misled, because the website clearly states that the estimate is based on 'the app + swab tests'.

3.6. On false positives in Covid-19 testing again

We are being misled over confirmatory testing (29 Dec 2020)

It has long been claimed that many of the COVID-19 'cases' reported (where a 'case' is simply a positive test result) are false positives. This short article addresses an aspect of the problem not widely discussed before and suggests that many of the very large number of new 'cases' reported amid great hysteria each day could be people who do not have COVID-19.

One of the biggest misunderstandings about the notion of accuracy for a type of test (such as a PCR test) is the idea that there is a (single) *false positive rate*, namely the probability that the test will be positive for a person who does not have the virus. The false positive rate at any particular time - and in any particular testing lab - will depend on multiple factors. Some of these factors relate to the lab doing the testing, which includes: experience of staff, pressure staff are working under, probability of contamination; the particular equipment and chemicals used; and, of course, the much discussed Ct-value threshold used. Other factors relate to the source of the samples being tested: for example, whether they were primarily from people with symptoms, whether they were primarily from people in hospitals, whether they were primarily from people who had been in recent contact with a COVID-19 positive person, etc. If any of these factors change, the false positive rate is likely to change. Without information about all these factors there is nothing we can conclude with any kind of certainty from counts of tests and positives alone.

However, as we previously explained, by far the biggest factor affecting the false positive rate is whether and how a positive test is repeated before actually declaring that a person has tested positive (this is called ***confirmatory testing***). Let us suppose that on any single test the current false positive rate is 0.01 (i.e. 1%). Then, if a lab does no confirmatory testing, 0.01 can be crudely assumed to be ***the*** false positive rate (meaning 1 in every 100 without the virus would wrongly test positive). However, if the lab does confirmatory testing whereby a new sample is taken from the person who tested positive, then it reasonable to assume that the two tests are 'independent' and in that case the probability a person who does not have the virus tests positive both times is 0.01 times 0.01 which is 0.0001, i.e. 0.01% (so only 1 in every 10,000 without the virus would wrongly be classified as testing positive).

Hence, for a Lab in which confirmatory testing is carried out rigorously, the false positive rate can be close to 0 even if 'the false positive rate' for individual tests is relatively high.

When we previously suggested that - due to pressure of massively increased numbers of tests - it might be possible that confirmatory testing was not always carried out - a number of indignant respondents on Twitter ridiculed the idea, insisting that confirmatory testing was always done. But, in the absence of any clear information about this everything points to the likelihood that rigorous confirmatory testing may not have been widely conducted at all since mass testing began in late summer.

The official NHS Guidance document on PCR testing says the following (page 7):

> Positive results that are sent by NHS England and NHS Improvement pathology network laboratories for confirmation to a PHE laboratory will be considered presumptive positives until confirmed. (see list –Appendix 2). Confirmation is not required if network laboratories are confident in the test they have adopted and assured of an accurate result. If in any doubt, samples can be referred to a PHE regional laboratory local to the NHS testing laboratory for confirmatory testing, for an initial period until the NHS network laboratory is assured their testing is robust, accurate and safe. After this time confirmation by local PHE laboratories will no longer be required. Presumptive positive/positive results will be notified to the co-ordination center for contact tracing, which will start immediately.

So, we know that confirmation was never ***required*** providing the labs were sufficiently confident that they could 'accurately test' first time round. Even if confirmatory testing is done there is also no definitive requirement to test a new sample, meaning that the second test may not be independent of the first; in that case there will not be such a great reduction in the false positive rate.

The simple anecdotal evidence that independent confirmatory testing is now unlikely to be done routinely is that we know many people who have got a positive test result (outside of hospitals) and they have never been asked to do a repeat test.

The Government website that produces the daily number of 'new cases' is supposed to only count 'confirmed' cases. In other words, it should **not include** any positive test where that was the first positive test for the person sampled. As we now know that this is no longer true it means that the published 'number of cases' are not all 'confirmed' cases. Hence, it will include a greater percentage of false positives than previous periods when more confirmatory testing was done.

The massive increase in testing since September means that it is very likely an increasingly smaller proportion of confirmatory testing has been done, which in turn means the false positive rate would have increased. Similarly, when testing is scaled back the false positive rate is likely to decrease. While there was also likely to have been a small resurgence of COVID-19 in September, the changes in false positive rate are likely to be the most significant causal explanation for the close correlation between number of tests and test positivity (% of test that are positive) that has been observed in all areas of the UK since September.

In contrast to the 'number of cases' which has risen steadily as more tests are conducted (and which cannot be considered as a reliable measure of the infection rate), the data on NHS triages for COVID - which includes all 999, 111 calls and 111-online reports also supports the hypothesis that the big increases in number of 'cases' since September is due in part to increase in false positives; while the greater availability of tests could explain some of the decrease in people using the NHS triage path, the data still provides evidence that, after a small resurgence in September, the number of people actually ill with COVID has remained quite steady and much lower than it was in the spring.

To give some idea of the impact of a changing false positive rate, let us suppose for illustration that (as above) the individual test false positive is 0.01 and that therefore the independent confirmatory false positive rate is 0.0001. Then, with confirmatory testing, if the population infection rate is 0.5% (1 in 200) then, assuming an 80% true positive test rate, it follows from Bayes Theorem that 97.6% of those testing positive really are positive. However, without confirmatory testing only 28.7% of those testing positive really are positive.

There is no getting away from the fact that the data on testing and cases provided by the Government is insufficient to make any definitive conclusions about the true status of Covid-19. We have previously listed the many additional pieces of information needed to make anything other than massively uncertain conclusions. We also need to know how many of the new 'cases' were subject to confirmatory testing. Given the incredible resources being spent on testing, if the Government cannot provide the additional information listed in Figure 10 (which all must be available somewhere) there really is no point in carrying out these tests.

COVID19 in the UK

Things we are told	Things we know (but are not often told)	Things we are not being told
"The problem is out of control because number of cases is increasing all the time"	A 'case' is just a positive test (usually PCR). Testing has massively increased and, as PCR testing produces false positives, this inevitably leads to an increase in 'cases'	How inaccurate and variable is the testing and how this has changed over time with mass testing
"Only people with symptoms or people at risk are being tested"	Lots of healthy people with no symptoms or recent contact with a symptomatic COVID positive person are routinely getting tested – and many are positive without ever being ill (example: college kids and footballers)	For the people tested without symptoms, what proportion are they of a) the total tested and b) those testing positive; and how this has changed since April
"The increase in numbers tested - along with increase in proportion testing positive - proves the problem is getting worse"	All other reporting indicators show number of people with COVID symptoms steady and much lower than the spring peak for months. The increase in proportion testing positive now correlates closely with the increase in testing.	The increase in proportion of people without symptoms getting tested. The increase in proportion of false positives that occur as testing increases.
"It is important to keep testing as many people as possible"	Mass testing has cost billions of pounds and is what is driving the lockdown decisions. It has caused massive distress and inconvenience, forced thousands of healthy, non-contagious people to quarantine unnecessarily	Whether mass testing has had any positive effect at all and whether there would still be a crisis if we had focused only on testing people genuinely ill with COVID symptoms
"Many hospitals are at - or close to – capacity and are struggling to cope with the pandemic"	There are always similar capacity problems at this time of year in parts of the NHS due to winter flu etc.	In these hospitals, how many healthy staff are absent simply because they tested positive after routine testing
"Mask wearing, handwashing and social distancing stop the spread of COVID. These measures also stop flu".	'Official' flu case numbers are now close to 0 (there would normally be thousands a month this time of year), suggesting (irrationally) that these measures completely eradicate flu, but actually fail to stop COVID.	How many flu cases are being misclassified as COVID.
"The number of COVID hospital admissions has been increasing"	Irrespective of reason for admission anybody with a positive COVID test before or after admission is classified as a COVID admission	What proportion of 'COVID hospital admissions' were admitted for a reason other than COVID.
"The number of COVID deaths has been increasing"	Irrespective of actual cause, anybody with a positive COVID test within 28 days of death is classified as a COVID death	What proportion of 'COVID deaths' were caused by something other than COVID.
"Lockdowns are necessary to control the virus"	Not a single person involved in advising/making lockdown decisions is at risk of losing their jobs as a result	The true cost of lockdowns (on health, economy and liberty)

https://probabilityandlaw.blogspot.com

Figure 10 what we need to know

There is also the issue of the difference between PCR test results and LFT test results. For example, in Scotland on 16 Dec 2020 it was reported that 2.02% of 10,545 healthy people tested by PCR were positive. But only 0.29% of 5,031 healthy people tested by LFT were positive. That is a sevenfold increase in positivity rate by PCR meaning that either or both testing methods is incredibly inaccurate.

3.7. The “1 in 3 people with Covid-19 have no symptoms” claim

We smash this claim (originally published 10 Feb 2021 then updated)

One of the most persistent and widely publicised claims made by the UK government and its scientific advisers about SARS-Cov-2 is that "1 in 3 people who have the virus have no symptoms” (Figure 11)

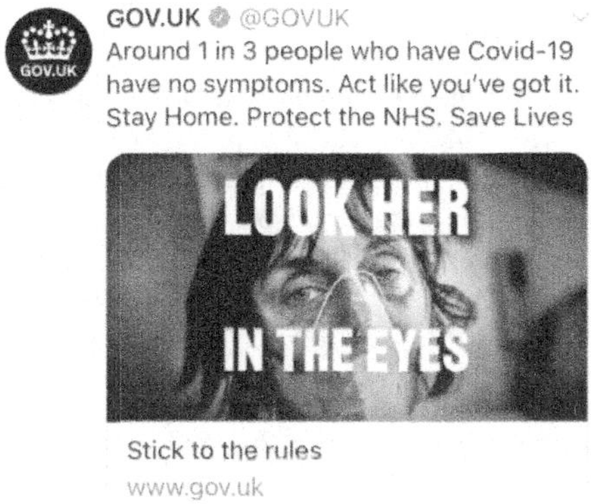

Figure 11 Fear tactics

However, using data from a study of asymptomatics at Cambridge we show that both the “1 in 3” claim and the Office for National Statistics (ONS) infection rate estimates are exaggerated. Here we provide a simplified summary and explanation of this full analysis [78].

The Cambridge study uses PCR tests on asymptomatic people, and a person is classified as having the virus if an initial positive test is confirmed in a follow-up test. Their data shows that, during a period when the ONS estimated the infection rate was 0.71%, an average of only 1 in 4,867 people (0.00205%) with no symptoms had the virus at any time. Although this does not tell us *how many people with the virus had no symptoms*, we can conclude the following:

Conclusion 1: If the ONS reported infection rate, 0.71%, is correct, then at most 2.9% (1 in 34) of people with the virus have no symptoms, and not 1 in 3 as claimed by the government.

Informal explanation: The population of Cambridge is 129,000. So, since only 1 in 4867 asymptomatics have the virus, the maximum possible number of asymptomatics with the virus is 27. If the ONS claimed infection rate is correct, then 0.71% of people in Cambridge would have the virus. This is about 916 people. Hence, at most 27 out of 916 with the virus had no symptoms. That is a maximum of 2.9% (27/916), 1 in 34.

But, on the other hand, it tells us:

Conclusion 2: If the government claim that "1 in 3 people with the virus has no symptoms" is correct, then the ONS reported infection rate must be at most 0.06%. This would mean the reported rate of 0.71% is at least 11 times greater than the true infection rate.

Informal explanation: We already noted that in Cambridge the maximum number of asymptomatics with the virus is 27. But if 1 in 3 people with the virus have no symptoms, then the maximum total number of people with the virus is three times that number, 81. That means a maximum of 81 out of 129,000 have the virus. Thus, the maximum infection rate consistent with the government's claim is 0.06% (81/129,000) and not 0.71%.

Hence, the UK government claim "1 in 3" claim and the ONS infection rate claim **cannot both be simultaneously true.**

What is the explanation for the government and ONS claims being mutually incompatible, and what *is* the likely virus infection rate and proportion of people with the virus who have no symptoms? The explanation lies in the impact of false positives. Unlike in the Cambridge study, the government assumes that a person who tests positive in a single PCR test has SARS-Cov-2 and they are very unlikely to be subject to confirmatory testing to determine whether this is a true or false positive. So, an estimated 0.71% infection rate is essentially an estimate that, if we randomly tested 100,000 people, we would expect 710 to test positive.

However, we also know from the Cambridge study that 3 in every 1000 people without symptoms will falsely test positive. Taking this, and all the other observed data into account we show that:

- The infection rate, for the period in question, was most likely to be 0.379% (95% confidence interval is 0.372% to 0.387%). We also performed a sensitivity analysis that showed that the results are robust against a range of prior assumptions; specifically, there is no reasonable scenario under which the maximum value for the infection rate was greater than 0.44%.
- The percentage of people with SARS-Cov-2, but no symptoms was most likely to be 5% (95% confidence interval is 4.4% to 5.4%). Again, we showed this result was robust under a sensitivity analysis. There is thus no reasonable scenario in which more than 1 in 18 people with SARS-Cov-2 had no symptoms.

So, we conclude:

- The government's "1 in 3" claim overestimates the percentage of people with SARS-Cov-2 who have no symptoms by at least 560%.
- The ONS's estimate of the infection rate (0.71%) is exaggerated by at least 80%.

We also considered the extent to which the government and ONS claims are exaggerated for different possible infection rates. As the infection rate drops, the extent to which the estimated infection rate is exaggerated increases, because the proportion of false positives inevitably increases. At the current estimated infection rate of 0.35%, it is likely that the actual infection rate is only around 0.1% meaning that the current estimated infection rate exaggerates the true rate by 250%. The percentage of people with SARS-Cov-2, but no symptoms is most likely to be 9.62%, about 1 in 10, not 1 in 3 as claimed.

One other interesting observation we found was that, when the ONS estimated infection rate is 1% the proportion of people testing positive who have no symptoms is approximately 1 in 3. Hence, the claim that "1 in 3 people with the virus have no symptoms" claim is approximately true in this case only if we replace "with the virus" with "test positive".

While the focus was on just one UK city there is reason to believe that the results apply generally throughout the UK, and it is therefore also reasonable to conclude that SARS-Cov-2 case numbers have been systematically exaggerated. It is also reasonable to conclude that mass testing of asymptomatic people (who have not been in recent contact with a person confirmed as having the virus) may be causing unnecessary anguish for minimal benefit at a very high societal and economic cost.

Chapter 4. More data shenanigans and censorship as the vaccine is rolled out

4.1. The Tiffany Dover (collapsing nurse) cover-up

1 February 2021

There could not have been a more dramatic early indication that the Pfizer vaccine was not safe than the case of critical care nurse, Tiffany Dover, from CHI Memorial Hospital in Chattanooga. On 17 Dec 2020 Tiffany collapsed on live television within seconds of being one of the first recipients of the Pfizer vaccine. We have been tweeting about this story because of the subsequent cover-up and concerted attempts by the mainstream media to confuse the public about what happened. Today the Independent has published [79] an article attempting to squash the 'conspiracy theories' by 'anti-vaxxers' including the claims that Tiffany Dover is no longer alive.

In fact, the only evidence that the Independent article provides is the fact that Tiffany was interviewed [81] shortly after feinting, saying she feels fine. The interview was on either 17 or 18 Dec 2020. But there has been no sighting of Tiffany since then and no public statement by her. The supposed 'evidence' that proves she is alive and well is more suggestive of a very clumsy cover-up. The supposed photographic evidence that she was alive on 21 Dec 2020 is a strange photo provided by the hospital of some masked nurses taken that day promoting the vaccine. They claim one of the nurses is Tiffany, but it is impossible to tell; many have pointed out it looks more like another nurse in the same unit.

What we do know is that until 17 Dec 2020 Tiffany had been a prolific social media user, posting often several times a day on her Facebook and Instagram accounts. She has not posted anything since and many people are rightly worried, especially as they want to know if whatever happened to her was caused by the vaccine. If Tiffany is alive and well, why doesn't she simply provide a video statement?

Updates to this story:

- Multiple mainstream sources produced articles 'disproving' the 'conspiracies' about Tiffany but curiously they all invariably linked to the Independent article as proof.
- The only ever update to Tiffany Dover's social media accounts was a single Instagram post on 26 Feb 2021 where 'she' wrote cryptically: "Meet me on the other side of paradise".
- Most bizarrely, in April 2022 NBC published to great fanfare a series of podcasts [82] titled, ironically "Tiffany Dover is dead", to 'prove' once and for all that the conspiracy theorists were wrong and that she was in fact alive and well. The only problem was that, despite all the wealth, power and influence of NBC, they were unable to get an interview with Tiffany Dover to prove that she was alive!

- This article [83] comprehensively catalogues what was known about the Tiffany Dover story up until August 2022. The author concluded that, although neither the Hospital nor Tiffany or any family member, had provided any proof, she was alive and well. He concluded that this was "part of the charade intended to discredit those who raised concerns about the rollout of the vaccines". He held her responsible for every one of the deaths and serious injuries resulting from the vaccines. He predicted that at some point in the next year Tiffany would show up, hence 'exposing' the 'conspiracy theorists' and 'anti-vaxxers'.
- Indeed on 10 April 2023 NBC did finally get an interview [84] and photoshoot with Tiffany Dover. In it Tiffany looks completely different to any of the previous images and videos of her prior to 19 Dec 2020 and the interview provided no clear explanation for why she was silent for so long.

4.2. Major problem with UK lighthouse laboratories testing

18 March 2021

We have recently discovered that UK laboratories have been routinely recording a significant proportion of Covid-19 test results as positive based on the presence of one target gene alone, when there should have been two or more, as required to comply with WHO rules and manufacturer instructions. Without diagnostic validation, for both the original virus and any variants, it is not clear what can be concluded from a positive test resulting from a single target gene call, especially if there was no confirmatory testing. Given this, many of the reported positive results may be inconclusive, negative or from people who suffered past infection for SARS-COV-2. Our full detailed report has been published [85]. Here we present a summary (which was also published in the BMJ [86].

The efficacy of mass population testing for SARS-COV-2 virus is critically dependent on the reliability of the test applied, whether it be a RT-PCR or lateral flow test. Given that many RT-PCR tests do not actually target all the genes necessary to reliably detect SARS-COV-2, the results of mass testing using RT-PCR need to be revisited and reanalysed.

The ONS publish a regular infection survey [87] that includes data from two UK lighthouse laboratories, where both use the same RT-PCR test kit to detect the SARS-COV-2 virus. This survey includes data on the cycle threshold (Ct) used to detect positive samples, the percentage of positive test results arising from using RT-PCR, and the combinations of the SARS-COV-2 virus target genes tested that gave rise to positives between 21 September 2020 and 1 March 2021 across the whole of the UK.

The kit used by the Glasgow and Milton Keynes lighthouse laboratories is the ThermoFisher TaqPath RT-PCR which tests for the presence of three target genes from SARS-COV-2 [88]. Despite Corman et al [89] originating the use of PCR testing for SARS-COV-2 genes there is no agreed international standard for SARS-COV-2 testing. Instead, the World Health Organisation (WHO) leaves it up to the manufacturer to determine what genes to use and instructs end users to adhere to the manufacturer instructions for use (IFU).

The WHO's emergency use assessment (EUA) for the ThermoFisher TaqPath kit [90] includes the instruction manual and contained therein (Table 6) is an interpretation algorithm describing an unequivocal requirement that two or more target genes be detected before a positive result can be declared. The latest revision of ThermoFisher's instruction manual contains the same algorithm [90] the WHO have been sufficiently concerned about correct use of RT-PCR kits that on 20 January 2021 they issued a notice for PCR users imploring them to review manufacturer IFUs carefully and adhere to them fully [91].

The ONS's report [87] lists SARS-COV-2 positive results for valid two and three target gene combinations and does the same in [92], for samples processed by the Glasgow and Milton Keynes lighthouse laboratories. However, it also lists single gene detections as positive results (See tables 6a and 6b). Over the period reported the maximum weekly percentage of positives on a single gene is 38% for the whole of the UK for the week of 1 February. The overall UK average was 23%. The maximum percentage reported is 65%, in East England in the week beginning 5 October. In Wales it was 50%, in Northern Ireland it is 55% and in Scotland it was 56%. The full data including averages and maxima/minima are given here [93].

Professor Alan McNally, Director of the University of Birmingham Turnkey laboratory, who helped set up the Milton Keynes lighthouse laboratory, contradicted what was stated in the ONS report in a Guardian newspaper article about the new variant. He reported [94] that all lighthouse laboratories operated a policy that adhered to the manufacturer instructions for use: requiring two-or-more genes for positive detection (this policy is also documented in [95], which defines the standard operating procedure reported in [87]).

In correspondence with Mr Nicholas Lewis about single gene testing, in February 2021, the ONS confirmed that they do indeed call single gene targets as positives in their Covid-19 Infection Survey and also confirmed that the samples are processed by UK lighthouse laboratories [96], [97].

As early as April 2020, the UK lighthouse laboratories were testing for single genes and discounted the S gene [98] as early as mid-May, months before the discovery of the new variant B1.1.7. Indeed, in Table 1 of [98] 18% of tests were positive on one gene only. Furthermore, in a Public Health England report on variants [88] published 8 January 2021, it states the goal of using one gene was explicitly to approximate the growth of the new B1.1.7 variant:

> "There has recently been an increase in the percentage of positive cases where only the ORF1ab- and N-genes were found and a decrease in the percentage of cases with all three genes. We can use this information to approximate the growth of the new variant."

Section 10 of this ONS Covid-19 Infection Survey report [99] on 8 January 2021 confirms that one gene is sufficient for a positive result.

Obviously, there is a higher risk of encountering false positives when testing for single genes alone, because of the possibility of cross-reactivity with other human coronaviruses (HCOVs) as well as prevalent bacteria or reagent contamination. The potential for cross reactivity has already been confirmed by the German Instand laboratory report from April 2020 [100] (note that Prof. Drosten, co-author of Corman et al is a cooperating partner listed in this report). The report describes the systematic blind testing of positive and negative samples anonymously sent to 463 laboratories from 36 countries and evaluated for the presence of a variety of genes associated with SARS-COV-2. They reported significant cross reactivity and resultant false positives for OC43, and HCoV 229E (a common cold virus) as well as for SARS-COV-2 negative samples, not containing any competing pathogen. Likewise, 70 Dutch laboratories were surveyed in November 2020, by the National Institute for Public Health and the Environment [101], with 76 diagnostic workflows reported as using only one target gene to diagnose the presence of SARS-COV-2 (46% of all workflows).

Without diagnostic validation it is not clear what can be concluded from a positive PCR test resulting from a single target gene call, especially if there was no confirmatory testing. Many of the reported positive results may be inconclusive, negative or from people who suffered past infection for SARS-CoV-2. Even with diagnostic validation of the single target gene call, the UK lighthouse laboratories appear not to be in strict conformance with the WHO emergency use assessment and the manufacturer instructions for use. Given this it is clear the ONS and the UK lighthouse laboratories needs to publicly clarify their use of, and justify the reasons for, deviating from these standards.

4.3. The Times attacks our vaccine scepticism

23 March 2021

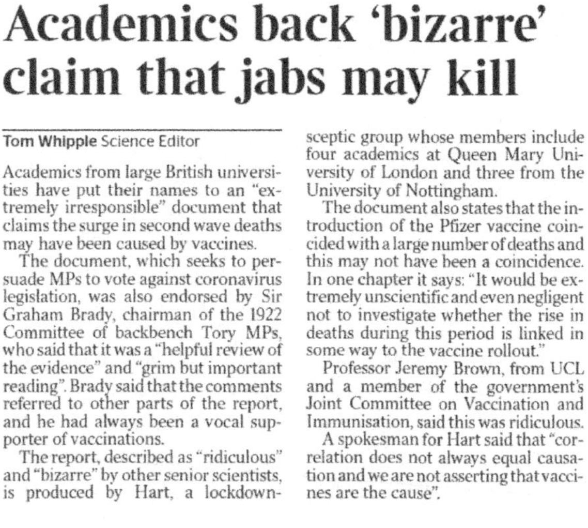

Academics back 'bizarre' claim that jabs may kill

Tom Whipple Science Editor

Academics from large British universities have put their names to an "extremely irresponsible" document that claims the surge in second wave deaths may have been caused by vaccines.

The document, which seeks to persuade MPs to vote against coronavirus legislation, was also endorsed by Sir Graham Brady, chairman of the 1922 Committee of backbench Tory MPs, who said that it was a "helpful review of the evidence" and "grim but important reading". Brady said that the comments referred to other parts of the report, and he had always been a vocal supporter of vaccinations.

The report, described as "ridiculous" and "bizarre" by other senior scientists, is produced by Hart, a lockdown-sceptic group whose members include four academics at Queen Mary University of London and three from the University of Nottingham.

The document also states that the introduction of the Pfizer vaccine coincided with a large number of deaths and this may not have been a coincidence. In one chapter it says: "It would be extremely unscientific and even negligent not to investigate whether the rise in deaths during this period is linked in some way to the vaccine rollout."

Professor Jeremy Brown, from UCL and a member of the government's Joint Committee on Vaccination and Immunisation, said this was ridiculous.

A spokesman for Hart said that "correlation does not always equal causation and we are not asserting that vaccines are the cause".

Figure 12 The Times 23 March 2021

On 23 March 2021 the Times published the article in Figure 12 by its 'Science Editor' Tom Whipple with the headline: "Academics back 'bizarre' claim that jabs may kill". While not explicitly mentioned in that version of the article, Norman and Martin were 2 of the 4 "Queen Mary" academics in HART, and Norman was singled out by name in the online version of the article published on 22 March 2021 (see Figure 13 screenshot) as documented here [102].

> The report, described as "ridiculous" and "bizarre" by other senior scientists, is produced by Hart, a lockdown-sceptic group whose members include four academics at Queen Mary University of London, and three from the University of Nottingham.
>
> Among the 41 academics named in its foreword, several of whom subsequently promoted it on social media, are Ellen Townsend, professor of psychology at Nottingham University, and the group's spokeswoman, Marilyn James, professor of health economics at the University of Nottingham, and Norman Fenton, professor of risk information management, Queen Mary University of London.

Figure 13 Screenshot from online version of The Times article, 22 March 2021

What is especially ironic is that the 23 March 2021 article appeared in the bottom right-hand corner of a double-page spread in The Times that hailed the AstraZeneca vaccine as 100% effective (Figure 14).

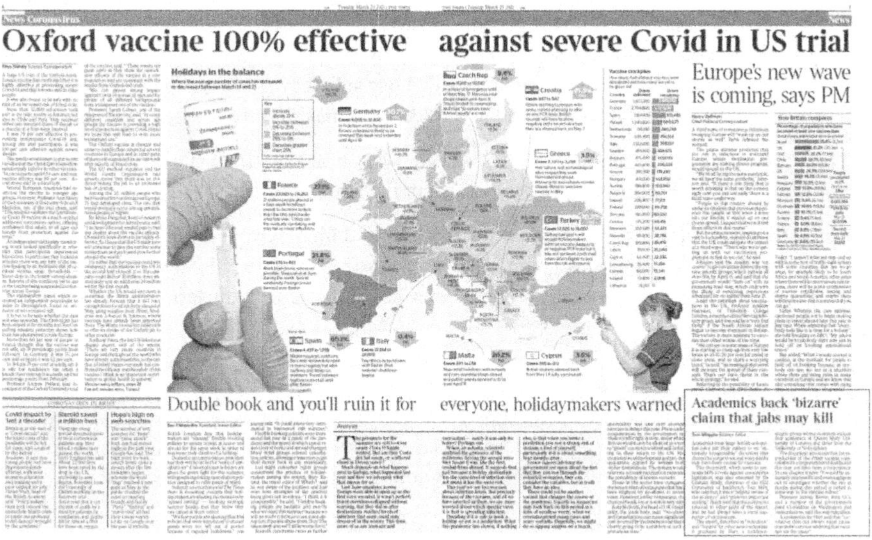
Oxford vaccine 100% effective against severe Covid in US trial

Holidays in the balance

Europe's new wave is coming, says PM

Double book and you'll ruin it for everyone, holidaymakers warned

Academics back 'bizarre' claim that jabs may kill

Figure 14 The Times double-page spread 23 March 2021

While we are proud that we did indeed raise the alarm about safety issues with the Covid-19 vaccines so early on, Whipple's article was inaccurate in many respects and yet also led to Norman's Wikipedia page being 'hacked' with the factually incorrect text shown in

Figure 15. The full details of this hacking and how a small number of activists also used Wikipedia to discredit anybody challenging the official covid narrative can be found here [102] .

COVID-19 [edit]

See also: COVID-19 misinformation

In March 2021, Fenton was one of several academics who put their name to a document seeking to persuade the British government not to pass COVID-19 legislation, suggesting that a large increase in deaths had been caused by the COVID-19 vaccination programme. Jeremy Brown of the Joint Committee on Vaccination and Immunisation said the document was "ridiculous" since the vaccines in question had an established safety profile, and virologist Jonathan Ball said it showed a "blatant disregard for the facts" and was "irresponsible in the extreme".[16]

Figure 15 The hacking of Norman's Wikipedia page

4.4. The barriers to academic publication

for work that challenges the 'official narrative' on Covid-19 (12 April 2021)

Our paper [103] about the "1 in 3 people with Covid-19 have no symptoms" claim has had (at time of writing this) 4093 reads since we posted it on ResearchGate on Friday, and 336,755 impressions to the tweet [104] about it. The video summary [105] has been watched by 7,422 people in 2 days. But this was the response we got less than 24 hours after we submitted it to the BMJ:

> "Thank you for sending us your paper. We read it with interest but I am sorry to say that we do not think it is right for the BMJ. In comparison with the many other papers we have to consider, this one is a lower priority for us. We do not send out for external peer review manuscripts whose subject matter, design or topic do not meet our current priorities and are unlikely to make it through our process."

Even more bizarrely, neither the medRxiv [106] or arXiv [107] sites (where we routinely post pre-prints of our research) would accept the paper. MedRxiv said:

> "Thank you for submitting your manuscript to medRxiv. We regret to inform you that your manuscript is inappropriate for posting. medRxiv is intended for research papers, and our screening process determined that this manuscript fell short of that description."

arXiv said:

> "Our moderators have determined that your submission is not of sufficient interest for inclusion within arXiv. The moderators have rejected your submission after examination, having determined that your article does not contain sufficient original or substantive scholarly research.
>
> As a result, we have removed your submission.Please note that our moderators are not referees and provide no reviews with such decisions. For in-depth reviews of your work, please seek feedback from another forum. Please do not resubmit this paper without contacting arXiv moderation and obtaining a positive response.

Resubmission of removed papers may result in the loss of your submission privileges"

Compare this with what happened in April 2020 when we first investigated the Covid-19 data. Whereas our latest work shows that Covid-19 'case' numbers have been exaggerated and that mass testing of asymptomatic people is counter-productive, at that time we were actually concerned that the numbers infected were being UNDERESTIMATED and the data were skewed by the fact that ONLY people with extreme covid symptoms were being tested (and hence we argued for the need for more random testing).

These views were not considered threatening to the "official narrative" and of course random testing WAS widely implemented after August. We had no problem getting those articles published in academic journals (see e.g. here [108] are some of our other articles on Covid-19. But things are completely different when you challenge the "official narrative". Given that even ResearchGate has been censoring such articles [109] it is possible that our latest paper may be removed. If so a copy can be found here [110].

4.5. NFL Covid-19 protocols

17 June 2021

Table 4 shows the new Covid-19 protocols [111] for NFL players. Eventually these kinds of differences will apply everywhere.

Table 4: Covid protocols for NFL players

Protocol Modifications for Vaccinated Individuals

Fully Vaccinated	Not Fully Vaccinated
• No daily testing required	• Testing required **every day**
• Masks not required at club facility or during team travel	• Masks required at club facility and during travel
• No physical distancing required in club facility with other vaccinated individuals	• Must remain physically distant from others in club facility
• No quarantine required after High Risk exposure to COVID	• Must quarantine after High Risk exposure to COVID
• No travel restrictions	• Travel restrictions in effect
• No capacity limits in weight room when all fully vaccinated	• 15 player limit in weight room
• May eat in cafeteria with other fully vaccinated individuals	• Players must be physically distanced in meal room; may not eat with teammates; • Staff must grab-and-go; no meals in the cafeteria
• No restrictions on social/media/ marketing/sponsorship opportunities	• No social/media/ marketing/ sponsorship activities permitted
• May use sauna/steam room	• May not use sauna/steam room
• May interact with vaccinated family/friends during team travel	• May not leave team hotel to eat in restaurants; may not interact with anyone outside of Team Traveling Party during team travel

Apart from the civil liberties issues, the fact that only unvaccinated will be routinely tested also means that data on vaccine effectiveness will be massively biased because the vast bulk of people being tested will be asymptomatic unvaccinated people. When real infection rates are low (as they are now) this bias will exaggerate vaccine effectiveness because almost all new 'cases' will be asymptomatics (i.e. unvaccinated) - most of which will be false positives. Yet, if infection rates are high the bias could ***underestimate*** vaccine effectiveness as the proportion of symptomatics among those tested will be higher for the vaccinated.

4.6. The problem with ALL studies into the risks/benefits of Covid-19 vaccines

26 June 2021

Here are some ***indisputable facts*** about the challenge of assessing the 'efficacy' – in particular, benefits and risks, of Covid-19 vaccines:

- Without an independent clinical assessment or post-mortem we can never be sure that the vaccine was the main or even a contributory factor if a person suffers an 'adverse reaction' or death after receiving the vaccine.
- All measures of 'effectiveness' used so far rely on comparing numbers of 'Covid-19 cases' of vaccinated v unvaccinated people where a 'case' is defined by a positive PCR test. But PCR tests are unreliable and so we can never be sure if a person does or does not contract Covid-19. Moreover, there is no uniformity in testing strategies between unvaccinated and vaccinated people.
- Even if we could accurately measure the true number of Covid-19 'cases' over time, we can never be sure of the main cause of any change in numbers (vaccines, lockdowns, heard immunity, seasonality, etc).
- The notion of whether or not there are 'excess deaths' (or excess illnesses) depends on multiple subjective criteria about previous years' of data which may be incomplete. Moreover, as with trends in case numbers, we can never be sure of the main cause of 'excess deaths'.

It follows that ***any study*** that claims to demonstrate benefits and/or risks of Covid-19 vaccines which assumes to ***know*** some or all of the following in its data is potentially flawed:

- a death/illness was or was not caused by the vaccine
- the difference in Covid-19 incidence for vaccinated v unvaccinated by using PCR testing
- decreasing or increasing 'cases' was or was not caused by the vaccine
- there is a known number of 'average' deaths that should be 'expected'

Until we have longer term data (especially on deaths for both vaccinated and unvaccinated) these problems can only be avoided by more independent clinical assessment, and a much more rigorous vaccine reaction yellow card reporting system. If Covid-19 'cases' really need to be considered to evaluate effectiveness, then only those where there is a clinical diagnosis with illness and symptoms should be counted. If Covid-19 is as dangerous as is generally assumed, then, in the longer term, the only criterion we need to determine if vaccines work and are safe is if the proportion of deaths and serious illnesses among the vaccinated is lower than that among the unvaccinated.

For the longer-term analysis, we can completely ignore: a) whether or not a death/illness is due to Covid-19; b) the notion of what is/not a Covid 'case'; c) any previous years' data. We just need to know the national (or large area) data as per Table 5 for a few fixed time periods (initially we could even ignore the serious illness data).

Table 5 Required data

	Vaccinated				Unvaccinated		
Age	Total	Deaths	Serious Illness		Total	Deaths	Serious Illness
<18							
...							
>85							

If the (proportional) number of deaths/illnesses overall are less in a vaccinated age group than the corresponding unvaccinated age group, then the vaccine is saving more lives than it is killing. It's as simple as that. No more and no less.

A full cost-benefit analysis should also add the cost of the vaccination programme (e.g. by using standard formulas that equate amounts of spending on healthcare with number of lives saved).

4.7. Simpson's paradox and vaccine effectiveness

26 June 2021

Some people are looking at today's Public Health England report and concluding the Case Fatality Rate for Delta positive cases is much higher for vaccinated compared to unvaccinated. But this is an instance of Simpson's paradox as shown in Table 6 (see a short video [112] explanation of Simpson's paradox).

Table 6 Data from Public Health England

	<50 category		
	Cases	Deaths	%
vaccinated	19693	2	0.010
unvaccinated	52846	6	0.011

	>50 category		
	Cases	Deaths	%
vaccinated	7499	68	0.907
unvaccinated	976	38	3.893

	Aggregated		
	Cases	Deaths	%
vaccinated	27192	70	0.257
unvaccinated	53822	44	0.082

In both age categories the rate among vaccinated is lower; but when the numbers are aggregated the fatality rate for the vaccinated is much higher. And it is simply because a much greater proportion in the older age group (in which most deaths occur) are vaccinated compared to the younger age group.

However, it is worth noting, the following:

- in the <50 age group there is little difference in fatality rate between the vaccinated and unvaccinated
- the data that is completely missing is that relating to deaths (or serious adverse reactions) of vaccinated v unvaccinated people who were NOT classified as having the Covid. So, there is no information on vaccine risks contained in this data.

In fact, as discussed in the previous article, we have general concerns about the usefulness and validity of all the studies and data published so far into the effectiveness and risks/benefits of Covid-19 vaccines. So, the above should certainly not be considered an argument in favour of the vaccine - in fact, we will shortly be producing a report (see next article) about deaths and adverse reactions from the vaccine. However, it is important to call out misrepresentation of data on 'both sides' of the argument.

We also wrote a comprehensive report [113] about the paradoxes and weaknesses to date of the vaccine efficacy studies.

4.8. Analysis of COVID-19 vaccine death reports from VAERS

30 June 2021

There have been multiple conflicting claims made about the safety of the COVID-19 vaccines that were rolled out world-wide from December 2020. However, there is no universally agreed system for reporting either deaths or serious side-effects for which these vaccines may have been the cause or a contributory factor, and hence, as a result, there are concerns about variability in the quality of reports and the credibility of the sources submitting them. Reports can be submitted by physicians involved in administering the vaccine or helping treat side effects that may have consequentially arisen, clinical and non-clinical health service employees, or pharmaceutical professionals involved in the investigation. Likewise, lay people, such as the patient or their family and friends, may have submitted a report independently of medical carers. It has been suggested that a third category of submission may have been made by members of anti-vaccine, or other groups, motivated by ill-intent, who may exaggerate case numbers reported.

Critics of safety reporting cite the fact that lay people, or those with malign intent, may form the bulk of reports and hence statistics on side effects must therefore be exaggerated because they come from non-credible sources. Set against this, research suggests that as few as 1% of the true adverse reactions ever get formally recorded.

In early April 2021 Scott McLachlan and colleagues downloaded the 2021 Vaccine Adverse Events Reporting System (VAERS) dataset (this is the US dataset) with the aim of analysing these reports to determine the range and frequency of health problems potentially caused by the vaccines as well as the quality of the reports and, by inference, the credibility of the reporters lodging them.

For each patient cited in a report, a clinically trained reviewer manually examined the report to determine its source and clinical credibility and to identify and record medical history, current illness, and symptoms. Each was then checked by a second reviewer. This process is ongoing, as there are 1644 deaths in the April VAERS deaths dataset that have been reported in patients who had recently received their first or second COVID-19 vaccination, and over 28,000 serious adverse events that did not result in death.

McLachlan, Fenton and colleagues have today published an interim report [114] (which by July 2024 had been read over 200,000 times) that presents the results of their analysis of the first 250 reported deaths that have been reviewed and coded by the team.

They identified health service employees as the reporter in at least 67% of the reports, while pharmaceutical employees were identified as the reporter in a further 5%. Lay people were identifiable as the reporter in only 28% of the reports. This suggests an intention for clinical applicability and usefulness and goes some way towards addressing the common disclaimer that many VAERS reports are made by aggrieved family members and anti-vaxxers, both with an axe to grind.

Regarding analysing the likely role of the vaccine in the reported deaths, the sample is heavily biased because these were all people vaccinated very early in the programme when only the elderly, those with significant or chronic health conditions and frontline health service staff were being vaccinated. The analysis shows that the patients can be grouped into three main types:

- those where the vaccine was most likely not a factor;
- those where the vaccine may have been a factor; and
- those where the vaccine was the most likely factor in their deaths.

Despite the sample bias, they found that in 34 of the 250 deaths (14%) a vaccine reaction could be ruled out as a contributing factor in their death; these were all patients either already bedridden and expected to die from a serious medical condition like lung cancer, or were described as at end of life or receiving palliative hospice care. For 203 of the 250 (81%) the vaccine may have been a factor in their death; however, many of these patients had one or more chronic or age-related comorbid conditions. Finally, for at least 13 of the 250 deaths (5%) the vaccine was the most likely cause of death; these patients had strong reactions soon after vaccination and died either on the same day, or during the next couple of days.

As a postscript the report received a lot of publicity within the covid sceptic community and got over 200,000 reads on ResearchGate. It is important to note that the more vicious personal attacks against us and our co-authors from mainstream journalists started with the publication of this VAERS work. Two comprehensive examples of these attacks are documented here [115] and here [116].

Chapter 5. The Lancet and the Pfizer study

5.1. Is the Pfizer vaccine as effective as claimed?

21 May 2021

There was massive media fanfare (see Figure 16) over the study [117] (published in The Lancet) in Israel on the effectiveness of the Pfizer vaccine.

Notwithstanding the fact that, in the paper's Declaration of Interests no less than 8 of the 15 authors (FJA, JMM, FK, GM, KP, JS DLS, and LJ) "hold stock and share options in Pfizer" the results look genuinely impressive and provide support for the hypothesis that the vaccine is effective in preventing infection.

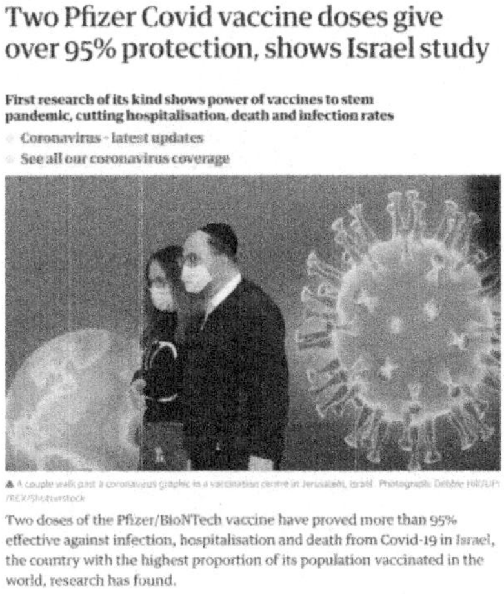
Two Pfizer Covid vaccine doses give over 95% protection, shows Israel study

First research of its kind shows power of vaccines to stem pandemic, cutting hospitalisation, death and infection rates

- Coronavirus - latest updates
- See all our coronavirus coverage

Two doses of the Pfizer/BioNTech vaccine have proved more than 95% effective against infection, hospitalisation and death from Covid-19 in Israel, the country with the highest proportion of its population vaccinated in the world, research has found.

Figure 16 Typical media coverage of the big Pfizer study

In particular, the authors claim that between 24 Jan 2021 and 3 April 2021 there were 109,876 'cases' of SARS-Cov-2 found among those unvaccinated compared to just 6,266 'cases' found among those vaccinated (although there seems to be an error in their table shown here in Figure 17 in that the total number of asymptomatic cases, 49,138, and symptomatic cases, 39,065, do not sum to 109,876.

The table also provides the 'incident rate per 100,000 person days' which is: 91.5 for unvaccinated compared to 3.1 for vaccinated.

Based on these data the (adjusted) 'vaccine effectiveness' measure (defined as: 100 times (1 minus the incident rate ratio where the incident rate ratio is approximately the incident rate of vaccinated divided by the incident rate of unvaccinated) is calculated as 95.3% (hence the headline figure picked up by all mainstream media).

There are, however, issues with the study and its analysis which mean the 95% effectiveness measure is exaggerated. In this article [118] Will Jones argues that the researchers have not adjusted for the declining infection rate during the study period and that when you do so, the effectiveness drops to 74% (in the over 65's).

	Unvaccinated		Fully vaccinated*		Vaccine effectiveness	
	Cases	Incidence rate per 100 000 person-days†	Cases	Incidence rate per 100 000 person-days‡	Unadjusted	Adjusted§
SARS-CoV-2 infection¶						
Age 16–44 years	84 611	95·1	1801	2·3	95·4% (94·0–96·5)	96·1% (95·7–96·5)
Age 45–64 years	18 579	86·1	2264	3·4	93·6% (91·4–95·3)	94·9% (94·2–95·5)
Age ≥65 years	5686	67·7	2201	3·8	93·4% (91·3–95·0)	94·8% (93·9–95·5)
All ages	109 876	91·5	6266	3·1	94·2% (93·2–95·1)	95·3% (94·9–95·7)
Asymptomatic SARS-CoV-2 infection						
Age 16–44 years	40 088	45·1	1174	1·5	92·8% (90·3–94·7)	93·6% (92·8–94·4)
Age 45–64 years	7414	32·6	1343	2·0	89·1% (84·7–92·3)	90·8% (89·6–91·9)
Age ≥65 years	1636	19·5	1115	1·9	85·9% (80·2–89·9)	88·5% (86·4–90·3)
All ages	49 138	40·9	3632	1·8	90·1% (88·0–91·8)	91·5% (90·7–92·2)
Symptomatic COVID-19						
Age 16–44 years	28 196	31·7	352	0·5	97·8% (97·0–98·3)	97·6% (97·3–97·8)
Age 45–64 years	7790	34·3	560	0·8	96·3% (95·0–97·3)	96·7% (96·3–97·0)
Age ≥65 years	3079	36·6	780	1·4	96·1% (94·8–97·1)	96·4% (95·9–97·0)
All ages	39 065	32·5	1692	0·8	96·6% (95·8–97·2)	97·0% (96·7–97·2)
COVID-19-related hospitalisation						
Age 16–44 years	2043	2·3	33	<0·01	98·1% (97·1–98·8)	98·1% (97·3–98·7)
Age 45–64 years	1687	7·4	112	0·2	97·6% (96·9–98·2)	97·6% (97·1–98·1)
Age ≥65 years	1826	21·7	451	0·8	96·6% (95·3–97·6)	96·8% (96·2–97·3)
All ages	5526	4·6	596	0·3	96·7% (95·5–97·6)	97·2% (96·8–97·5)
Severe or critical COVID-19-related hospitalisation						
Age 16–44 years	644	0·7	7	0·01	98·8% (97·3–99·5)	98·9% (97·6–99·5)
Age 45–64 years	1132	5·0	62	0·1	98·1% (97·2–98·6)	98·1% (97·5–98·5)
Age ≥65 years	1425	17·0	295	0·5	97·2% (95·9–98·1)	97·3% (96·8–97·8)
All ages	3201	2·7	364	0·2	97·2% (95·9–98·1)	97·5% (97·1–97·8)
COVID-19-related death						
Age 16–44 years	36	0·04	0	0·0	100	100
Age 45–64 years	125	0·5	14	<0·01	96·2% (92·6–98·0)	95·8% (92·6–97·6)
Age ≥65 years	554	6·6	124	0·2	96·8% (94·6–98·1)	96·9% (96·0–97·6)
All ages	715	0·6	138	0·1	96·6% (93·9–98·1)	96·7% (96·0–97·3)

Numbers and incidence rates of outcomes are shown for unvaccinated and fully vaccinated individuals. Vaccine effectiveness estimates are % (95% CI). *Defined as people for whom at least 7 days had passed after the second dose of BNT162b2 vaccine. †Total person-days for all outcomes were 88 938 455 for age 16–44 years, 22 734 025 for age 45–64 years, 8 403 760 for age ≥65 years, and 120 076 240 for all ages. ‡Total person-days for all outcomes were 77 280 720 for age 16–44 years, 67 027 505 for age 45–64 years, 57 573 640 for age ≥65 years, and 201 881 865 for all ages. §Model is adjusted for age group (16–24, 25–34, 35–44, 45–54, 55–64, 65–74, 75–84, and ≥85 years), sex, and calendar week. ¶Includes asymptomatic and symptomatic infections, as well as cases with positive SARS-CoV-2 tests for which the symptom interview portion of the epidemiological investigation was not completed.

Table 2: **Estimated effectiveness of two doses of BNT162b2 (≥7 days after the second dose) against laboratory-confirmed SARS-CoV-2 outcomes by age group (Jan 24 to April 3, 2021)**

Figure 17 Table 2 from the paper

A different problem with the study (that we focus on here) arises from the statement found on page 8 of the paper (shown in Figure 18).

What this is saying is that, whereas unvaccinated people continued to be regularly and routinely subject to PCR tests, vaccinated people no longer had to be. The number of 'cases' stated in Table 2 is, of course, simply the number of positive PCR test outcomes (which includes false positives). If you stop testing vaccinated people, then you are not going to find any 'cases' among them. The paper says that 19% of the tests were, however, on 'exempted', i.e. vaccinated people. But, this still means unvaccinated people were much more likely to be tested than vaccinated people, so we have to take account of the absolute number of tests performed on both vaccinated and unvaccinated.

> symptoms later). Although we made efforts to avoid this type of misclassification by excluding the small number of people who were initially reported to be asymptomatic but were later hospitalised for or died from COVID-19, some presymptomatic individuals who later developed symptoms without being hospitalised or dying might still have been included. This type of misclassification, however, was probably uncommon and would be unlikely to substantially influence the vaccine effectiveness estimate against asymptomatic infection.
>
> Notably, Israel's SARS-CoV-2 testing policy was different for unvaccinated and vaccinated individuals during the study period. At 7 days after the second dose, vaccinated individuals were exempt from the SARS-CoV-2 testing required of individuals who either had contact with a laboratory-confirmed case or returned from travel abroad. This testing policy might have resulted in a differential bias that would cause overestimation of vaccine effectiveness against asymptomatic infection (ie, asymptomatic people who received two doses were less likely to be tested than unvaccinated asymptomatic people). However, 19% of the 4·4 million PCR tests conducted during the study period were done on exempted individuals (MoH, unpublished data). Additionally, symptomatic individuals might have been reluctant to report symptoms for fear of being blamed for infecting other individuals, in which case asymptomatic vaccine effectiveness would also be overestimated. Conversely, individuals who were hesitant to receive a COVID-19 vaccine might also have been reluctant to seek SARS-CoV-2 testing, which would lead to underestimation of vaccine effectiveness against asymptomatic infection. Further studies are needed to confirm the magnitude of BNT162b2 protection against
>
> 8 www.thelancet.com **Published online May 5, 2021 https://doi.org/10.1016/S0140-6736(21)00947-8**

Figure 18 Crucial statement in paper

We know that there were 4.4 million PCR tests and that 19% of these were on vaccinated people. Hence, we can conclude that there were:

- 836,000 tests on vaccinated people (of whom therc were 4,714,932, making up 72.1% of the population; so on average approximately one in six vaccinated people received a PCR test);
- 3,564,000 tests on unvaccinated people (of whom there were 1,823,979; so, on average, each unvaccinated person received two PCR tests)

So, the number of 'cases' per 1000 tests were:

- 30.8 for unvaccinated people (109,876 divided by 3,564,000 times 1000)
- 7.5 for vaccinated people (6,266 divided by 836,000 times 1000)

Using the simple 'cases per 1000 tests' (rather than the biased 'incident rate per 100,000 person days'), results in an approximate 'vaccine effectiveness' measure of 75.7%. While this is much less than the 95% headline figure, it is still impressive, so it is strange why the study failed to account for the difference in proportions tested.

It appears that the failure to adjust the vaccine effectiveness calculation for different testing protocols for vaccinated and unvaccinated people is not restricted to this Pfizer study in Israel. The data in the FDA briefing document [119] on the Pfizer vaccine (dated 10 Dec 2020) suggests there was a similar problem with the phase 3 trial of the vaccine. This was a randomized, double-blinded and placebo-controlled trial of the vaccine in 44,000 uninfected participants. It similarly reports a 95% effectiveness measure based on the fact that (post injection) there were 162 confirmed Covid-19 cases among the placebo participants compared to just 8 among the vaccinated participants. However, the study also reports that there were a much larger number of 'suspected but unconfirmed' cases and that these were more evenly spread between placebo participants (1,816 such cases) and vaccinated participants (1,594 such cases). This seems to suggest that a disproportionately small number of vaccinated participants with symptoms received PCR tests compared to placebo participants with symptoms.

Clearly the failure to properly adjust for both a decreasing infection rate and different testing protocols for vaccinated and unvaccinated people casts doubt on the validity of the studies.

It is also worth noting that, even if we ignore all of the above issues and accept as undisputed the number for 'COVID-19 related deaths' in the Israel study (715 among the unvaccinated and 138 among the vaccinated), then the absolute percentage increase in risk of death for an unvaccinated person is just 0.036%. That means that, even if we accept the 95% effectiveness measure, for every 10,000 unvaccinated people, about 3 or 4 would die as a result of not being vaccinated. And this brings us to the final (and critical) problem with the study. It does not provide any information about the number of adverse reactions - in particular the number of deaths - due to the vaccine. Hence, it does not provide the necessary information to make an informed decision about the overall risk/benefit of the vaccine.

We submitted the following 250-word response to The Lancet on 13 May summarising the above concerns about the article.

> "The article [117] provides impressive support for the effectiveness of the Pfizer vaccine, but important limitations in the overall analysis mean the results over-estimate vaccine effectiveness. One is that the study does not adjust for declining infection rate [118]. But there is also failure to properly adjust for the different testing protocols for vaccinated and unvaccinated people (page 8 of the paper). Whereas unvaccinated people continued to be regularly and routinely subject to PCR tests, vaccinated people no longer had to be. Although 836,000 (19%) of the 4.4 million PCR tests were on vaccinated people, 3,564,000 were on unvaccinated.
>
> So, using the Table 2 data (109,876 cases among unvaccinated, and 6,266 among vaccinated) the number of 'cases' per 1000 tests were: 30.8 for unvaccinated; 7.5 for vaccinated
>
> Using 'cases per 1000 tests' results in an approximate 'vaccine effectiveness' measure of 75.7%, compared to the 95% headline figure.
>
> Failure to account for different testing protocols is also evident in the phase 3 trial of the Pfizer vaccine [119]. It similarly reports a 95% effectiveness measure based on 162 confirmed cases among placebo participants compared to just 8 among vaccinated participants. However, the study also reports a much larger number of 'suspected but unconfirmed' cases more evenly spread between placebo participants (1,816) and vaccinated participants (1,594). This suggests a disproportionately small number of vaccinated participants with symptoms received PCR tests compared to placebo participants with symptoms."

There were additional fundamental flaws in the study, such as the fact that it ignored all the covid cases reported for people who had received either just a single dose or a second dose less than 7 days previously (such people were not considered 'fully vaccinated') - and this inevitably leads to a significant exaggeration of vaccine effectiveness. The consequence of this deliberate miscategorisation is reported in our analysis [120] of official UK government data , and is explained here [121].

With hindsight our concerns, about the study have absolutely been borne out by events. We now have confirmation [122] of how wildly exaggerated Pfizer's 95% effectiveness claim was and evidence of manipulation [123] of official statistics used to support claims of vaccine effectiveness, resulting in our formal complaint [124] to the UK Statistics Regulator.

After three weeks without reply we prompted the editors who said they were waiting for the authors to respond before they could publish the letter. The response finally came 20 months later in January 2023 .... and caused an internet sensation.

5.2. The curious case of Dr Sharon Alroy-Preis

..and the claims of safety and effectiveness of the Pfizer vaccine (10 January 2023)

After 20 months (yes you read that right) on 8 January 2023 we finally got this response from The Lancet:

> **From:** The Lancet Team
> **Sent:** 08 January 2023 13:30
> **To:** Norman Fenton
> **Subject:** Your Submission THELANCET-D-21-03671
>
> Manuscript number: THELANCET-D-21-03671
> Title: Study on effectiveness of Pfizer vaccine overestimates its effectiveness
>
> Dear Professor Fenton,
>
> Happy new year. I hope you've had a good start to 2023 so far.
>
> Here at The Lancet editorial office, we have begun the new year by sorting through dated submissions in our online manuscript management system, Editorial Manager. I am sorry to see that this submission of yours from 2021 is still open.
>
> We had invited Dr Sharon Alroy-Preis and co-authors of the published article to consider your letter, but I am sorry that we never received a formal reply from them and therefore have not been able to pursue an exchange. But I am even more sorry that I didn't communicate a decision with you in a timely manner.
>
> I will now close your submission, but I thank you for supporting post-publication debate in The Lancet.
>
> Yours sincerely
>
> Josefine Gibson
> Senior Editor
> *The Lancet*

So, because the lead author Dr Sharon Alroy-Preis (SA-P) did not respond to our short (just 250-word) letter, they have decided – after 20 months - not to publish it. But who exactly is Dr Sharon Alroy-Preis? Well, if you look at the authors' declaration of interests in the paper you will find that, while 8 of the 15 authors hold stock and stock options in Pfizer, SA-P is not among them and, indeed **declares no conflict of interest at all**.

9.1 Publications.

9.1.1 PFIZER and MoH will jointly prepare and publish the Results in submission(s) for publication, to peer-reviewed scientific or medical journals. Nothing in this Agreement shall prevent the MoH from continuing to disseminate Project Data or other data collected by the MoH, other than Results of the Project objective

[redacted]

specified in Section 2.1, to the public on a regular basis or as required for public health reasons and according to Israeli laws, or prevent MoH from possessing and analyzing such data, independent of this agreement and making publications thereof. Nothing in this Agreement shall prevent PFIZER from making publications using publicly available data. All publications involving the Project, will acknowledge the role of MoH and Pfizer in the Project.

Without derogating from the generality of the above, to the extent that PFIZER and MoH cannot agree on a joint publication within a reasonable time, or to the extent that PFIZER or the MoH wishes to make further publications of data and results from this Agreement other than a joint publication, each Party will provide to the other Party with a copy of the publication [redacted] days prior to the date of submission for publication or of public disclosure to review such material. During its review period, the other Party may provide input, make factual corrections, and request the deletion of any reference to the other Party's Confidential Information from the proposed disclosure or publication. All disclosures and publications must expressly acknowledge the other Party, unless such Party objects to such acknowledgment. To the extent the Parties cannot resolve disputes regarding publications they shall escalate such matters to a good faith discussion between PFIZER's [redacted] and Sharon Alroy-Preis, MD, MPH, MBA.

Figure 19 Israel-Pfizer agreement

But it turns out that SA-P just happens to be the Head of Public Health Services at the Israeli Ministry of Health (IMOH) (here [125]).

It is also well known that, through the IMOH, Israel essentially became 'the laboratory for Pfizer' as reported by the Times of Israel in September 2021 (here [126]):

> "Philip Dormitzer, the chief scientific officer at Pfizer, made the comments to a Zoom gathering of academics last week. They were first reported by Channel 12 news on Friday night.
>
> "Early in the pandemic we established a relationship with the Israeli Ministry of Health where they used exclusively the Pfizer vaccine and then monitored it very

closely," Dormitzer told the gathering, "so we had a sort of laboratory where we could see the effect."

Indeed, the collaboration between Pfizer and the IMOH (which started 6 Jan 2021, i.e. 4 months *before* the SA-P article in which she declared no conflict of interest was published) is clearly laid out in this (partially redacted) collaboration agreement [127]. Section 9.1 of this Israel-Pfizer agreement provided for the parties to jointly approve any publication, and **SAP is explicitly named as the IMOH's representative in resolving any differences** (Figure 19).

So, SA-P was leading the IMOH's collaboration with Pfizer all along.

The Lancet article provided no information at all about the number of Covid-19 vaccine adverse reactions which we now know are substantial, and so it is also relevant and timely to point out SA-P's role in the emerging IMOH scandal [128] relating to the system for monitoring serious adverse reactions to the Pfizer vaccine. In her presentation to the FDA expert committee about the booster, SA-P claimed Israel monitors safety closely, whereas we now know they did not in fact have a functioning system until the end of 2021 - as was exposed in a leaked video from an internal meeting of the IMOH that they do not want anybody to see (here [129]).

And, it is also worth pointing out that SA-P has called [130] doctors who dare to question the IMOH policies on covid and the vaccines 'covid deniers'.

5.3. The Lancet has become a laughing stock

14 January 2023

We tweeted [131] The Lancet's response and within 24 hours it got over one million impressions. We also published a substack article [132] highlighting the fact we were now aware of additional problems with the paper relating to SA-P's relationship with Pfizer.

On 10 January 2023 we got the following unsolicited email from Josefine Gibson:

> **From:** Gibson, Josefine
> **Sent:** Tuesday, January 10, 2023 3:50 PM
> **To:** Norman Fenton
> **Subject:** The Lancet - Your letter from May 2021.
>
> Dear Professor Fenton,
>
> Thank you for bringing your letter from May 2021 back to our attention. We are looking into next steps and will get back to you as soon as we can.
>
> Kind regards,
>
> Josefine
> Josefine Gibson, Dr. rer. nat. Senior Editor, Correspondence | THE LANCET

On 11 January 2023 (at 10:58) we sent the following email to The Lancet's Editor-in-Chief Richard Horton:

Dear Prof Horton

I received the response below 20 months after first submitting a very short response to an article that appeared in The Lancet in May 2021 (the article claimed 95% effectiveness of the Pfizer vaccine in Israel).

I posted this response on twitter (along with a link to a blog piece we wrote in May 2021 containing more detailed concerns about the article):

https://twitter.com/profnfenton/status/1612110949279752194

That tweet gained over a million impressions within 24 hours, with many people expressing their disgust with The Lancet in response.

But it turns out that we have since discovered further concerns regarding undeclared conflicts of interest with the lead author of the article.

These concerns are summarised in a substack article we have just produced:

https://wherearethenumbers.substack.com/p/alroy-preis

I would be grateful to hear if, in the light of the damage to the credibility of The Lancet, you have any plans to highlight the concerns we have raised about the article especially given the damage it has done with respect to misinformation about vaccine effectiveness.

Yours

Norman Fenton

On 11 January 2023 (at 11:21) we got an email from Josefine Gibson apologising for the 'sub standard experience' we had with The Lancet. She said that, after discussing it with Horton, they were now inviting us to publish the original letter or an update to it, suggesting the update 'reflect more current experience with the vaccine'.

From: Gibson, Josefine
Sent: Wednesday, January 11, 2023 11:21 AM
To: Norman Fenton
Subject: The Lancet - invitation

Dear Professor Fenton,

I am writing to offer my sincerest apologies for the substandard experience you've had with *The Lancet*.

We have very specific processes for submitted letters that respond to our published content, and these are designed to ensure that an outcome is reached in a timely manner. I regret that I was unable to uphold those processes for your letter.

Having discussed this unfortunate situation with my Editor in Chief, Richard Horton, I would like to offer publication of your original letter. Alternatively, we could publish a new letter that reflects more a current experience with the Pfizer vaccine. We defer to your best judgement of what would best serve the medical community.

We very much hope you'll accept this offer. Rest assured that your submission will be handled by a colleague with upmost priority.

Kind regards,

Josefine

We responded (at 12:00 on 11 Jan) as follows:

From: Norman Fenton
Sent: Wednesday, January 11, 2023 12:00 PM
To: Gibson, Josefine

Subject: RE: The Lancet - invitation

Josefine

Thank you for this. If we go with the new letter option what is the word limit?

Yours

Norman Fenton

At 22:46 on 11 Jan, Josefine responded:

Dear Professor Fenton,

If you choose to write in response to published content, the word limit is 250 words. If you'd like to write a more general letter, the limit is 350 words. In both cases, please limit the number of references to five.

Thank you.

My best wishes,

Josefine

At 16:26 on 12 Jan, we sent the following letter (349 words):

"Misleading Claims in study of Pfizer vaccine effectiveness
Norman Fenton and Martin Neil, 12 Jan 2023
An article about Israel's experience with the Pfizer Covid-19 vaccine was published in The Lancet in May 2021, [1]. We wrote a response letter, [2], explaining why its claim of 95% effectiveness was exaggerated, pointing out that the study failed to adjust for a declining infection rate, and for the very different testing protocols applied to vaccinated versus unvaccinated people. The study also ignored all covid cases reported for people who had received either just a single or a second dose less than seven days previously; such people were not considered 'fully vaccinated', inevitably leading to an exaggeration of vaccine effectiveness [3].

These concerns expressed 20 months ago, have been borne out by data confirming how exaggerated the effectiveness claim was.

The Lancet sent our letter to the lead author of the study, Sharon Alroy-Preis (SA-P), for comment but she did not respond to the criticisms, so the Lancet did not publish it.

We have further concerns about the integrity of the article. SA-P was not among the 8 of 15 authors who declared holding share and stock options in Pfizer; she also declared no conflict of interest. Yet, she is Head of Public Health Services at the Israeli Ministry of Health (IMOH) during the period when Israel became the 'laboratory for Pfizer' [4]. The relationship between Pfizer and the IMOH (starting 6 Jan 2021, four months before the Lancet article was published) is laid out in their collaboration agreement [5] which makes clear results cannot be made public without both parties' approval, and names SA-P as the IMOH appointee responsible for managing this relationship with Pfizer.

> The Lancet article provided no information about the vaccine's adverse reactions which we now know are substantial. In her presentation to the FDA expert committee about the booster, SA-P claimed Israel monitors safety closely, whereas we now know they did not have a functioning system until the end of 2021 [4].
>
> Hence, we feel that the paper's findings – which led many to believe the Pfizer vaccine was extremely safe and effective - are severely compromised and that the article should be retracted."

Three hours later Josefine replied "Thank you very much, Norman. I shall share this with Richard Horton now, and I expect I'll be back in touch with you re next steps tomorrow." But at 15:24 on 13 Jan she sent the following email rejecting the letter:

> From: Gibson, Josefine (ELS-LOW)
> Sent: 13 January 2023 15:24
> To: Norman Fenton
> Subject: RE: The Lancet - invitation
>
> Dear Professor Fenton,
>
> Thank you for submitting your letter for consideration.
>
> We have discussed the points you raise among The Lancet's Editorial Team and have decided against publication for the following reasons:
>
> 1. Given existing evidence about the effectiveness and safety of the Pfizer vaccine, it is factually incorrect – indeed, it is misinformation - to say that reported adverse reactions are "substantial".
> 2. Author Dr Sharon Alroy-Preis clearly gives her affiliation with the Israel Ministry of Health (IMoH) in the paper – "Correspondence to: Dr Sharon Alroy-Preis, Public Health Services, Israel Ministry of Health, Jerusalem 9101002", and we do not consider her position an undeclared conflict of interest or a challenge to the integrity of the data.
>
> We regret the delayed correspondence regarding the status of your letter and fully accept your criticism of our editorial processes in this regard.
>
> Sincerely,

Josefine

So, there you have it. We are dubbed misinformation spreaders because The Lancet have unique access to the truth, and furthermore the integrity of the Israeli trial data is placed beyond question even though the Israeli public health apparatchik, SA-P, who is supposed to be independent of corporate interests, is legally bound to publish results approved by Pfizer.

Of course, our experience is just one of many cases [133] of corruption by The Lancet. But it gets worse….

5.4. The Lancet heavily redact response to our subject access request

14 March 2023

Following that fiasco, we submitted a subject access information request to Elsevier (who publish The Lancet) asking for all internal correspondence between editors and reviewers relating to the submission (and ultimate rejection) of our letter.

After a lengthy delay we received the response today. First their cover letter [134] and the very lengthy response [135] (but massively redacted - by them).

It is remarkable that most of the details are redacted even though it clearly is not done solely for the legitimate protection of the names of third parties. Clearly, we were being discussed in a negative light as they were referring to Norman as 'an ongoing issue'. It is also clear that they only reached out after we publicised their initial delayed rejection letter on twitter (they were getting a lot of heat as a result of that). See Figure 20.

- **Delayed email response to a letter reject** – A disgruntled Prof Norman Fenton shared [redacted] response on Twitter. His tweet has attracted significant engagement, [redacted]

Figure 20 Redacted response

It is disturbing to realise how much effort was spent to ensure that an obviously flawed study promoting the Pfizer vaccine was not challenged.

Despite most of it being redacted there are still some alarming unredacted highlights (imagine what the redacted stuff says about us!) First, they seem to reluctantly concede that Norman has a legitimate academic appointment, as shown in Figure 21.

[redacted]

Subject: RE: FYI – Ongoing issues monitoring

[redacted] have investigated him a little and he does seem to have a legitimate academic appointment. Let's see how he responds to your email.

Figure 21 Redacted response doubting Norman's academic credentials

In Figure 22 they mention 'helpful background on Fenton'. Did they try to dig up dirt on Norman on their own or did the 77th brigade furnish them with my dossier?

To: [redacted]
Cc: [redacted]

Subject: FW: FYI – Ongoing issues monitoring

[redacted]

There has been further development on the Fenton Twitter case. This includes an additional tweet by Fenton this evening, and helpful background on Fenton [redacted]

Figure 22 Redacted response doubting Norman's academic credentials

They are worried about the proximity of vaccine misinformation sources! See Figure 23.

Subject: RE: FYI – Ongoing issues monitoring

[redacted] pass on this message

[redacted] a source of vaccine misinformation is an academic prof based right around the corner from our Lancet offices.

Figure 23 Redacted response revealing proximity concerns

Next, they accuse Norman and (most likely) Martin of retweeting 'anti-vaxx posts on Twitter'. We'd be interested to know precisely who they are referring to and what posts (see Figure 24).

They also refer to 'holding off further email' suggesting their offer to consider the letter was not genuine, as shown in Figure 25.

We are not happy about the scale of the redactions in the Elsevier response. If the Lancet editors were not making disparaging comments about us, then there should be no reason to redact them. What do they have to hide?

Subject: RE: FYI – Ongoing issues monitoring

[redacted]

[redacted] Fenton's additional tweet this afternoon: (16) Prof Norman Fenton on Twitter: "After .@TheLancet delayed response to our complaint about the paper claiming Pfizer vaxx 95% effective in Israel, we did some digging on the lead author (who failed to reply to our complaint). Makes .@TheLancet response even more scandalous: https://t.co/S61vArJsXZ" / Twitter

Both Fenton [redacted] have retweeted anti-vaxx posts on Twitter, and their Substack articles are worth a scan (Archive - Where are the numbers? (substack.com). [redacted]

Figure 24 Redacted response about anti-vaxx posts on twitter

[redacted]

[redacted]ecommend holding off on further email response to Fenton until you've confirmed the above, especially given that anything you say directly to Fenton has the potential to be shared on social media. [redacted]

Figure 25 Redacted response noting social media concerns

The redactions suggest Elsevier have not acted in good faith, and neither have they acted in the spirit of FOIA. Hence, we have informed Elsevier that if they are unable to provide a proper and full response with most of these comments unredacted, we will no choice but to report them to the Information Commissioner's Office (ICO).

This is not the first disgraceful episode in the recent history of the Lancet where, under Richard Horton's leadership, clearly flawed papers promoting the 'official narrative' on covid have been published. Remember LancetGate [136] when they published a fraudulent study that effectively stopped the use of hydroxychloroquine (HCQ) to treat covid patients. At least that paper was eventually retracted. In this case, rather than even allow a proper response to a flawed study, they have instead attacked their critics, accusing them of being spreaders of misinformation and 'anti-vaxxers'.

It is worth noting that (as shown here [137]), The Lancet is by no means the only major academic journal routinely rejecting any articles/letters that in any way question the accuracy of studies claiming vaccine effectiveness or safety. It is now fair to conclude that not a single major peer-reviewed study claiming vaccine effectiveness and/or safety can be trusted to be valid.

Chapter 6. The 'safe and effective' vaccine narrative crumbles

6.1. Comparing vaccinated and unvaccinated mortality rates

Using rates in England's age adjusted all-cause mortality data (23 Sept 2021)

As explained in Figure 26, we have argued that the most reliable long-term measure of Covid-19 vaccine effectiveness/safety is the age adjusted all-cause mortality rate.

Why all "all-cause mortality" is the most appropriate measure for overall cost-benefit analysis of Covid vaccines

- If Covid is as ***dangerous*** as claimed - and if the vaccine is as ***effective*** as claimed - we should by now have seen many more Covid related deaths among the unvaccinated than the vaccinated (in each age group).
- If the vaccine is as ***safe*** as claimed then there should have been very few more deaths from causes unrelated to Covid among the vaccinated than the unvaccinated (in each age group).
- So, the count of all-cause deaths should be higher among the unvaccinated than the vaccinated (in each age group), confirming that the benefits of vaccination outweigh the risks.
- Counting all-cause deaths completely bypasses the problem of defining what constitutes a 'Covid case' or a 'Covid related death' (definitions which can be easily manipulated to fit different narratives).
- We define a person as 'vaccinated' if they have received at least one dose. As we are not interested in whether a person becomes a 'Covid case', any other definition is flawed as it will fail to acknowledge that adverse reactions (including death) from vaccines are most likely to occur shortly after vaccination.
- The fact that the CDC now counts a person as 'unvaccinated' if they die within 14 days of the second dose, or after just one dose, might make some sense if we are interested only in the vaccine's ability to stop infection. But in the context of death attribution it is nothing less than fraudulent.

Figure 26 Why we focus on all-cause mortality

If, over a reasonably prolonged period, fewer vaccinated people die, from whatever cause, including Covid-19, than unvaccinated people then we could conclude that the benefits of the vaccine outweigh the risks. We also pointed out that, to avoid the confounding effect of age, it is critical that data for each age category are available, rather than the aggregated data because, clearly, aggregated data might exaggerate vaccine mortality rates if more older people, with shorter expected mortality, are included. The UK roll out of the vaccine was executed in descending age order, from older to younger, except very early on in the vaccination programme when the vulnerable young were vaccinated along with the very elderly. As the programme progressed those vaccinated were, on average, older than those who remained unvaccinated and as the roll out proceeded a progressively higher proportion of the residual unvaccinated population are younger.

The latest Office for National Statistics report [138] on mortality rates by Covid-19 vaccination status provides data on all deaths – Covid-19 related and non-Covid related for the period Jan-July 2021 for the unvaccinated and the different categories of vaccinated ('within 21 days of first dose', '21 days or more after first dose', 'second dose'). The ONS data for Covid-19 mortality, is given in Table 4 of the ONS spreadsheet [139] and the ONS data for all-cause mortality excluding Covid-19, is given in Table 5 of [140] the same spreadsheet. Both tables are reproduced in this report [141].

We believe there are severe weaknesses and possible errors in the ONS data:

- It does not provide the raw age categorised data.
- The age standardised score used by ONS relies on the 2011 census data to determine the population proportions in each age category. These proportions have changed since 2011 and, as we noted in this article [142], these differences can significantly change the results.
- (As we discovered and clarified in subsequent articles) the ONS dataset is only a (highly biased) subset of the England and Waled population consisting of those people who were both included in the 2011 census and registered with a GP in 2019.
- The rates in the unvaccinated on 8th Jan are lower than the double vaccinated in summer. Also, on 8th January only 12% of over 65-year-olds had been vaccinated, so the unvaccinated population should have had a death rate very similar to background levels.
- The wildly increasing weekly age adjusted mortality rates (for non-Covid related deaths) for the 38 million unvaccinated population in January are totally inconsistent with weekly changes in previous years. Although this population excludes the under 18s and the 1.2 million (mainly over 65s) who had by then received their first dose, we would not expect the mortality rate for this population to be drastically different to the mortality rate for England seen in recent years as reported in a different ONS report [143].
- Ultimately, we need to exclude unnatural deaths such as murders, accidents and suicides since these may introduce bias between the cohorts, especially in the young age categories where the overall death numbers are small.

But importantly, while it does not provide the raw age categorised data, it ***does*** provide "age standardised" mortality rates (see this report [144] and this explanatory video [145]). This means the ONS have calculated the overall mortality rate in a way which (they believe) adjusts for the confounding effect of age, and this is 'baked into' the mortality rates they have published. However, while they report this age adjusted mortality rate for each of the three separate categories of vaccinated people, they do not report it for the combined set of vaccinated people. In our analysis, and in the absence of the actual age stratified data, we compute a population weighted age adjusted all-cause mortality rate by using the ONS's published population sizes for each of the three categories of vaccinated. This is not ideal because the ONS age adjusted rates are so opaque and are not 'absolute numbers'. However, in the absence of detailed data this should provide a reasonable estimate of what the ONS age adjusted all-cause mortality rate would be for all unvaccinated if they had bothered to report it. We will call this the 'weighted vaccinated mortality rate'. All the relevant data from ONS and charts we produced can be found in the full article [141].

It turns out that, even using this age adjusted mortality rate, the death rate is currently higher among the vaccinated than the unvaccinated. The chart for age adjusted mortality rates for vaccinated against unvaccinated for weeks 1 to 26 of 2021 shows that, over time, the weighted mortality rate for the vaccinated has steadily increased and by week 16 (23 April 2021), surpassed that for the unvaccinated. The chart suggests a normal seasonal mortality trend for the unvaccinated, with a winter peak on week 6, 12 February 2021, and a steady decline toward summer. In contrast, the pattern for the vaccinated is completely different. From week 24 onwards the mortality rates for the vaccinated and unvaccinated appear to be converging as summer begins.

As the ONS breaks down the data over time for the three categories of vaccinated (those within 21 days of first dose, those 21 days after first dose, and those after two doses), we also plotted mortality charts for each of these categories. The mortality rate, for week 26, up to 2 July, for the unvaccinated is around 25 deaths per 100,000. But there are big differences between the mortality rates for the different categories of vaccinated deaths. For example, for those after 21 days of first dose, the comparable mortality is around 89 deaths per 100,000 people (a number which has drastically increased since January), while for those vaccinated with two doses there were approximately 15 deaths per 100,000 in the same July period.

The trends for the different vaccination categories are also concerning. In contrast to the unvaccinated, the mortality rates for the vaccinated have initially increased from very low initial values, but then have increased, whilst that for the unvaccinated has decreased. Since 19 March the double dose vaccination mortality rate has increased week-on-week more or less consistently. The mortality rate for those more than 21 days after first dose increased drastically in the spring (at week 14) and remained high thereafter. Mortality within 21 days of vaccination initially increased but looks to have stabilised, albeit with some noise. We will leave it to clinical colleagues to explain why there are such different patterns.

Because of the limitations and possible errors in the ONS data, there are many caveats that need to be applied to our crude analysis. But we can conclude that the ONS's own data do not support the claims made for vaccine effectiveness/safety.

It is also important to note that the population of vaccinated people is becoming sufficiently large and representative that the criticality of age adjustment becomes much diminished. We will be doing a follow-up analysis that takes account of this.

This article and the subsequent comprehensive research paper [144] we published on it (with an updated version here [146]) attracted enormous interest. Because it was considered a sufficient challenge to the narrative it also came to the attention of the self-appointed 'fact checking' organization fullfact.org. A representative of fullfact contacted Norman on 5 Oct 2021. The correspondence [147] demonstrates how fullfact work and also how incompetent they are. They search for somebody on twitter who is trying to discredit the claim they wish to say is false and assume that such a person is an authoritative source. The fact that twitter hides critical responses to this 'authoritative source' compounds their confirmation bias.

6.2. Is vaccine efficacy a statistical illusion?

14 November 2021

To evaluate the risk/benefit of a vaccine for treating a virus, such as Covid-19, we can compare the all-cause mortality rate of vaccinated against unvaccinated people on a periodic basis. If the mortality rate for those vaccinated is consistently lower than that for unvaccinated then we might conclude the vaccine must be beneficial.

6.2.1. Placebo Vaccination

Imagine that a placebo rather than a vaccine is quickly rolled out to a population of one million people of similar age and health. Let's assume the weekly non-virus mortality rate for this population is 15 per 100,000 (100k), so we would expect about 150 out of the million to die in any given week. Because the placebo changes nothing, the mortality rates for both vaccinated and unvaccinated average the same 15 per 100k, each week every week. Hence, on average, what we should observe – as the 'vaccination' programme rolls out to most of the population - is shown in Table 7. Notice that the placebo vaccine roll-out programme is enacted at pace and the cumulative percentage of the population vaccinated rises to 98% within 12 weeks. We assume no population growth and each week the total population reduced by previous week's deaths.

Table 7 Roll out of placebo 'vaccine'

			Vaccinated			Unvaccinated		
Week	Population	Cumulative Percentage vaccinated	Deaths	Population	Mortality rate	Deaths	Population	Mortality rate
1	1,000,000	0.5	1	5,000	15	149	995,000	15
2	999,850	1	1	9,999	15	148	989,852	15
3	999,700	2	3	19,994	15	147	979,706	15
4	999,550	4	6	39,982	15	144	959,568	15
5	999,400	7	10	69,958	15	139	929,442	15
6	999,250	14	21	139,895	15	129	859,355	15
7	999,100	28	42	279,748	15	108	719,352	15
8	998,950	45	67	449,528	15	82	549,423	15
9	998,801	65	97	649,220	15	52	349,580	15
10	998,651	80	120	798,921	15	30	199,730	15
11	998,501	93	139	928,606	15	10	69,895	15
12	998,351	98	147	978,384	15	3	19,967	15
13	998,201	98.5	147	983,228	15	2	14,973	15
14	998,052	98.6	148	984,079	15	2	13,973	15
15	997,902	98.7	148	984,929	15	2	12,973	15
16	997,752	98.9	148	986,777	15	2	10,975	15
17	997,603	99	148	987,627	15	1	9,976	15
18	997,453	99.1	148	988,476	15	1	8,977	15
19	997,303	99.2	148	989,325	15	1	7,978	15
20	997,154	99.3	149	990,174	15	1	6,980	15

Now suppose there is a one-week delay in the reporting of deaths. Such delays are routine in statistical reporting of mortality and vaccine data. Then the data reported by the authorities is different from reality, here shown in Table 8, which is the same as Table 1 but where the death totals are simply 'shifted' down one week.

Suppose we want to examine and compare the mortality rates of the unvaccinated and vaccinated cohorts based on the data in Table 8. Figure 27 shows this comparison, and we can see that the mortality rate is consistently lower for the vaccinated than that for the unvaccinated throughout the roll out of the vaccination programme and it reduces as soon as vaccination nears population saturation at close to 100%.

Table 8 Death reporting delayed by one week

			Vaccinated			Unvaccinated		
Week	Population	Cumulative Percentage vaccinated	Deaths	Population	Mortality rate	Deaths	Population	Mortality rate
1	1,000,000	0.5	-	5,000	-	-	995,000	-
2	999,850	1	1	9,999	7.50	149	989,852	15.08
3	999,700	2	1	19,994	7.50	148	979,706	15.16
4	999,550	4	3	39,982	7.50	147	959,568	15.31
5	999,400	7	6	69,958	8.57	144	929,442	15.49
6	999,250	14	10	139,895	7.50	139	859,355	16.22
7	999,100	28	21	279,748	7.50	129	719,352	17.92
8	998,950	45	42	449,528	9.33	108	549,423	19.64
9	998,801	65	67	649,220	10.39	82	349,580	23.57
10	998,651	80	97	798,921	12.19	52	199,730	26.25
11	998,501	93	120	928,606	12.91	30	69,895	42.86
12	998,351	98	139	978,384	14.24	10	19,967	52.51
13	998,201	98.5	147	983,228	14.93	3	14,973	20.00
14	998,052	98.6	147	984,079	14.99	2	13,973	16.07
15	997,902	98.7	148	984,929	14.99	2	12,973	16.16
16	997,752	98.9	148	986,777	14.97	2	10,975	17.73
17	997,603	99	148	987,627	14.99	2	9,976	16.50
18	997,453	99.1	148	988,476	14.99	1	8,977	16.67
19	997,303	99.2	148	989,325	14.99	1	7,978	16.88
20	997,154	99.3	148	990,174	14.99	1	6,980	17.15

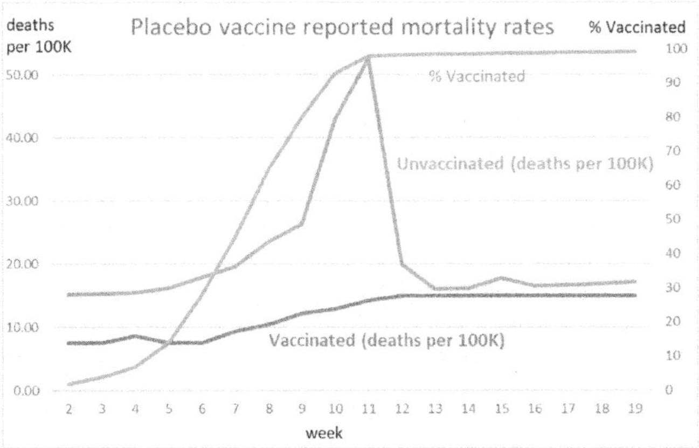

Figure 27 Reported weekly mortality rates vaccinated against unvaccinated

We might conclude that those who remain unvaccinated look to be suffering much higher levels of mortality than the vaccinated. The reporting delay therefore creates a completely artificial impression that the vaccine must be highly effective. In fact, it looks like a magic 'cure all' wonder drug!

The fact that the mortality rate of the unvaccinated peaks when the percentage of those vaccinated peaks should ring some alarm bells that something strange is going on (unless there is independent evidence that the virus was peaking at the same time).

6.2.2. ONS data on Covid-19 Vaccination

While the placebo vaccine example was purely hypothetical, Figure 28 shows the vaccinated against unvaccinated mortality using the data in the latest ONS report [149] on mortality in England by Covid-19 vaccination status (weeks 1 to 38), complemented by NIMS vaccination survey data (up to week 27 only). Here we show other-than Covid-19 mortality to remove the virus signal.

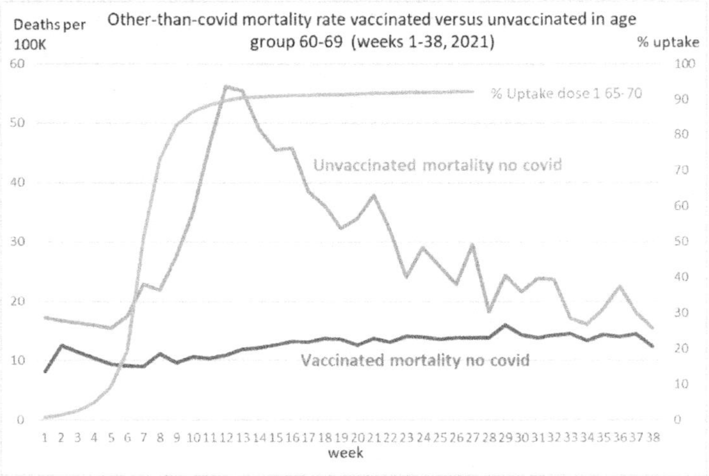

Figure 28 Reported weekly other-than Covid-19 mortality rates for vaccinated versus unvaccinated for 60-69 age group for weeks 1-38 2021

Note that we see the same features as the shifted graph in Figure 27. In other words, a perfectly reasonable explanation for what is observed here could be that there is no difference in mortality rates between vaccinated and unvaccinated and the mortality differences are simply a result of a delay in death reporting. Moreover, given we have removed Covid-19 deaths (which were only a small percentage of all-cause deaths in the reported data) we get a near identical result for non-covid mortality to that which would result if the vaccine were a placebo! Thus, we appear to have created a statistical illusion of vaccine efficacy.

It is important to note that we are not claiming the death reporting is delayed in the ONS data. In fact, our work on this is ongoing and we believe that the most plausible explanation is misclassification and underestimation of proportion of unvaccinated.

If this is not a statistical illusion, how is it possible that the unvaccinated are dying from non-covid causes at a higher rate than vaccinated? Also how is it possible that, at the time vaccination rates are ramped up to nearly 100% of the population, the nonvaccinated are dying from non-covid deaths at almost twice the rate of those who are vaccinated?

These same patterns are also observable in the 70-79 and 80+ age groups (with the mortality peaks for the unvaccinated appearing at different weeks because these age groups received vaccinations earlier). This strongly suggests that what we are observing is a genuine statistical illusion unexplainable by any real impact of the vaccine on mortality rates.

6.2.3. Consider a deadly placebo

It is also important to note that even if the actual mortality rate for the vaccinated was higher than that of the unvaccinated, where the vaccine was causing death, as a side effect, we would still likely observe the same illusion.

To see this effect let's revisit our placebo vaccine example and make a small change to Table 1 where instead of a mortality rate of 15 per 100k for the vaccinated, suppose it is 17 per 100k (a rise in mortality of approximately 13%). So, the placebo vaccine is killing two more people per 100k and gives no mortality benefit otherwise. Even here we see the illusion that the mortality rate for the vaccinated is lower than unvaccinated. Both scenarios are the opposite of reality, and both look interchangeable. This means the chance of picking up a vaccine side effect signal is close to impossible and instead the illusion is created of vaccine efficacy.

6.2.4. The illusion of declining vaccine efficacy

Finally, it is important to note that the same statistical illusion applies to all measures of vaccine efficacy whether they be cases, hospitalisations, or deaths.

This reporting bias is one type of bias that might be called 'reporting lag censoring', a phenomenon whereby structural or process factors systematically interfere when data is handled and reported with the consequential effect that it is then misinterpreted, leading to false conclusions.

A 25-minute video lecture demonstrating this work and its background and context can be found here [150].

6.3. Impact of miscategorising deaths when evaluating vaccine safety

The same statistical illusion, (1 December 2021).

In the previous section we showed that if there was a one-week delay in reporting deaths then a vaccine that was a placebo would be seen to have a decreased mortality rate for the vaccinated compared to the unvaccinated. In other words, an illusion of effectiveness is created by the one-week delay in reporting. The new hypothetical example provided in our new article [148] compares the correct figures to the reported figures based on a one-week delay assuming that in a population of 10 million people there is a (constant) weekly mortality rate of 50 deaths per 100,000 people. Each week the population reduces by the number of deaths the previous week. All death numbers (which are simply the relevant population multiplied by 50/100000) are rounded to whole numbers.

It turns out that, under the same hypothetical assumptions, the same results arise if, instead of a one-week delay in death reporting there is a misclassification of newly vaccinated deaths; specifically, any death of a person occurring in the same week as the person is vaccinated is treated as an unvaccinated, rather than vaccinated, death. A proof of why the results are equivalent (except for week 1) is provided here [148].

The plot resulting from either reporting error shows the apparently clear life-saving benefit of the 'vaccine' with the mortality rate in the unvaccinated peaking at about the same time as the vaccine programme reaches its peak. But this is an obvious indication that these results are not real.

As we reported in the previous section, it turns out that the plots for mortality rates from the ONS report [149] (weeks 1-38) for the Covid-19 vaccination programme in each of the older age categories look remarkably similar to the plots from our hypothetical example, i.e. with the same peaks in unvaccinated mortality coinciding with when the vaccination programme reached its peak for this age group.

Why are the theoretical results important? Because they at least partly explain how the strange observed ONS results could occur even if the mortality rate of the vaccinated was the same (or even higher) than that of the unvaccinated. While it seems that deaths in the ONS report are being reported by date of death (hence are not delayed), newly vaccinated deaths are being classified as unvaccinated. Indeed, it is likely that any death within the first 14 days of vaccination may be classified as unvaccinated.

Moreover, as we will explain in the full analysis that we are currently preparing, the ONS data provides other clues that suggest different types of errors in reporting. For example, even at the end of the reporting period (when errors such as death misclassification should be minimal and indeed the plots converge) the non-covid mortality rate for the vaccinated is still consistently lower than that of the unvaccinated. This suggests that the proportion of unvaccinated must be systematically underestimated.

6.4. Further concerns about systematic miscategorisation

3 December 2021

Our research team (which senior clinicians and other researchers who remain anonymous to protect their careers) have now analysed the ONS England November mortality data. We conclude that, despite seeming evidence to support vaccine effectiveness, this conclusion is doubtful because of a range of serious inconsistencies and anomalies. Our detailed report is here [151].

The data appear to show lower non-Covid mortality for the vaccinated compared to the unvaccinated. Odd. Also unvaccinated mortality rates peak at the same time as the vaccine rollout peaks for the age group, then falls and closes in on the vaccinated (as shown in Figure 28 above). This is not natural. Consider what we are witnessing here. We have a vaccine whose recipients are suffering fewer non-covid deaths and hence are benefitting from improved mortality. And the mortality rates look to differ significantly from historical norms, as evidenced in mortality lifetables.

Correlating unvaccinated mortality with vaccine roll out we also find curious patterns The unvaccinated are dying after NOT getting the 1st dose and the single dosed are dying after NOT getting the 2nd dose.

There is plenty of evidence that the vaccinated who die within 14 days of vaccination may be categorised as unvaccinated. Then someone who dies within 14 days of first dose is miscategorised as unvaccinated and a similar thing could occur post second dose.

Miscategorisation might explain odd phenomena in ONS mortality (as explained in the previous two sections). To correct the error, we can take the difference between the expected mortality for the unvaccinated and the data, and re-allocate this unexpected excess mortality to the vaccinated to get new ADJUSTED estimates.

The early spikes in mortality that appear to occur soon after vaccination may be caused by the infirm, moribund, and severely ill receiving vaccination in priority order and thus simply appearing to hasten deaths that might otherwise have occurred later in the year.

Turning to Covid-19 mortality, at face value, there appears again to be clear evidence of vaccine effectiveness.

But after vaccination people endure weakened immune response for a period of up to 28 days and may be in danger of infection from Covid-19 or other infectious agent at any time in that period. It therefore makes sense to examine infection date rather than date of death registration.

We adjust for this using a temporal offset and see a large spike in mortality for all age groups during the early weeks, when Covid-19 prevalence was high, and when the first dose vaccination rollout peaked.

After our offset adjustment we observe no significant benefit of the vaccines in the short term. They appear to expose people to an increased mortality, in line with what we know about immune exposure or pre-infection risks,

Whatever the explanations for the observed data, the ONS data is both unreliable and misleading. Absent any better explanation Occam's razor would support our conclusions. The ONS data provide no reliable evidence that the vaccines reduce all-cause mortality.

Postscript: On 2 Feb 2022 we reported [152] how the British Medical Journal (BMJ) rejected an updated version of our paper without review or any explanation why it would not be reviewed. The paper had, at the time, over 300,000 reads on ResearchGate.

6.5. New ONS report on deaths by vaccination

Serious anomalies and the 'healthy vaccinee effect' (24 December 2021)

The latest ONS report [149] on deaths by vaccination status has serious anomalies (as in their previous report which we analysed in this paper [153]). The most obvious one is that their analysis claims age standardised non-covid mortality rate is TWICE as high in the unvaccinated as the vaccinated.

This is not credible. If it were really true, then this would mean either

a) healthier people got vaccinated and/or very sick people did not get vaccinated. But then this would mean that all ONS estimates of vaccine effectiveness are massively exaggerated due to the confounding effect of prior health status; or

b) the Covid-19 vaccines are full of magic fairy dust that cures non-Covid illness and increases your life expectancy.

The report does indeed claim that a) is true (Page 5):

> "The all-cause ASMRs for the year-to-date were lower in the first three weeks after a vaccine dose than in subsequent weeks after that dose. This could be because of a "healthy vaccinee effect" where people who are ill (either due to COVID-19 or another relevant illness) are likely to delay vaccination. Therefore, the people who delay vaccination have been recently vaccinated are, in the short term, in better health than the general population. The same is true for deaths involving COVID-19 after the second dose. This is likely because the healthy vaccinee effect where people who know or suspect they have COVID-19 delay vaccination until recovered, has a bigger effect here than the difference in protection offered by the vaccine within and following the first three weeks after vaccination."

The healthy vaccinee effect is the hypothesis that people closer to death are too ill to be vaccinated and so become concentrated in a shrinking unvaccinated population, thus increasing the group's mortality rate. However, this contradicts NHS guidance [154] report ("Joint Committee on Vaccination and Immunisation: advice on priority groups for Covid-19 vaccination", Page 3), which is explicit in ensuring that the most at-risk and vulnerable get **priority** for vaccination)

> There is clear evidence that those living in residential care homes for older adults have been disproportionately affected by COVID-19 (20-23) as they have had a high risk of exposure to infection and are at higher clinical risk of severe disease and mortality. Given the increased risk of outbreaks, morbidity and mortality in these closed settings, these adults are considered to be at very high risk. The Committee's advice is that this group should be the highest priority for vaccination. Vaccination of residents and staff at the same time is considered to be a highly efficient strategy within a mass vaccination programme with the greatest potential impact (see below).

It is also contradicted by the ONS in the very same report in three different places:

> (Page 2): Changes in non-COVID-19 mortality by vaccination status are largely driven by the changing composition of the vaccination status groups because of the prioritisation of clinically extremely vulnerable and people with underlying health conditions, and differences in timing of vaccination among people who were eligible.

on page 8 of their same report:

> (Page 8) ...the vaccination roll-out was also prioritised by health status of individuals, with the extremely clinically vulnerable and those with underlying health conditions being vaccinated earlier...
>
> (Page 8) The higher non-COVID-19 mortality rate for 18 to 39-year-olds who had received a second dose is likely to be explained by the prioritisation of the clinically vulnerable for vaccination

There is also anecdotal evidence that even terminally ill patients got the vaccine early. So, if the healthy vaccinee effect hypothesis (a) is false then, since the magic fairy dust hypothesis (b) is false, as we claimed in our previous article, there is miscategorisation in the data; specifically, many of those dying shortly after vaccination are being classified as unvaccinated.

But even if a) is true the effect is the same: without the necessary adjustments to the data that we applied in our article, the data is worthless in terms of evaluating the effectiveness and safety of the vaccines.

In fact, in a subsequent article [155] (13 Jan 2022) we debunked the hypothesis that the "healthy vaccinee" effect explains anomalies in ONS mortality data and produced a new and significantly updated report [156] accordingly.

If the ONS hypothesis was correct, then we would see:

> a) The percentage of the unvaccinated in poor health rise as vaccine rollout progresses
>
> b) A steady non-Covid mortality rate among the unhealthy (because they are dying at same rate as they always have done).

To support their claim the ONS released the percentage of 70-79 age group with "very poor" health in each vaccination category. Yet, we showed that the vaccinated population contains a higher percentage of those in very poor health and this increases over time. Surprisingly the unvaccinated population has the LOWEST concentration of the unhealthy and the percentage declines over time. In this unhealthy sub-population we found the non-Covid mortality rate for the unvaccinated is HIGHER than for the vaccinated. Both rates should be equivalent. Again, we see unnatural spikes in non-Covid mortality just after vaccine roll out as seen before in whole population.

Therefore, those in poorest health were NOT more likely to remain unvaccinated. Also, there is a rise in non-Covid mortality, coincidental with vaccine rollout that is not only seen in the population as a whole but is also seen in those with the poorest health.

We conclude that the "healthy vaccine effect" cannot explain the anomalies we discovered in the ONS data and believe it is up to advocates for this hypothesis to now prove their case using the released data.

6.6. Covid-19: Definitions matter - and these are real

29 December 2022

Norman posted a graphic on twitter summarising Covid-19 definitions:

Fred, who has no Covid-19 symptoms, tests positive in a PCR test for work. He doesn't go on to develop any symptoms. Fred is classified as a Covid-19 case.

13 days after his PCR test Fred is critically injured in a car crash and rushed to hospital. Fred is classified as a Covid-19 hospital admission.

2 weeks after being taken to hospital Fred dies from his injuries. Fred is classified as a Covid-19 death.

Jane gets a Covid-19 vaccine and 13 days later tests PCR positive with symptomatic Covid-19. Jane is classified as an unvaccinated Covid-19 case.

Peter gets a Covid-19 vaccine and dies the next day. Peter is classified as an unvaccinated death.

The usual useful idiots said it was all false without offering any evidence. But the UK Government Covid-19 dashboard website from today on definitions of Covid-19 cases [157] and deaths [158] confirms these definitions. For example, for deaths it states:

> "Deaths in United Kingdom: Number of people who died within 28 days of their first positive test for COVID-19."

It is also important to note that having a positive PCR test within 28 days of deaths is not the ONLY way to be counted as a Covid-19 death. In fact, the dashboard also plots

> "Daily deaths with COVID-19 on the death certificate: Daily numbers of deaths of people whose death certificate mentioned COVID-19 as one of the causes, and 7-day rolling average. There is a lag in reporting of at least 11 days because the data are based on death certificates."

If proper analyses of cause of death were undertaken, then clearly this number should be much lower than the number who died within 28 days of a positive test. Unfortunately, the numbers are consistently HIGHER - as of today the cumulative total of deaths within 28 days of a positive test is 148,089 whereas the cumulative total with Covid-19 on the death certificate is 171,801. This means that, in addition to all of those classified as a Covid-19 death by virtue of a positive test within 28 days, another 23,000 deaths have been added. We suspect that many are like that of this twitter responder:

> It's so strange my uncle was in hospital suffering from a stroke when the pandemic hit, moved to care home and later passed away, but because the home had a few cases of covid he also was classified as a covid death although he was never tested to confirm it?

And (as the dashboard website has recently removed the definition of a Covid-19 hospitalisation) here is the definition in the NHS England Report [159]:

Definition of confirmed Covid-19 patients:

- For all relevant data items: a confirmed Covid-19 patient is any patient admitted to the trust who has recently (i.e. in the last 5 days) tested positive for Covid-19 following a polymerase chain reaction (PCR) test or LFD.

- Patients who have been diagnosed via X-ray and assessment rather than a positive test should be counted as suspected (and not confirmed) Covid-19 patients.

- Report a patient as a confirmed Covid-19 patient in the sitrep for as long as they are being treated as a Covid-19 patient – so either they are being treated for Covid-19 caused symptoms or the trust is still taking the precautions they would take with a Covid-19 positive patient.

- A patient who has previously but not recently – (i.e. not in the last 5 days) had a positive Covid-19 test and is admitted for non-covid related treatment should not be counted as a confirmed Covid-19 patient.

For the CDC definition of a vaccinated and unvaccinated person see this report [160] (all the various studies of vaccine efficacy and safety from around the world that we have previously reported on use these definitions):

> "Persons were considered fully vaccinated ≥14 days after receipt of the second dose in a 2-dose series (Pfizer-BioNTech or Moderna COVID-19 vaccines) or after 1 dose of the single-dose Janssen (Johnson & Johnson) COVID-19 vaccine; partially vaccinated ≥14 days after receipt of the first dose and <14 days after the second dose in a 2-dose series; and **unvaccinated <14 days after receipt of the first dose of a 2-dose series or 1 dose of the single-dose vaccine** or if no CAIR2 vaccination data were available."

This CDC report also has the US definitions of cases, hospitalisations and deaths. The only difference to the UK definitions is that anybody dying **within 60 days** of a positive PCR test is classified as a Covid-19 death:

> "COVID-19–associated deaths were defined as deaths occurring ≤60 days after the date of a first laboratory-confirmed SARS-CoV-2 infection or deaths with COVID-19 listed as a cause of or contributing condition to death."

6.7. Undercounting of deaths in first two weeks of vaccination

3 March 2022

Our new research (full paper 0[161] with first author Clare Craig available on ResearchGate) has discovered over 26,000 Covid-19 and non-Covid deaths expected to have occurred within two weeks of first dose vaccination have been omitted from the latest UK ONS deaths by vaccination status report [162]. This is after accounting for the fact that the ONS only uses a subset of the England and Wales population in its dataset.

The ONS data also fails to include millions of people categorised in the UK NIMS database as 'within 21 days vaccination' status. Our analysis compares expected deaths in the ONS dataset to those that have occurred in the whole population. We only use data from UK government sources including data from NIMS and UKHSA. We found implausibly low numbers of non-covid deaths in the 'within 21 days of first dose' category.

The ONS dataset only includes the number of non-covid deaths equivalent to the number expected to have occurred in the third week after vaccination only. So, the expected deaths for the first two weeks post first dose vaccination are missing. This is the case for all age groups 60+.

For Covid-19 deaths the same patterns are evident, across all age groups 60+. This is a significant and rather troubling anomaly warranting an explanation. The peaks in the graphs are synchronised with the vaccine roll out for each age group and hence are not natural or due to random error. Errors appear systematic and strongly suggest that deaths have been miscategorised as hypothesised in our previous paper on the ONS data [163].

Numerous factors could have led to deaths being omitted, including miscategorisation, reporting lags and data handling or transcription errors. Hence, we believe that the dataset is corrupted, making any inferences about vaccine efficacy or safety, reliant on the data, moot.

We have presented these findings to the ONS and they have acknowledged in correspondence that our analyses are valuable and important. They have also promised to release all raw data to allow independent analysis and to investigate the serious anomalies reported by our paper.

6.8. Why are UKHSA obfuscating data on stillbirths by vaccine status

Just another statistical illusion? (3 March 2022 with updates)

The latest UKHSA Feb 2022 Covid-19 vaccine surveillance report [154] suggests that there is no increased risk of stillbirth from vaccination. This seems like good news but, as pointed out by Hamish Soutar [165], instead of simply comparing outcomes of vaccinated women against unvaccinated it uses the categories:

- One or more doses in pregnancy
- No doses in pregnancy

So, women vaccinated prior to pregnancy are included in "no doses in pregnancy".

This is an outrageous piece of obfuscation. Even though the rest of the report contains quite a lot of detailed raw data, there are no raw data provided to answer the simple question:

> is the stillbirth rate higher for those unvaccinated than those vaccinated (before or during pregnancy)?

The only way to answer this question is to know the number of women and stillbirths in each of the following four categories:

1. Unvaccinated pre pregnancy and unvaccinated during pregnancy
2. Unvaccinated pre pregnancy but at least one jab during pregnancy
3. At least one jab pre pregnancy but unvaccinated during pregnancy
4. At least one jab pre pregnancy and at least one jab during pregnancy

By assigning realistic but hypothetical numbers for these categories in the full version of this article [164] we show how easy it is to come to the UKHSA conclusion that there is no difference in stillbirth rates between the "one or more doses in pregnancy" and the "no doses in pregnancy" even though stillbirth rates are significantly ***higher*** in the vaccinated.

In fact, it is not hard to produce hypothetical examples in which the vaccine appears to ***reduce*** risk of stillbirth using the UKHSA 'method', while the stillbirth rates are significantly higher in the vaccinated. This is explained in a 4 minute video [166].

The subsequent (21 April 2022) UKHSA Covid-19 surveillance report [167] continued with the same obfuscation. As a very timely example of the problems with the UKHSA reporting, on 22 April 2022 Britain's greatest ever female athlete Laura Kenny who won gold at the Tokyo Olympics in August 2021 revealed [168] she suffered a miscarriage in November 21 and an ectopic pregnancy in mid-January 2022. She says:

> "Since the Olympics we haven't had much luck and it's been the hardest few months I've ever had to go through. Jason and I fell pregnant immediately after the games and we were absolutely chuffed to bits. But unfortunately in November when commentating at the track champions league I miscarried our baby at 9 weeks. I've never felt so lost and sad. It felt like a part of me had been torn away. I grabbed for my safety blanket, bike riding! I found myself back in my happy place training again. I then caught Covid in mid January and found myself feeling really very unwell. I didn't have typical covid symptoms and I just felt I needed to go to hospital. A day later I found myself in A&E being rushed to theatre because I was having an ectopic pregnancy. Scared doesn't even come close. I lost a fallopian tube that day. I've always known I was tough, but sometimes life pushes you to an unbearable limit."

While it was apparently not a mandatory requirement for all countries' athletes to be vaccinated to attend the Tokyo Olympics, it ***was*** mandatory for all British athletes to be fully vaccinated [169]. Hence, Laura would have to have got double vaccinated shortly before the games to be allowed to take part. While there may be no reason to suspect the vaccination had anything to do with her two unfortunate pregnancy outcomes, both would be classified in the UKHSA "no doses in pregnancy" category.

On 28 March 2024 - after Laura Kenny announced her retirement – Norman posted a video to his YouTube channel about this story. Within minutes of posting it YouTube removed the video [170] and gave Norman's channel a strike.

On 30 Sept 2022 we published another article [171] related to this one about how 'survivor bias' in vaccine pregnancy studies can lead to flawed claims of better outcomes for vaccinated women (the article also contains a video explanation). Specifically, those women in a study who are vaccinated late in pregnancy must have already avoided early miscarriages, which is when most pregnancy failures occur.

Indeed, those claiming that the vaccine is safe and effective for pregnant women point to studies such as this [172] which even seem to show the miscarriage and still birth rates of vaccinated women to be lower than that of unvaccinated women. But these studies do not properly factor in the stage during pregnancy when the vaccine was taken. To understand the scale of the problem, in article [171] we produced another hypothetical, but realistic, example of how, using the UKHRA classification the foetal death rate for the "one or more doses in pregnancy" was much lower than that for the "no doses in pregnancy" even though the foetal death rate for the never vaccinated is significantly lower than each of the possible different categories of vaccinated. The possible categories of vaccinated were:

- vaxxed pre pregnancy only
- vaxxed both pre pregnancy **and** early pregnancy (i.e. 0-20 weeks) **or** early pregnancy only
- vaxxed both pre and/or early (i.e. at least once before 20 weeks) **and** late (i.e. after week 20)
- vaxxed late only (i.e. after week 20)

Note that for every woman in the latter two categories, the pregnancy must have survived the first 20 weeks (hence survivor bias).

6.9. The Bangladesh Mask Study

Provides no evidence that masks reduce Covid-19 infection (2 May 2022)

A very large trial, whose results were published [173] in Science, carried out in Bangladesh between 2020 and 2021 has been widely acclaimed as providing the most convincing evidence yet that masks work in reducing Covid-19 transmission and infections. However, the media grossly exaggerated the authors' own conclusions, and sceptical researchers have identified weaknesses in various aspects of the trial and statistical analysis which cast doubts on the significance of the results.

We conducted an analysis [174] to determine what can really be learned about the impact of mask wearing on Covid-19 infections from the data in the trial. Using a novel Bayesian causal modelling approach, we found that the claimed benefits do not hold up when subject to this rigorous analysis. At best, one can conclude that there is only a 52% probability that the seropositivity rate among people subject to a mask intervention campaign is lower than those who are not, while there is a 95% chance that a mask intervention campaign would result in anything between 19,240 fewer positives and 18,500 more positives in every 100,000. This means there was no discernible effect of the mask intervention on Covid-19 infection.

On 2 May 2022, Norman sent the following letter to the Editor of Science (note: he sent his analysis to the lead author of the study - Jason Abaluck - before making the report public and the report contains some changes following communication with him).

> Dear Sir/Madam
>
> You recently published the article "Impact of community masking on COVID-19: A cluster-randomized trial in Bangladesh". Science, 375(6577), by Abaluck et al which contained the summary statement:
>
> "A randomized-trial of community-level mask promotion in rural Bangladesh during COVID-19 shows that the intervention tripled mask usage and reduced

symptomatic SARS-CoV-2 infections, demonstrating that promoting community mask-wearing can improve public health."

As explained in the attached report, this statement grossly exaggerates the actual findings of the study and – unsurprisingly - has been widely used by the media to argue that the study provides the most convincing evidence yet of the effectiveness of masks in preventing covid-19 transmission and infection. More worryingly, the article has been cited explicitly to justify continuing or reintroducing aspects of mask mandates in the USA, UK and elsewhere. Because the paper provides no evidence that mask wearing reduces covid transmission or infections, it needs to be corrected or withdrawn.

Yours sincerely

Professor Norman Fenton

We never received a response to this letter.

6.10. Why did Frontiers publish a flawed study?

Massively exaggerating Covid-19 risk to children (14 July 2022)

Before publishing this article we sent it to the Editors of Frontiers in Pediatrics asking if they wished to correct any inaccuracies or provide any updates, giving them several days to respond. They did not acknowledge or respond.

In September 2021 Frontiers in Pediatrics published an article [176] by members of the Indonesian Pediatrician Association (IDAI) claiming that the case fatality rate (CFR) for children with 'suspected' Covid-19 in Indonesia was 1.4% (i.e. 1 in 71) with a CFR of 0.46% (1 in 217) for those with 'confirmed' Covid-19. No such high Covid-19 fatality rates for children have been observed elsewhere in the world. In fact, worldwide the infection fatality rate was estimated (at the time the IDAI paper was published) to be 1 in 37,000 for those aged under 20. [177]

The IDAI authors also made the startingly claim that, of the 175 'confirmed Covid-19 deaths' of children in their study, 62 had no existing comorbidities. But again, elsewhere in the world cases of Covid-19 death in children without serious comorbidities are almost unheard of. For example, in the UK in the whole of 2020, a deep analysis [178] of ALL child deaths with Covid-19 (there were 28 in total) revealed only 8 were confirmed as likely caused by Covid-19 and that all 8 had a comorbidity recorded, seven of whom had a life-limiting condition.

An article by Ted Hilbert [179] written shortly after the IDAI article was published highlighted the major problems with the study. While the claims in the paper were startling, in June 2021 the IDAI (through its chairman) exaggerated the paper's findings even further, claiming to the media that Indonesia has the highest child mortality rate (CFR) in the world, 3% to 5%. This article [180] provides the full details of the obviously fraudulent claim and includes the police report that was filed in response.

However, the massively exaggerated claim was used by IDAI to justify vaccinating children in Indonesia, and indeed a recommendation letter from IDAI to the government, based on the flawed study and claims about it, has been used as the main justification by the Indonesian government to issue the EUA and related policies for vaccinating children.

In the paper, the IDAI authors did not provide the raw data from which their conclusions were drawn, so Hilbert wrote to them requesting it. He received no reply (despite a statement by the authors that "The raw data supporting the conclusions of this article will be made available by the authors, without undue reservation") and so wrote to the Editors of Frontiers on 23 Oct 2021 to request the data. The Editors finally replied on 11 Nov 2021 stating that they would contact the authors requesting the data and finally on 30 Nov 2021 the "Research Integrity Specialist" at Frontiers sent this link [181] to the data.

After analysing the data with other experts including pathologists, a group of authors wrote an 8-page detailed response [182] to Frontiers on 15 Dec 2021 pointing out multiple flaws in the study and inaccuracies in the data.

Hilbert has been promised several times that a review by the editors will take place but (as of today 14 July 2022) this has never happened despite several follow up requests by Hilbert. The paper, with its flawed conclusions that have led to Indonesia's child vaccine policy, remains published and unchanged.

Frontiers can hardly be accused of not responding to complaints about papers on Covid treatments. But it seems only complaints against papers showing benefits of alternative treatments are taken seriously. In May 2021 Frontiers in Pharmacology published an abstract of a study by Pierre Kory on ivermectin for Covid-19 that had passed peer review with an expert panel of reviewers including senior reviewers from the FDA; but shortly before the full paper was due to be published in a special issue edited by Robert Malone - it was pulled [183] due to a third-party complaint, with no chance for resubmission.

Chapter 7. How the BBC and ONS pushed a false narrative about the unvaccinated

7.1. The BBC claim of "8% unvaccinated against Covid"

7 July 2022

On 6 July 2022 the BBC website announced a new documentary [184] (hosted by mathematician Prof Hannah Fry) that:

> "seeks to understand why eight percent of the population remain unvaccinated against Covid-19."

(For reasons that will become clear they subsequently changed the wording on the website, but screenshots capturing the original and revised versions can be found here [185]).

But, as pointed out by Clare Craig [186], the latest UKHSA Covid-19 surveillance report [187] (dated 7 July 2022) reports something very different. Their Table 5 shows that almost 30% of the population of England eligible for the vaccine ***has not had a single dose of the vaccine***. Even if we ignore those aged under 18 it is almost 20% without a single dose and almost 40% who have not had 3 doses.

We have shown in several of our own research articles, (see for example here [188] and here [189]) and also in this a short video [221] why accurate estimates of the proportion of people who are unvaccinated is critical in determining both vaccine efficacy and vaccine safety.

To see why suppose, for illustration, we know that in a given period there were one million people in a specific age group of whom one thousand died. Then the overall all-cause mortality rate is 1 in 1000. Suppose we know that 800 of those who died were vaccinated while 200 were not. Then:

- If the true proportion of unvaccinated is 10% that means 200 out of 100,000 unvaccinated died (that's a mortality rate of 1 in 500), while 800 out of 900,000 vaccinated died (that's a mortality rate of 1 in 1,125). *So the mortality rate in the unvaccinated is* ***much higher*** *than that of the vaccinated.*
- If the true proportion of unvaccinated is 30%, that means 200 out of 300,000 unvaccinated died (that's a mortality rate of 1 in 1,150), while 800 out of 700,000 vaccinated died (that's a mortality rate of 1 in 875). *So the mortality rate in the unvaccinated is* ***much lower*** *than that of the vaccinated.*

Our reports showed clearly that many of the claims by the Office for National Statistics (ONS) about vaccine efficacy and safety are based on flawed data, which includes not just misclassifying some of those who die shortly after vaccinated as 'unvaccinated', but also underestimating the true proportion of unvaccinated.

The 8% unvaccinated claim by the BBC is wrong and it clearly has a major impact in exaggerating any claims about vaccine safety and efficacy. Having previously co-presented a BBC documentary with Hannah Fry [189], Norman is well aware of the extent to which what presenters say is scripted by others. So, we would be interested to know if Hannah is comfortable presenting such obviously inaccurate statistics.

Within 2 hours of us posting this article (the original is here [185]) and tweeting it, the BBC updated their website article, replacing the 8% statement above with:

> "seeks to understand why a portion of the population remain unvaccinated against Covid-19."

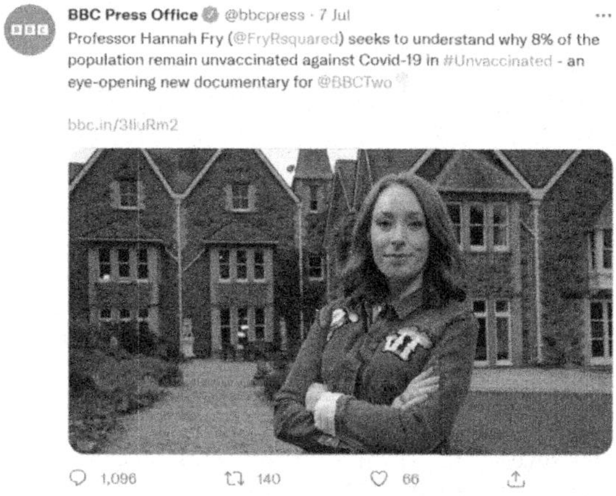

Figure 29 Tweet announcing the programme

The heavily 'ratioed' tweet [190] shown in Figure 29 was, however, still left up (until it was deleted some weeks later).

So, while it was a small success of sorts, we asked "How about an apology by the BBC for misleading the public again and also an explanation for how they came to get it so wrong. Who are the 'experts' they relied on for the data and are they the same 'experts' who will be scripting the programme with a biased narrative?"

7.2. BBC's biased 'vaccine experts'

18 July 2022

As previously reported [191] the BBC is screening a documentary on 20 July in which mathematician Prof Hannah Fry - with the help of 'experts' - attempts to convince 7 members of the public (who have so far refused) to take the Covid vaccine. As we pointed out the BBC (in the publicity for the programme) already signposted the likely extreme bias in the programme by massively underestimating the number of unvaccinated people in the UK, hence trying to present such people as a tiny extreme fringe.

This newspaper article about the Programme [192] unwittingly provides more evidence of just how biased the programme is going to be. To give just one example, we have this:

> "As for concerns about how exactly the jab works, the group travelled to meet Professor Adam Finn, a paediatrician from the University of Bristol who has been instrumental in Covid vaccine research."

So, who exactly is Prof Finn? What the article (and subsequently the documentary itself) failed to reveal was that he just happens to be the leader of the Pfizer Centre of Excellence for Epidemiology of Vaccine-preventable Diseases [193]- set up with an initial £4.6 million investment in May 2021.

And then we have this about the 'expert' Asma Khalil from the article:

> "To address concerns about fertility, Prof Fry introduces Chanelle and Naomi – both concerned about female fertility – to Asma Khalil, a professor of obstetrics and maternal-foetal medicine at St George's University Hospital in London, who has conducted research into the effect of the jab on pregnant women.
>
> Her latest review, looking at the outcomes of nearly 120,000 jabbed pregnant women, concluded that vaccination in pregnancy was safe."

So, who exactly is Asma Khalil? What the article (and subsequently the documentary itself) failed to reveal was that, that in the review "of nearly 120,000 jabbed pregnant women" she declares that she just happened to be the "PI of the Pfizer Covid in pregnancy trial". Also, as long ago as 2015 she declared the following paid conflicts of interest as a member of the NICE Quality Standards Committee [194]:

> Collaboration with commercial companies, such as USCOM®, Roche Diagnostics®, Alere Diagnostics® and proact medical Ltd® (research equipment and/or consumables)

It is also important to note that the review "of nearly 120,000 jabbed pregnant women" is only a meta-analysis of what appears to be cherry-picked studies (many of which have obvious biases and flaws).

But that's not all regarding Asma Khalil. It turns out the she was a participant in the Bill and Melinda Gates Foundation funded simulation "Preparing for Disease X: Ensuring Vaccine Equity for Pregnant Women in Future Pandemics" - the results of which are reported in this paper [195] that she co-authored: In the funding and COI statement at the end of that paper there is no declaration by Khalil. This requires an explanation. Nor does Khalil declare any COI's in her other recent publications.

7.3. Critique of BBC2 documentary 'Unvaccinated'

22 July 2022

Our pre-screening articles and tweets about the forthcoming programme were very widely read, and one of the participants Nazarin Veronica [202] contacted us to express her serious concerns about the way the programme was made – and how it might be edited – and to confirm that the participants were indeed not informed of the experts' conflicts of interest (this is covered well in this article by threadsirish [203]). Her subsequent tweets, such as one on 19 July 2022, made clear her extreme concerns about the programme even before it was screened:

> "They have completely fucked it. There were six days of filming. That's 6 days of real debating of sharing both sides' reasons for choosing to get it or not, sharing statistics from both sides, sharing science from both sides, having scientists and doctors come into the house to try to brainwash us into changing our minds. Still after all the coercion no one chose to take it in the end so that says a lot. Yet they seem to have mostly included the small moments where people slipped up, out of the entire 6 days of proper debating. There were times where Hannah slipped up too, but I can guarantee that won't be in there. I knew they would edit it in a way that would make us look stupid, pick out the parts which discredit what each individual is saying and twist our words, but I wasn't expecting the manipulation to be this obvious.
>
> I have warned them that if I watch the documentary and I feel, misrepresented in any way I will go to the Press with my version of events, with evidence and witnesses. I have evidence of how the debate really went, where we made a comment or asked a question and Hannah had nothing to say in response. I have evidence of us being told we're not allowed to say certain things on camera. I have evidence of them shutting me up mid-sentence. I have evidence of their Doctor not being able to answer some of my questions which I already knew the answers to. I have evidence of them lying to us multiple times. I've explained to them that they still have 3 days to re-edit the documentary in a way which accurately represents what happened in those 6 days of filming and if I feel it's in accurate any way I'm going straight to the press with everything. If you play with fire, you get burned."

The programme turned out to be every bit as bad and biased as feared. Many of the problems have been highlighted by the especially vocal participants Nazarin and Vicky Borman [204] (see the interview [205] of them and Norman on Maajid Nawaz's show). Below we summarise our key concerns and what was missing:

Claim of 4 million UK adults unvaccinated: Despite us alerting the BBC to this error (which led them to change their website description [206]) this claim (i.e. that only 8% of adults were unvaccinated) was right up front. It set the context suggesting that this was only a tiny, crazed minority. But what was really interesting is that the presenter Hannah Fry stated that, as part of the programme research, they did a survey of 2,500 people about their views on vaccination, and she was surprised to discover that 600 were unvaccinated. If the sample was representative of UK adults (and there was no suggestion it was not) then that means 24% of UK adults are unvaccinated, which is even higher than the figure we estimate, and blows apart the BBC's ludicrous 8% claim. In fact, the survey was indeed representative of the population [207] and the actual number never vaccinated was 664 out of 2570 - i.e. 26%. This provides further evidence of what we have claimed for a long time: The ONS is massively underestimating the proportion of unvaccinated.

Failure to disclose the Pfizer links of the two key experts (Finn and Khalil) on the programme: As feared the programme did not inform either the participants or the viewers of the major conflicts of interest of the key experts detailed in our previous article [201].

Failure to disclose background to FullFact.org: The CEO Will Moy was brought in to claim that vaccine hesitancy was all due to online 'misinformation'. But fullfact have received massive funding by organisations like Google and Facebook to present precisely the biased narrative that all the covid 'misinformation' is coming from 'antivaxxers and conspiracy theorists' and they have shown no interest in pointing out the far greater volume of misinformation put out by governments, the pharma companies and their supporters. They only 'fact check' information that counters the 'standard narrative' and avoid checking obvious misinformation claims of vaccine efficacy and safety. For some background on how bad fullfact are see this article [208].

No challenge to the many explicit false claims made: Among the most outrageous and demonstrably false claims that went unchallenged were: 1) Adam Finn claimed that people had stronger immunity from the vaccination than from having been infected; 2) Asma Khalil claimed the vaccination was not only completely safe for pregnant women but actually reduced the risk of miscarriage by 15% (but look at what was in the Pfizer trial [209] with more here [210]).

The jellybeans game: Hannah Fry tried to create the impression that only 1 in 33,000 had a serious adverse reaction by mischievously picking that number as the incidence of myocarditis, which she claims was by the most common serious adverse reaction. Showing what 33,000 jellybeans looked like – only one of which was 'bad' – was supposed to show how 'rare' adverse reactions to the vaccines were. But the most recent relevant data (from the German government [211]) actually suggest as many as 1 in 300 serious adverse reactions ***per dose*** after the vaccine. Assuming independence between doses this means that a triple vaccinated person has an approximate probability of 1 in a 100 of getting a serious adverse reaction and for a person double boosted this rises to 1 in 75. And, as somebody on twitter said "what if all the bad jelly beans were in one big batch and all the others weren't 'good jelly beans' – we just didn't know yet".

No mention of the failure of the vaccination to stop infection or transmission of covid

Failure to humanize any actual vaccination victims. The programme spoke about actual unvaccinated people dying from covid, but used the bad jelly beans to represent vaccination victims. Why didn't they mention actual victims like the BBC's own Lisa Shaw? [212] or Vicky Spit's husband Zion [213]?

The ludicrous and misleading MMR vaccination anecdote: In response to the 9-page Pfizer report of adverse reactions, Hannah Fry used a bizarre anecdote to downplay its impact. This imagined a Doctor about to give the MMR jab to a child when the phone rings; there is a 50:50 chance he picks up the phone before giving the jab. He picks up the phone and during the call the child has a fit. Saying there was a 50:50 chance the doctor picks up the phone or gives the jab deliberately creates the false impression that there is also a 50:50 chance any adverse reaction after a vaccination is purely coincidental.

No challenge to the powerful claim that 20 out of 21 ICU patients at St Georges hospital in Dec 2021 were unvaccinated: all evidence of national ICU data suggests vaccinated are now disproportionally hospitalised with covid, so this claim was either false/exaggerated or an unbelievable outlier. Much more likely, the 'unvaccinated' were defined as 'not fully boosted' rather than 'never vaccinated as was implied.

Failure to mention reported data on adverse reactions: Systems like VAERS in the US and YellowCard in the UK make it difficult to report adverse reactions and so are widely believed to massively underestimate true numbers. Yet, in VAERS alone (mainly US) as of 8/7/22 there were 1,341,605 covid vaccine adverse reactions of which 29,460 were deaths[214]. In all 32 years of VAERS reporting a total of only 9,754 deaths (and 878,053 adverse events) were recorded for ALL OTHER vaccines combined. So, in just 18 months, 3 times as many deaths for covid vaccines have been recorded than in 32 years combined for all other vaccines.

No mention of the true risk of covid based on worldwide data: Except for those with multiple comorbidities (who are not given appropriate early treatments) Covid poses very little risk of hospitalisation and death. Young people are at essentially zero risk of dying due to Covid.

No mention of the way covid data are by definition fixed to exaggerate cases numbers, hospitalisations, deaths as well as vaccine efficacy and safety. Specifically: any person admitted to hospital who had a PCR positive within 14 days prior – or who tests PCR positive after hospitalisation' – is classified as a covid hospitalisation even if the reason for hospitalisation was unrelated to covid; any person who dies within 28 days of PCR positive test is classified as a covid death irrespective of the true cause of death; any person who contracts covid or who suffers adverse reaction inside 14 days of vaccination is classified as 'unvaccinated'.

No mention of lack of long-term safety data: In particular, the failure of the Pfizer trial to provide this was glossed over suggesting that their people were so dedicated that the worked much faster than for any previous vaccine to ensure a high quality and safe product.

No mention of all the protocol violations now known in the main Pfizer trial. Even with the violations, Pfizer's their own data showed more deaths in vaccine arm than placebo arm and the risk of serious adverse event in the vaccinated was greater than risk of covid hospitalisation in the unvaccinated.

No mention of international data showing strong evidence the vaccine is neither effective nor safe: Countries with lowest vaccination rates have lowest covid death rates [215]; spikes in all-cause deaths happen after vaccination dose rollouts [216]; countries with highest vaccination rates have highest covid rates [217] and are experiencing non-covid excess death increases; and falling birth rates. There is no reliable evidence anywhere in world that vaccinated people have lower all-cause mortality than unvaccinated.

What was Hannah Fry's involvement in the stat/maths modelling: Near the start of the programme Hannah stated that she had been involved in the stats/math modelling that 'helped get us out of lockdown'. This was a surprising claim. It's the first we had heard that such modelling was formally used to get us out of lockdown. If she was involved in such modelling, she was presumably also involved in the modelling that took us INTO lockdown (curiously nobody wants to be associated with that any more given we know it was so wrong with disastrous consequences). What exactly was her involvement in this modelling – are there papers describing it other than this one [218]?

7.4. BBC response to our complaint about 'Unvaccinated'

3 August 2022

Two weeks ago we submitted a complaint to the BBC about its "Unvaccinated" documentary based on the details in the previous article [219]. Today we received the following pathetic response.

> Dear Prof Fenton, Thanks for contacting us about 'Unvaccinated', broadcast on 20 July. With UK Covid infections on the rise, this programme sought to understand why some people remain unvaccinated against Covid-19.
>
> To fully explore this debate a group of unvaccinated strangers, each with their own different reasons for not getting the vaccine, were brought together to discuss their views and the programme fairly represented what happened over the 6 days of filming. As the programme said, there are still around four million adults who remain unvaccinated - this is based on government figures and Office for National Statistics estimates.
>
> To assist with the science, the programme included Professor Finn of the University of Bristol and Professor Khalil of St George's University Hospital (University of London). In his capacity as an employee of the University, Professor Finn leads a research group within the Pfizer Vaccine Centre of Excellence - where his work in relation to Covid-19 vaccines is independent of Pfizer and he did not lead or conduct any trials of the Pfizer Covid-19 vaccine. Similarly, Prof Khalil is an employee of St George's Hospital and in that capacity is the Principal Investigator of Preg-CoV - the largest clinical trial in the UK, funded by the government, investigating the best gap between first and second COVID-19 vaccine doses for pregnant women. Professor Khalil has not conducted any independent paid consultancy work for Pfizer or any other pharma company relating to Covid-19 vaccines and her position at St George's is not dependent on Pfizer funding. Professor Khalil receives no payment or benefit directly from Pfizer. The programme acknowledges that in some rare circumstances the vaccine has been shown to cause harm. Your feedback is valued and has been seen by the 'Unvaccinated' team. Thanks again for taking the time to contact us. Kind regards,
>
> BBC Complaints Team

The response completely fails to address most of the points in our complaint, choosing to focus only on the concerns we raised about a) the undeclared conflicts of interest of Prof Finn and Prof Khalil and b) the accuracy of the "4 million unvaccinated adults" claim.

Note that they try to downplay Prof Finn's Pfizer association by saying he "leads a research group within the Pfizer Vaccine Centre of Excellence" whereas - as the announcement [193] on his own University's website announced on 28/5/2021 – states that Finn **leads the whole Centre** which was set up then with an initial investment of £4.6 million from Pfizer.

As for Prof Khalil, they seem to be claiming no Pfizer association at all, but in the Nature article she co-authored she declares in "competing interests" that she is PI of the **Pfizer** COVID in pregnancy trial. We already pointed out those details, so we are not sure why the BBC is trying to ignore and/or downplay these conflicts of interest.

Finally, regarding our complaint about the "4 million unvaccinated adults" claim - which amounts to just 8% of the adult population. They claim "this is based on government figures and Office for National Statistics estimates." Well we already pointed out to them that we knew this figure was based on ONS estimates, but we know they are wrong, not least because they are completely contradicted by data from another government agency - the UKHSA - which estimates 20% of adults are unvaccinated. If the BBC choose to ignore the "government figures" of UKHSA , then why do they at least not trust the extensive survey of a representative sample of 2570 adults carried out explicitly for the programme [207]. Of these 664 were unvaccinated, which is 26%. Based on that survey, **there is essentially zero probability that the true population unvaccinated percentage is less than 20%.** In fact, there is a 99.973% probability the proportion of unvaccinated is at least 23%.

7.5. More updates on BBC2 documentary 'Unvaccinated'

15 August 2022

Following previous reports Norman produced a video [220] which looks at the large representative ICM survey that was commissioned for the programme.

Contrary to the BBC claim that only 8% of the UK adult population is unvaccinated (based on the ONS data), in the survey the proportion was 26%. The video looks at the full survey data and shows that it is very highly representative of the UK adult population in every respect against ONS population data - except mysteriously the proportion unvaccinated which is completely different. We would love to know how the BBC and ONS explain that. Using a proportion of 8% when it is really over 20% means any claims of vaccine efficacy and safety are massively exaggerated.

This video [222] from PennyDrop Films highlights yet more problems with the documentary. Note especially the claim about the fake NHS consent form pushing 'absolute nonsense':

Further revealing insights by Iain Davis into the undisclosed conflicts of interest are revealed in this documentary [223].

7.6. BBC response to our follow-up complaint

28 August 2022

First of all it is worth noting that if you look at the BBC's complaints summary [224] for the week following the programme's screening, it was the second most complained about programme with 133 complaining about "Bias in favour of vaccinations". The only programme with more was the BBC 1 Prime Minister's debate. Given the relatively low number of viewers for a BBC2 documentary compared to the big debate, in terms of *complaints by viewer numbers* we suspect "Unvaccinated" might be one of their most complained about programmes for a long time –In many months there is NO programme for which they receive more than 100 complaints.

The BBC's response to Norman's initial complaint was discussed in the previous article [225]. Norman decided to make a follow up complaint (based on the arguments used in the blog post [226]) and received the following second response:

> Dear Prof Fenton
>
> Thanks for your further correspondence.
>
> We're sorry to learn you were unhappy with our response. You previously raised concerns regarding two of the experts who featured in the documentary and we have discussed your further complaint on this point with the programme production team again.
>
> With regard to Professor Finn, the programme pointed out he has been involved in Covid 19 vaccine research. Prof Finn and his work in relation to Covid-19 vaccines is independent of Pfizer and he did not lead or conduct any trials of the Pfizer Covid-19 vaccine.
>
> Regarding Professor Khalil, it was stated in the programme that Prof Khalil works at one of the largest vaccine and pregnancy trials in the UK. Professor Khalil has not conducted any independent paid consultancy work for Pfizer - or any other pharmaceutical company relating to Covid-19 vaccines - and Professor Khalil receives no payment or benefit directly from Pfizer.
>
> The programme included a range of experts to talk about the latest scientific understanding of the vaccine and, in line with BBC Editorial Guidelines, it appropriately reported the latest science and statistics.
>
> With regard to your follow up complaint about the statement 'there are still around four million adults who remain unvaccinated', we stand by this as accurate. This is based on adults eligible for the vaccine and eligible adults who had taken up the vaccine. Official figures at the time were:
>
> UK ONS 16+ population estimate: 54,353,665 England 16+ vax: 42,415,586 Wales 16+ vax: 2,408,063 Scotland 16+ vax: 4,162,392 NI 16+ vax: 1,372,456 = around 4 million adults who remain unvaccinated
>
> If you remain unhappy, you can now contact the BBC's Executive Complaints Unit (ECU). The ECU is Stage 2 of the BBC's complaints process. You'll need to explain why you think there's a potential breach of standards, or if the issue is significant and should still be investigated. Please do so within 20 working days of this reply.

Most people who take the trouble of formally complaining do not bother with a follow-up and certainly do not bother with a second follow up if - as in this case - they are fobbed off with the same nonsense as they got first time. But given that they provided a unique link for Norman to contact the ECU he has now made the following response:

My original complaint was detailed fully in my blog posting here:

In summary …. <the key points were listed>

The BBC responses have focused on the first two points (the number of unvaccinated and the failure to disclose Pfizer links of Finn and Khalil). Even if we ignore the fact that the BBC has not addressed the other complaints, the BBC response to the first two points is totally inadequate and flawed.

The BBC is quoting ONS data for the estimate of adult unvaccinated (they estimate 8%) but fails to acknowledge that this is just one (extremely biased) estimate. Another UK Government agency UKHSA estimates 20% adult unvaccinated (see this article) and as I made clear in my complaint the large representative ICM survey commissioned for the programme itself revealed 26% adult unvaccinated. This is explained in detail in this video I made.

To continually quote only the obviously flawed ONS figure as 'the truth' is contemptible but fits the biased narrative that the documentary wished to create, namely that while a 'large' number of adults remained unvaccinated they still only represent a tiny fringe minority.

Regarding the BBC response on the failure to disclose the Pfizer links of Finn and Khalil, this is also laughable. To claim that there was no need to disclose any links because they are not directly paid by Pfizer is more ludicrous than claiming a season ticket holder of a Premiership Football Club can give an unbiased opinion of their Club's ability as they are not paid by the Club. The fact is – as you must be well aware – being the LEADER of the Pfizer Centre of Excellence for Epidemiology of Vaccine-preventable Diseases (set up with an initial £4.6 million investment by Pfizer in May 2021- means that Finn cannot possibly be assumed to provide an unbiased opinion on the Pfizer vaccines. Similarly, Khalil being the PRINCIPAL INVESTIGATOR of the Pfizer funded vaccination in pregnancy trial means she cannot possibly be assumed to provide an unbiased opinion on the Pfizer vaccines. Irrespective of whether the claims made by Finn and Khalil were correct or not, the failure by the BBC to inform both the participants and the public of their Pfizer associations is a disgrace.

7.7. Did the documentary breach regulations?

On advertising and promoting medicines (30 August 2022 with updates)

What we were not aware of was that the programme likely breached regulations governing advertising of prescription medicines.

A group of scientists and clinicians (who have given us permission to reproduce this) have written to the Advertising Standards and Outreach Unit of the Medicines and Healthcare products Regulatory Agency [229] arguing that the programme was 1) promoting medicinal products as defined in the MHRA Regulations applying to advertisements relating to medicinal products (*"The Blue Guide, Advertising and Promotion of Medicines in the UK*

(Updated 2020)" and 2) failed to comply with the legal requirements for such promotion and advertising.

The full letter of complaint is an extremely comprehensive and carefully written explanation of exactly how the programme was in breach of the legal requirements. The summary says:

> Society demands that advertising of any commodity, service or anything that may be of interest to the consumer, should be of a high standard. It should not include anything that could cause serious or widespread offence, create unrealistic expectations in the consumer or be misleading. Furthermore, UK law recognises that medicines should not be treated as an ordinary general commodity by placing specific restrictions on them. There is recognition in this approach that potentially vulnerable, sick people and their carers could be affected or even targeted by such promotional activities.
>
> Therefore, over and above the general legislation and controls on advertising, there is additional specific legislation that applies to the advertising of medicines. All advertising and promotion of medicines, both for self-medication and to healthcare professionals where medical prescription is required, must be responsible and of the highest standard. All means and media used in the promotional marketing of medicines are subject to the legislation controlling advertising. This includes academics, journalists and broadcast media.
>
> The television programme "Unvaccinated" broadcast by the BBC and still available on its iPlayer streaming service meets the definition of an advertisement for a medicinal product as set out in the Advertising Regulations. As such it is therefore in breach of these regulations as it is promoting specific POMs to the general public. It also fails to meet the required quality standards for the advertising of medicinal products as set out in these regulations as, on a number of counts, it fails to encourage the rational use of the products by presenting them objectively and without exaggerating their qualities, it is misleading and it also describes them as "safe".
>
> We would be grateful if you would take the necessary steps to ensure that these breaches of the UK legislation are dealt with appropriately.

Unfortunately, the response [230] from the Head of Advertising (Healthcare Quality and Access) at MHRA does not address any of the detailed concerns raised in the letter and was ludicrously dismissive:

> Although the documentary cites some Covid-19 vaccines by name, I consider that this is done in a factual and informative way throughout without highlighting particular qualities of a medicine (i.e, without use of any product claims)

It asserted that the Programme fell outside the scope of the definition for an advertisement for a particular medicine as defined in the (MHRA) Regulations and advised the letter signatories to refer their concerns to the Advertising Standards Authority (ASA):

I am therefore of the view that a programme that investigates and reports on attitudes and behaviours of members of the UK general public to taking up a public health medical intervention—i.e., vaccination—to prevent illness from an infectious disease would not be within scope of the definition for an advertisement for a particular medicine as defined in the Regulations.

On 4 Sept 2022 the same group of scientists and clinicians sent this appeal [231] of the initial MHRA response. Despite the MHRA 20-day response time they like to quote, and follow-up requests from the scientists, there was no response until 5 Nov 2022.

The MHRA response (pdf) [232] to Dr Black on 5 Nov simply doubled-down on the original. As Dr Black says:

Unsurprisingly the MHRA have doubled down on their initial decision and refused to engage with any of the details of the complaint because they continue to assert that the programme was not promotion. They originally said it was not promotion because it did not contain any product claims. So, I sent them a list of product claims made in the programme and this was their latest response:

"We consider the examples listed in your follow-up letter about "vaccine" are factual statements, not product claims." This is of course a risable response and begs the retort "When is a product claim not a product claim? Answer: When it's made by the BBC, then it becomes a 'factual statement' !"

Their other reason for continuing to deny that the programme promoted the use of the vaccines was "the documentary cannot have led members of the public to request a prescription-only medicine because the decision of which product(s) to deploy is one made by public health officials." This so ridiculous a response that it's difficult to know where to start.

They appear so desperate to get this out of their in-tray that they are now volunteering to send it to the ASA on our behalf. In my opinion, I think it would be a mistake to accept this offer. I doubt the ASA are geared up to deal with a complaint with such potentially serious PH implications. We have insisted that this is a job for the MHRA and I think we should stick to our guns. Their decision not to investigate our complaint is now on the record and hopefully they will be held to account for it one day.

7.8. About that ONS estimate of only 8% adults unvaccinated

18 October 2022

As explained here [235] Norman produced a detailed analysis [236] of the true proportion of unvaccinated in the UK as of May 2022. As was now becoming routine, the preprint servers arXiv and medrXiv refused to publish the article.

The analysis noted that the ONS estimate of 8% adults unvaccinated is, like all its covid data, based on a special (biased) subset of the England population (namely those people who were both registered in the 2011 census and registered with a GP in 2019). Other independent estimates for the whole of the population in May were higher: the UK Health

Security Agency (UKHSA) estimated 20%, while the large independent survey by ICM [207] found 26%.

Assuming the ONS estimate is correct for its subset of the England population and that the other independent estimates of between 20 and 26% for the whole population are also correct then between 69% and 99.6% of adults missing from the ONS sample are unvaccinated. This would mean the ONS sample is unrepresentative of the whole England population and any conclusions about vaccine take-up, efficacy and safety based on the ONS data may not be relevant to the population as a whole. So, however they spin it, the ONS estimate of only 8% adults unvaccinated compromises all of their conclusions on vaccine safety.

7.9. BBC's final response

23 November 2022

Like the MHRA, the BBC also failed to meet its own response deadline to my follow-up complaint [233] of 26 August to them about the programme, despite them having sent an acknowledgement on 27 August stating that: "The ECU will investigate your complaint and aim to reply within 20 working days of receiving it, though some complaints take longer than others to investigate. A target of 35 working days applies to those complaints that require longer or more complex investigation."

Jeremy Hayes The BBC Complaints Director has finally provided their response (8 pages pdf file) [234] Unsurprisingly it's a complete whitewash. He fails to properly address the complaint that the "8% unvaccinated" was a massive underestimate and argues (without any explanation for the discrepancy) that the highly representative survey they used (which unfortunately for them showed 26% unvaccinated) "*was not intended to estimate the take-up of the vaccine across the population of the UK.*"

Regarding the fact that the programme failed to mention that Prof Finn was the leader of the Pfizer Centre of Excellence for Epidemiology of Vaccine-preventable Diseases at Bristol University, Hayes says he does "*not think that his position at the University of Bristol in a research centre on epidemiology sponsored by a company which produces a Covid vaccine itself was information which could have materially altered the perception of his observations*".

Regarding the fact that the programme failed to mention that Prof Khalil was the Principal Investigator of the Pfizer-BioNTech Covid-19 vaccine trial in healthy pregnant women, Hayes says: "*The fact that the trial was sponsored by the manufacturer is not a reason in my judgment to question Professor Khalil's expertise in maternal vaccinations or require disclosure in the context of her contribution*".

All the other defences he uses against the misinformation presented in the programme are based on simply cherry-picking flawed studies that support what was said while ignoring the overwhelming evidence of the contrary. But the most telling and also particularly amusing response was the defence of the ludicrous claim by Dr Patel that 20 out of 21 ICU patients at St George's hospital in Dec 2021 were unvaccinated. He says:

"I have approached the programme makers for information about the data which were quoted by Dr Patel. I have been advised that ***the figures were compiled by Dr Patel himself*** *for the purposes of research".*

Chapter 8. More Lies, cover-up and censorship over vaccine safety

8.1. Is the vaccine safe for pregnant and breastfeeding women?

UK Government website says it is not (29 August 2022)

A twitter user called TracyK2017 has alerted people today to the fact that the UK Government has a website page with this document [237] that was "updated on 16 August 2022" (Figure 30). She was almost immediately permanently suspended from Twitter.

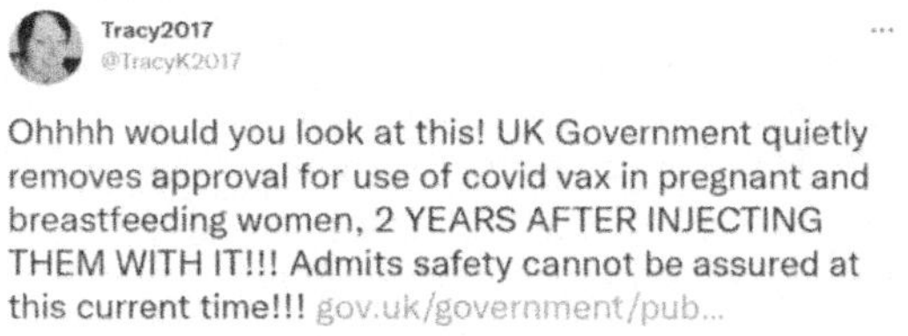

Figure 30 Tracy2017's tweet (she was almost immediately suspended for this)

The relevant text (which we can confirm is in the document at the end of Section 3.4) is:

> "In the context of supply under Regulation 174, it is considered that sufficient reassurance of safe use of the vaccine in pregnant women cannot be provided at the present time"

and

> "Women who are breastfeeding should also not be vaccinated."

Tracy also noted that people are pointing out that the document has not in fact been recently updated; apparently the wayback machine shows no changes since March 2021. However, this would make things even worse as it means that the Government officials and the NHS have been recommending pregnant women get the vaccine *against the official Government document advice*. Also, Tracy's pinned tweet dated 6 May 2022 linked to an archived version [238] of a similar but different document. That document does not have the section titled 'Toxicity conclusions' in it, although it does contain the following statement in Section 4.6:

> "Administration of the COVID-19 mRNA Vaccine BNT162b2 in pregnancy should only be considered when the potential benefits outweigh any potential risks for the mother and foetus."

But Sajid Javid (and many other Government and NHS officials) have been saying the exact opposite for months. And look what this Government webpage says [238] (screenshot at 18:19 on 29 August 2022):

> "COVID-19 vaccination is strongly recommended for pregnant and breastfeeding women.
>
> The COVID-19 vaccines available in the UK have been shown to be effective and to have a good safety profile. It is important to have your COVID-19 vaccinations to protect you and your baby."

And indeed, the ***current*** advice given to NHS staff is to strongly encourage all pregnant women to get vaccinated as soon as possible. So, as of now we have directly contradictory recommendations on the Government website.

This all also raises further alarms about the BBC who, in its documentary Unvaccinated had Prof Asma Khalil stating the vaccine was not only safe and effective for all pregnant women but that it 'reduced the risk of miscarriage by 15%' [240].

Viki Male (one of the staunchest advocates for vaccinating pregnant women) has responded to this by arguing that there is no contradiction because the Summary of the Public Assessment Report refers only to the Pfizer report and does not take account of new UK data (which, incidentally, have never been made public). When we asked her to confirm when the crucial changes were made to the Summary Report she referred us to this link [241]. This list of updates does not include the crucial "Toxicity Conclusions" paragraph. However, the very existence of this update list introduces new confusion. Why does the wayback machine insist that the document has never been changed?

A retired healthcare professional has sent us this [242] government document issued to UK Healthcare professionals in December 2020. Section 4.6 on "Fertility, pregnancy and lactation" states the following:

> "**Pregnancy**: There are no or limited amount of data from the use of COVID-19 mRNA Vaccine BNT162b2. Animal reproductive toxicity studies have not been completed. COVID-19 mRNA Vaccine BNT162b2 is not recommended during pregnancy. For women of childbearing age, pregnancy should be excluded before vaccination. In addition, women of childbearing age should be advised to avoid pregnancy for at least 2 months after their second dose.
>
> **Breast-feeding**: It is unknown whether COVID-19 mRNA Vaccine BNT162b2 is excreted in human milk. A risk to the newborns/infants cannot be excluded. COVID-19 mRNA Vaccine BNT162b2 should not be used during breast-feeding.
>
> **Fertility**: It is unknown whether COVID-19 mRNA Vaccine BNT162b2 has an impact on fertility."

There was enormous fallout over this story (documented here [243], with the usual 'fact checkers' and pharma apologists going into overdrive to convince people (but failing abysmally) that there really was nothing to be concerned about.

8.2. Does ONS have data for accurate assessment of vaccine safety?

No – they admit they do not (4 September 2022)

A mouse has just alerted us to this response (dated 11 Feb 2022) [244] by the Office for National Statistics (ONS) to an FOI request asking:

> "I want to know how many pregnant women end up in ICU each year starting from the year 2015 to dec 2021 and how many resulting in deaths and discharges?
>
> And then second chart or table split into vaccinated and unvaccinated pregnant women that end up in ICU resulting in death and discharge?"

The response from the ONS is that they do not have this data, but the part that is especially striking is this statement:

> "Vaccination status is not recorded on the death certificate and can only be linked to mortality data through complex data linkage with NHS vaccination and test and trace data. We do not hold information showing deaths by vaccination status and if the person was pregnant."

We had been raising concerns about the reliability of the ONS analyses on vaccine safety - which rely totally on having accurate data on the vaccine status of all deaths - in the Spring of 2021 when the ONS first started publishing its vaccine surveillance reports on vaccine safety and efficacy. We produced this article [245] in Sept 2021 showing that the ONS data were clearly inaccurate. Yet, when we raised these concerns directly with ONS, we were continually assured by them that they had all the relevant data and they ***was*** accurate. These assurances continued, despite subsequent additional evidence that their data were not accurate (see here [246] and here [247], for example). We even produced a report [248] that provided a detailed explanation of why it was likely that so many errors could be made in the data (see especially Section 7). Now it appears that the ONS is admitting that it is, indeed, too hard to get the necessary data.

So, it is worth repeating what we said at the end of the abstract in [248]:

> "The dataset is therefore corrupted, making any inferences about vaccine efficacy or safety that are reliant on the data, moot. Accordingly, the ONS should publicly withdraw their dataset and call for the retraction of any claims made by others that are based upon it."

8.3. Are vaccinees especially healthy or especially unhealthy?

Our detractors need to decide as they have claimed both (29 September 2022)

One of the key findings [249] in our various analyses of the ONS (Office for National Statistics) vaccine mortality surveillance data was that there were spikes in non-covid mortality in the unvaccinated that coincided with peak vaccine rollouts. We demonstrated that the main plausible explanation for such an obvious anomaly was that people dying shortly after vaccination were being wrongly classified as unvaccinated deaths. Whether through policy or error this certainly happens (indeed in Sweden a reply [250] to an FOI confirms that those dying within 14 days of vaccination are routinely counted as unvaccinated).

Once the ONS data were adjusted for these anomalies there was no evidence that the vaccines reduced all-cause mortality.

Our detractors (mainly from the 'mutton crew' [251]), who are always desperate to suppress any data suggesting the vaccines were not as safe and effective as claimed, said that there was an alternative explanation for the anomalies They argued that the anomalies were the result of especially ill people being denied the vaccine; so, there was, they claimed, a 'healthy vaccinee effect' (or equivalently a 'moribund unvaccinated effect'). Figure 30 shows one of the key mutton crew repeating that explanation this week (while attacking the recent paper [252] by Dr Aseem Malthotra exposing problems with the covid vaccines):

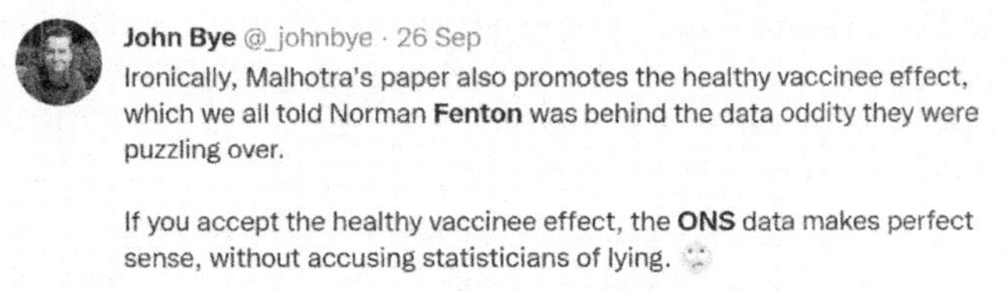

Figure 31 Healthy vaccinee effect claim

The ONS also stated the 'healthy vaccinee effect' as an explanation in a subsequent report [253] after we identified the anomalies in their data. But the notion of the 'healthy vaccinee' was contradicted by the NHS guidelines (which required the most critically ill people to be ***prioritised for the vaccine***, not denied it) and we know that even terminally ill patients in care homes were given the vaccine as a priority. Moreover, the observed data could not be theoretically simulated by a 'healthy vaccinee' effect.

Another problem with the ONS claim that its data shows [254] lower (age standardised) mortality rates in the vaccinated is that it is based on a subset of the England population which likely massively underestimates [255] the true national proportion of unvaccinated and hence underestimates the mortality rate of the vaccinated. Using the UKHSA and NIMS data [20] on the number of unvaccinated results in higher (age standardised) mortality rates. In fact, there is increasing evidence now that the vaccinated have the higher mortality rates. And that brings us to a very interesting comment by one of the people - 'Health Nerd' (@GidMK on twitter) - who has been especially vocal in trying to delegitimise our work, and who is the key source of authority for the mutton crew. He, like John Bye, has been outspoken in trying to delegitimise the recent paper by Dr Aseem Malhotra. In a long twitter thread [257] he wrote the comment in Figure 32.

So, in contrast to the previously claimed 'healthy vaccinee' effect used to explain the non-covid mortality spikes, the same people are now claiming an 'unhealthy vaccinee' effect to explain the higher age-standardised mortality rates of the vaccinated.

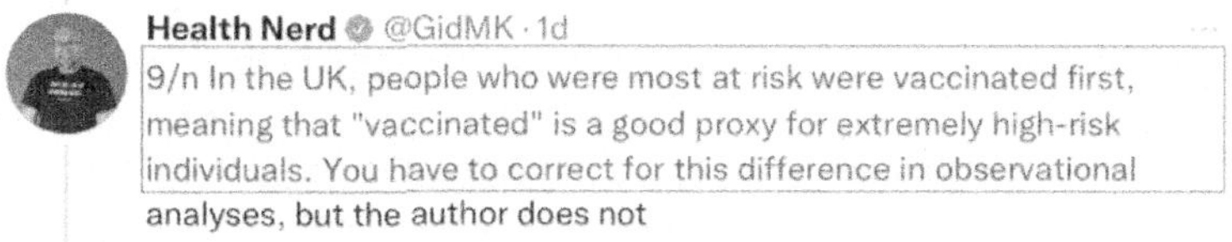
Health Nerd @GidMK · 1d
9/n In the UK, people who were most at risk were vaccinated first, meaning that "vaccinated" is a good proxy for extremely high-risk individuals. You have to correct for this difference in observational analyses, but the author does not

Figure 32 Unhealthy vaccinee effect?

Can these people please make up their minds as to whether vaccinees are especially healthy or especially unhealthy?

As an update, @jikkyleaks reported [258] that the UKHSA vaccine surveillance report of March 2022 [259] showed that in each age group (except under 18s) the 'unadjusted' covid infection rate among the unvaccinated was lower than that among the fully vaccinated.

Table 9 UKHSA vaccine effectiveness report

Vaccine effectiveness data UKHSA 2022 week 13 report, p45

	Unadjusted rates among persons vaccinated with at least 3 doses (per 100,000)	Unadjusted rates among persons not vaccinated (per 100,000)	Vaccine effectiveness
Under 18	1454.0	1711.7	15%
18 to 29	3118.8	941.6	-231%
30 to 39	4324.7	1085.6	-298%
40 to 49	3957.8	955.3	-314%
50 to 59	3303.4	779.8	-324%
60 to 69	2814.9	572.8	-391%
70 to 79	2161.5	532.1	-306%
80 or over	2023.7	775.6	-161%

After that they stopped publishing the infection rates! But guess what they offered (page 39) as a possible explanation for the higher infection rate among the vaccinated? The unhealthy vaccinee effect:

> "Many of those who were at the head of the queue for vaccination are those at higher risk from COVID-19 due to their age, their occupation, their family circumstances or because of underlying health issues."

8.4. ONS data on vaccine mortality not fit for purpose

11 November 2022

Following on from our latest report [260] highlighting multiple anomalies in the most recent ONS covid vaccine mortality surveillance report [261] we have written the following self-explanatory letter to the Statistics Regulator.

"Dear Sir/Madam,

Since the ONS began producing its covid vaccine mortality surveillance reports in 2021, we have been highlighting various anomalies in their datasets. This includes strong evidence that many of those dying shortly after vaccination were being misclassified as unvaccinated [262] and systematic undercounting of deaths occurring within first two weeks of vaccination [263].

We are especially concerned about the latest [261] ONS dataset and have produced a detailed analysis [260] which highlights the multiple glaring anomalies in it.

We show that, in addition to further definitive evidence of the misclassification and missing deaths, there is: a) gross underestimation of the population proportion unvaccinated, and b) mortality rates that are both nonsensical in various categories and completely incompatible with historical rates.

We believe that there are multiple violations of your code of practice [264]. In particular, the dataset breaches the Quality and Value criteria numbered: Q 1.1, Q1.4 – 1.7, Q 2.4, Q 2.5, Q 3.2 – 3.5, V 1.1, V 3.2 – 3.3.

All of the anomalies in the dataset introduce bias in favour of analyses supporting vaccine 'safety and efficacy'. The fact that these data are being used as continued justification for the efficacy and safety of the covid vaccines is therefore now a matter of national concern and scandal. We believe that an investigation into how and why the ONS dataset is so flawed and corrupted is required. In the meantime, we call for

1. the public withdrawal of the ONS dataset and
2. the retraction of any claims made by others that are based upon it.

Yours

Norman Fenton, Martin Neil, Clare Craig and Scott McLachlan"

A slightly updated version of our report (with more detailed reference citations than the version on ResearchGate) is here [265].

On 20 Jan 2023 we received the formal response [266] and it is on the Regulator's website. They agreed with our recommendation to ignore any claims of vaccine safety based on ONS deaths by vaccination status data. They also agree that the ONS underestimates the true population proportion unvaccinated.

While there are aspects of the response that we are unhappy with, the crucial point is that they have completely accepted our main recommendation (to ignore any claims of vaccine safety based on ONS deaths by vaccination status data) because they say:

> "Overall, then, our view is that the Deaths by Vaccination Status publication does not provide information on vaccine effectiveness or vaccine safety, and should not be used in this way."

Many researchers and news organisations have made claims of vaccine efficacy and safety based on the ONS reports. We therefore now call on all those who have made such claims to publicly retract them.

It is also important to note that the Regulator agreed with our conclusions that the ONS population sample was biased - with those excluded much more likely to be unvaccinated.

> "We consider that it is therefore likely that the sample used in the Deaths by Vaccination Status publication is not representative of the general population. Those who are missing are, we think, more likely to be younger and unvaccinated."

We therefore call on all of those - including especially the BBC - who have used the ludicrously low estimates from the ONS [267] to publicly withdraw all material based on these estimates, as they have been deliberately used to represent the unvaccinated as a tiny fringe minority.

The not-so-good news is that, as expected the Regulator has gone to extreme lengths to defend the integrity of the ONS. In particular, they are putting forward the 'healthy vaccinee effect' which we have previously dealt with [262] and which we will be further dismantling in the next few weeks.

Our analysis of the most recent ONS report on deaths by vaccination status is here [260]. That report was published in July 2022 with the most recent data up to May 2022. Despite promises to do so, the ONS (as of 20 Jan 2023) had not provided any updates to it since.

8.5. About those estimates of '20 million lives saved' by the vaccine

27 November 2022

A paper [268] published in The Lancet claims the covid vaccines saved 20 million lives in the first year alone. Even without considering the flawed modelling in the paper there is the obviously fundamental problem with their conclusions in that the least vaccinated countries in the world also happened to be the ones that suffered the fewest covid deaths. The authors acknowledge that this compromises their conclusions, but they bizarrely address this by insisting that such countries need to vaccinate more:

> "COVID-19 vaccination has substantially altered the course of the pandemic, saving tens of millions of lives globally. However, inadequate access to vaccines in low-income countries has limited the impact in these settings, reinforcing the need for global vaccine equity and coverage. "

There is also the problem that the study was funded by none other than the WHO; Gavi, the Vaccine Alliance; and the Bill & Melinda Gates Foundation.

How did they get to the 20 million lives saved? They used a flawed model that exaggerated the predicted number of lives lost to covid if there had been no vaccination and simply subtracted the subsequent observed number of lives lost from that as shown in Figure 33. The analogy in Figure 34 shows how ludicrous this type of modelling is.

Unfortunately, the Lancet paper claim is being used to shut down debate about vaccine injuries and deaths. After all, if the 'prestigious' Lancet says the vaccine saved 20 million lives then we have to prove that the vaccine killed at least this number to show that the risks outweigh the benefits.

For example, Iskra Reic, AstraZeneca EVP, shown in the video in this article [269], uses the Lancet study to shut down the debate in the EU Parliament. She also wrote this OpEd [270] on 1 July 2021 demanding everyone in the world be vaccinated as she says "Everyone now recognises no one is safe until we are all safe." She is, of course, listed with the World Economic Forum (WEF).

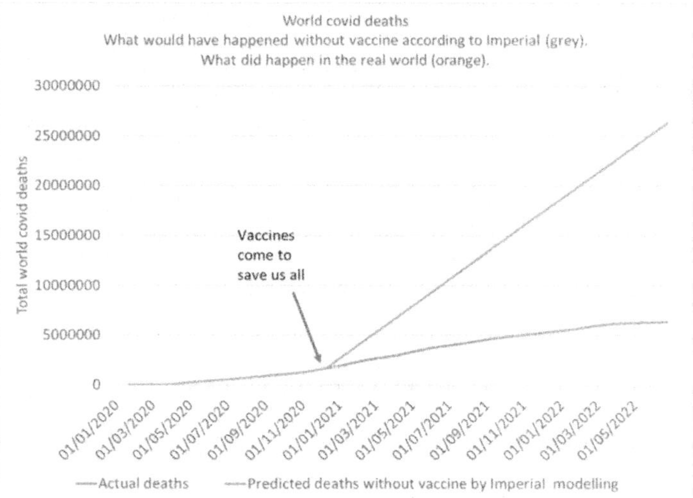

Figure 33 Predicted deaths without vaccines

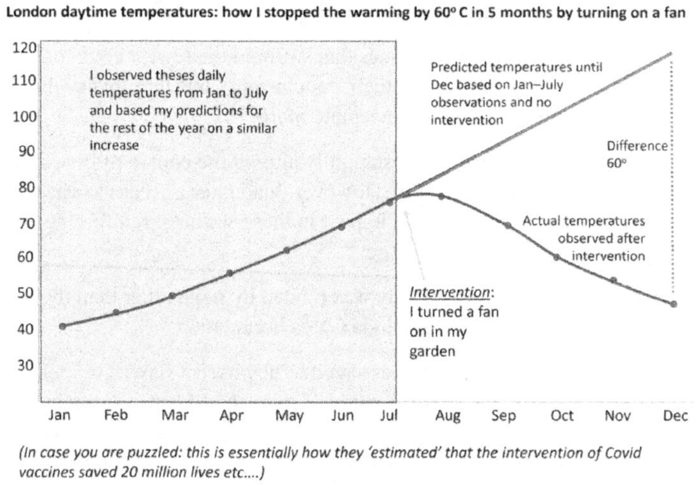

Figure 34 Saving 20 million lives analogy

8.6. A Study in Stupidity

16 December 2022

It's fair to say that people who do no regular exercise are less likely to be involved in an accident in a gym than those who exercise regularly. But we certainly wouldn't conclude that not doing regular exercise is good because it decreases your chances of being injured in a gym.

But that conclusion is essentially no different to the claims made in a study [271] just published (in The American Journal of Medicine) into the link between injuries in car accidents and vaccine status. As this video [272] shows the study is laughably flawed.

The video draws on the observations [273] of the likes of Igor Chudov, Law, Health and Technology [274]: and Clare Craig [275]. One of the problems with the study is that it is almost certain it relies on an estimated proportion of the population who are unvaccinated. And we have shown [276] how important and difficult it is to get an accurate estimate.

8.7. Scientific paper preprint sites censor submissions

17 December 2022

The whole point of research paper preprint sites like medRxiv and arXiv is that they are supposed to enable researchers to publicise their work prior to any formal review process. It used to be the case that, providing the material passed automated checks for plagiarism and offensive language, then it would be published within a couple of days.

But all that changed in the covid era. We have reported many times how all of our covid papers, that in any way challenge the 'official narrative', are now routinely rejected by both medRxiv and arXiv. This censorship of papers that do not toe the party line is now openly stated by medRxiv:

> "Are submissions to medRxiv scrutinized before posting?
>
> All articles are screened on submission for plagiarism, non-scientific content, inappropriate article types, and material that could potentially endanger the health of individual patients or the public. The latter may include, but is not limited to, studies describing dual-use research of concern and works that challenge or could compromise accepted public health measures and advice regarding infectious disease transmission, immunization, and therapy."

By way of our most recent example, we submitted this paper [277] containing a detailed analysis of the latest ONS vaccine mortality surveillance data to medRxiv on 9 November 2022. This is the response we got on 10 November 2022.

> "We regret to inform you that your manuscript is inappropriate for posting. medRxiv is intended for research papers, and our screening process determined that this manuscript fell short of that description."

At the same time (9 November 2022) we submitted the paper to arXiv. As is usual with arXiv we received a reply within hours stating that the paper would be published at 00.00

the next day, but (again as usual) this did not happen, and the paper appeared as 'pending' on the arXiv dashboard. When this happens, we always know it will be rejected by the censors. Often, they never reply at all, and it is left pending forever or is simply removed from the dashboard. However, this time we eventually got this email from arXiv Support on 9 December 2022

> "Thank you for submitting your work to arXiv. We regret to inform you that arXiv's moderators have determined that your submission will not be accepted and made public on [|http://arxiv.org][arXiv.org|http://arxiv.org]. Our moderators have determined that your submission is on a topic not covered by arXiv or that the intended audience for your work is not a community we currently serve."

So, they rejected the paper as being out of scope. Which is curious given the enormous number of papers they have on covid data analytics (including a few of ours before we were writing stuff that challenged 'the narrative'). But what is particularly curious in this case is that just 2 days earlier (7 December 2022) we got the following rejection (after several weeks) for a paper [278] that focused on one particular part of the paper they rejected on 9 December, namely the statistical implications of the different estimates of proportion unvaccinated:

> "Thank you for submitting your work to arXiv. We regret to inform you that arXiv's moderators have determined that your submission will not be accepted and made public on [|http://arxiv.org][arXiv.org|http://arxiv.org]. Our moderators determined that your submission does not contain sufficient original or substantive scholarly research and is not of interest to arXiv."

So, even though both papers addressed the same topic, one was rejected on the basis that it was not sufficiently original, while the other was rejected on the basis it was out of scope.

This activity is a variant on a theme as we reported [279] about Wikipedia, and Norman was interviewed by Bret Weinstein, on the Dark Horse podcast [280] about this experience. Fortunately (for the time being at least), it seems ResearchGate has not been censoring papers on covid and hence we have had no difficulty in putting our papers there.

8.8. How many lives did the Covid-19 vaccines really save?

3 January 2023

Steve Kirsch asked the following question:

> "Based on your analysis, what is the decrease in all-cause mortality from Covid specifically attributable to the vaccines? For an average society like America. So, will it save on average one life per 10,000? One life for 20,000? What would be your best guess? Or did you do absolutely nothing and not saved any lives at all?"

Before we answer we'd like to clarify some ambiguity in the question. All-cause mortality following a vaccine roll-out is the only rational way to assess the efficacy of the vaccine because it tells us whether the benefits of the vaccine outweigh the risks; if all-cause mortality rates are lower in the vaccinated then we can conclude that the vaccine must be saving more people from dying from the disease than it is killing from adverse reactions to it.

Any claims about the vaccine reducing the number of covid deaths are therefore irrelevant in assessing efficacy without considering the overall impact on all-cause mortality. Even if the vaccines really did save 20 million from covid deaths then it would not be effective if it led to more than 20 million deaths from adverse events.

In fact, not only is there now strong evidence of an increase in all-cause mortality among the vaccinated, but we do not believe there is any objective reliable evidence that the covid vaccines saved any PREVENTABLE deaths from Covid-19.

There are nine reasons for coming to this conclusion:

1. No properly conducted randomized trial has provided evidence of any covid deaths avoided

They were never designed [281] to do so. Even if we accept the flawed Pfizer study results of efficacy based on 162 out of 22,000 placebo recipients getting covid compared to only 8 out of 22,000 vaccine recipients not even one of those 162 placebo recipients in the trial who got covid died of covid**.

2. The Pfizer trial actually provides some evidence of increased all-cause mortality in the vaccinated

Although the numbers are too small to be statistically significant, in the 6-month Pfizer follow up [282] there were more all-cause deaths in the vaccine group than the placebo group (15 vs 14 deaths, later 21 vs 17) with just 3 people in total having covid listed as a cause of death (1 in vaccine group, 2 in placebo group). Moreover, the Pfizer trial [283] exhibited a 36 % higher risk of serious adverse events in the vaccine group.

3. Anecdotal evidence: Our own experience shows the vaccines are neither effective nor safe

Since the vaccination programme started, we have observed that it is our vaccinated friends and colleagues who are almost exclusively getting ill from covid. And it is also the vaccinated who we see dying unexpectedly. This anecdotal evidence [284] of increased all-cause mortality in the vaccinated is backed up by the only independent survey evidence attempting to determine the difference in all-cause mortality.

4. Official government statistics claiming vaccines reduce covid mortality cannot be trusted

The gatekeepers of such data have a major vested interest in claiming success of the vaccine programme. They therefore do not allow access to the raw data and frequently manipulate the data [285]. Moreover, these data are compromised by the flawed definition of what constitutes a covid death ('anybody dying of any cause within 28 days of a positive PCR test') and defining a person getting covid within

14 days of vaccination as 'unvaccinated' (here [286] & here [287]). These various corrupt definition and data integrity problems all create bias in favour of vaccine efficacy and are also evident in all observational studies claiming vaccines reduce covid mortality.

5. Official government statistics claiming vaccines reduce all-cause mortality are demonstrably flawed

In addition to all the definition and data integrity problems, official data (for example from the UK's office for National Statistics, here [288], are further compromised in that 1) many deaths shortly after vaccination are misclassified as unvaccinated and 2) grossly underestimate the population proportion of unvaccinated, which inflates the true mortality rate of the unvaccinated (here [289]). When adjusted for these biases, the data show that since the start of 2022, all-cause mortality in the ever-vaccinated is higher than the never vaccinated in all-age groups (here [290]).

6. Artificially inflated covid death numbers

Many deaths classified as covid deaths were not caused by covid, and many of those that were could have been prevented if demonstrably successful alternative early protocol treatments were provided. Moreover, many covid deaths may ultimately have been caused by denial of antibiotics to treat the resulting bacterial pneumonia that was the ultimate cause of death (here [291] and here [292]).

7. National comparisons suggest the vaccines do not reduce covid mortality

Even with the built-in biases relating to the definition of covid death and vaccination classification, those regions of the world with the lowest vaccination rates also have the lowest covid mortality rates (there are 906 times more covid deaths in most vs least vaccinated countries). These differences cannot be explained by inherent population differences (such as countries with younger populations being less at risk from covid death).

8. The claims that millions of covid deaths were prevented by the vaccines are based on flawed models and/or assumptions

Specifically, they were either based on models that subtract the actual number of covid classified deaths since the start of the vaccination programme from the number predicted to die, assuming there was no vaccination programme, and the mortality rate would simply increase nevertheless; or based on the flawed assumption that the vaccines were 95% effective at stopping infection.

9. Independent evidence points to an increase in all-cause mortality among the vaccinated

It is because of the inherent problems with the definition of 'a covid death' that we have always argued that vaccine safety and efficacy can only reliably be assessed by all-cause mortality. If covid is as deadly as claimed and if the vaccines are as safe and effective as claimed by their proponents, then we should be seeing higher all-cause mortality in the unvaccinated. But increasingly we see evidence to the contrary (here [293]). In all the heavily vaccinated countries we should have seen lower all-cause mortality in the period since mid-2021 (by which time the majority of the population was vaccinated in these countries) than the main covid period Feb 2020 to mid-2021. But what we have seen is the opposite; almost all such countries are now showing consistent and significant increases in excess deaths. Vaccine proponents have tried to explain this mainly by the effects of lockdowns and 'long covid', but publicly available data (even with all its in-build biases in favour of the vaccine safe and effective narrative) shows the vaccines as the most plausible explanation for the increases (here [294]).

8.9. The CDC's data on covid vaccine safety signals

4 January 2023

Compared to all previous non-covid vaccines there are many worrying signals in the Pfizer and Moderna vaccines.

A standard way to determine whether there is a genuine concern that a new vaccine may be causing a particular type of serious adverse event (SAE), such as 'myocarditis', is to compare the proportion of adverse event reports associated with the new vaccine that include myocarditis with the proportion that include myocarditis in other vaccines.

For example, suppose hypothetically that in Vaccine Adverse Event Reporting System (VAERS):

- For the new vaccine there are 1000 reports of SAEs of which 300 include myocarditis.
- For all other vaccines there are 2000 reports of SAEs of which 100 include myocarditis.

Then 30% of the reports for the new vaccine include myocarditis compared to just 5% for all other vaccines. This is used to calculate the proportional reporting ratio (PRR) which is simply 30% divided by 5% in this case, and here the PRR is equal to 6 for a myocarditis SAE. The fact that there is a much greater proportion of myocarditis events in the new vaccine compared to previous vaccines should be concerning.

To be considered a potential 'safety signal' by the Centers for Disease Control and Prevention (CDC), the PRR must be at least 2 and must also have a chi-square test statistic value of at least 4. The chi-square test statistic is a classical statistical test of significance that takes account of the total number of events and reports.

In our hypothetical example the chi-square is 361 which is highly significant; but if, say we divide the values in the example by 100 (so 3 out of 10 compared for the new vaccine and 1 out of 20 for all other vaccines), then although the PRR is still 6, the chi-square value is just 1.9 which would not be significant under the CDC's rule.

The CDC conducted a PRR analysis of adverse events reported in the VAERS system for the Pfizer and Moderna covid vaccines for the period Dec. 14, 2020, to July 29, 2022. For each different type of adverse event reported, the CDC calculated the PRR of every SAE for each of the two covid vaccines against all other non-covid vaccines. They also computed the PRR of every SAE for Pfizer against Moderna.

Zachary Stieber of the Epoch Times obtained the results of the CDC analysis through a Freedom of Information Act request after the CDC refused to make the results public. Zach sent the spreadsheets with the results to Norman and colleague Josh Guetzkow asking for comments. Zach has now published his article on this - with links to all the data - including some of the comments that Josh and I provided. The article [296] is also published on the CHD website. Josh has also now published his own extensive article [297].

For completeness, here is the full list of comments we made to Zack (these were made these after seeing Josh's comments and so are in addition to what he had already covered):

- Since these PRRs are just the ratio of the proportions what it means of course is that all that it is 'measuring' is the extent to which there are different categories of SAEs between the covid vaccines and other vaccines. There must therefore be a whole bunch of SAE categories not listed here for which the PRR > 2 for the non-covid vaccines (meaning the non-covid vaccines are relatively more dangerous with respect to those SAEs).

- Now while it is still important to determine the extent to which specific SAEs are much more prevalent in the covid vaccines, ultimately what matters most is simply the overall proportion of reports that are classified as serious.

    - For the 18+ age group the proportions are: 11.1% for the covid vaccines (73,178 out of 660,643) compared to 5.5% for non-covid vaccines (13,287 out of 242,091). That is a very important signal especially as this age group is where the vast majority of reports are. It is a highly significant difference. Therefore, if the CDC wish to claim that the probability of SAEs with the covid vaccines is not significantly higher than that of other vaccines the onus is on them to provide an alternative causal explanation for this difference.

    - For the 12-17 age group: 6% for covid (1,893 out of 31,447) compared to 5.3% for no-covid (1,598 out of 30,084). This is a statistically significant difference.

    - For the 5-11 age group: 2.6% for covid (319 out of 12,329) compared to 3.8% for non-covid (1,111 out of 27,960) (surprising as this too is a significant difference in the opposite direction).

- Of course, we must also compare the total numbers of SAEs reported. The total number of SAE reports for the Pfizer and Moderna covid vaccines in just 19 months (73,178) is over five times the total number of SAE reports for all other non-covid vaccines (13,278) in 163 months (since 1 Jan 2009).

- Another incredibly important statistic is the proportion of deaths (which is only given for the 18+ age group) which is 14% in the covid vaccines (10,169 out of

73,178) compared to just 4.7% (618 out of 13,278) in non-covid vaccines. If the CDC wish to claim that the probability a covid vaccine adverse event results in death is not significantly higher than that of other vaccines the onus is on them to come up with some other causal explanation for this difference.

- Note that there are many instances of differently named SAEs that really should be merged because they might be obfuscating the scale of some of the problems. For example, in the serious 18+ age group worksheet we have separately: cardiac failure acute, cardiac failure, infarction, myocardial strain, myocardial fibrosis – but not simply 'myocarditis'. These are not mutually exclusive categories and spreading the same condition between categories obviously reduces the frequency counts per category, resulting in an underpowered chi-square test and a reduced chance of triggering a significant PRR under the CDC's rule.

- Likewise, 'myocarditis' does not appear in the 18+ age group serious worksheet but it is in the serious 12-17 age group worksheet where it is the most serious after 'chest pain' (ignoring the covid specific material and generic stuff like 'intensive care'). Presumably, in the older age group cases of myocarditis are simply subsumed within the other cardiac failure SAEs.

Josh commented on this:

> "Keep in mind though that if a certain type of SAE was reported less than 3 times for all other vaccines, it will not show up as a safety signal here even if it was reported a million times. So it could be that there are many other cardiac failure AEs for 12–17-year-olds that simply don't show up because they were never reported in the past. It's a huge blind spot with this method."

- In the 18+ age group, non-serious AE, worksheet there are two categories "Menstruation irregular" and "Heavy Menstrual bleeding" both with a lot of cases and high PRR. Presumably these should have been merged (as there may be some overlap between them) but the key question is why these are not included at all in the serious categories? On a related note, since neither still birth nor miscarriage appear anywhere here does this mean they did not meet the threshold of N>=3, PRR>2 and chi-squared>4?

Josh commented on this:

> "Yes, I agree about merging. There are other menstrual categories as well. Assuming there are few or no serious issues with the women reporting menstrual issues, then there is no reason it would show up in the serious reports (see definition in my previous e-mail as to what counts as a serious report). Regarding miscarriages (aka spontaneous abortions), yes that is my inference. I am assuming they did this for every AE/PT that had been coded from the reports, but we don't know for sure because we don't actually know what methodology they used."

- For most of the SAEs considered the chi-squared is so high that, from a Bayesian perspective, the probability that the true rate of the SAE of the covid vaccines is not higher than that of the non-covid vaccines is essentially zero. So, it is up to the regulators to come up with some other causal explanation for the difference if they wish to claim the probability of any of these SAE's is not increased with the covid vaccines.

- Regarding the difference between Moderna and Pfizer: By far the most important difference is in the overall proportions of serious cases: for Moderna the proportion is 9.6% (33,003 out of 342,456) compared to 12.6% for Pfizer (40,193 out of 318,346). This is a highly significant difference that cannot be ignored (in fact, if you remove the many serious AEs that are specifically connected with injection site – for which Moderna has overwhelmingly more than Pfizer - then difference would be much greater still). So again, the onus is on the regulators to come up with some other causal explanation for the difference if they wish to claim the probability of a serious AE with Pfizer is not significantly higher than that of Moderna. Ideally, we would also like to compare these with all previous vaccines.

- The only other really interesting difference between Moderna and Pfizer is – as mentioned above - that there is a significantly higher rate of injection site SAEs with Moderna.

We do not believe that the PRR is an ideal method for finding safety signals because it only identifies significantly new, different or unexpected SAEs compared to other vaccines and does not consider underlying population rates for the SAE conditions. However, there are so many red flags for the two covid vaccines the CDC analysed that they should reconsider their decision not to halt further roll-out of these vaccines until these SAEs are more thoroughly investigated.

Chapter 9. The Iatrogenesis Hypothesis

9.1. The deadly spring 2020 Covid-19 wave

14 February 2023

It has long been hypothesised that deadly health policies were a major factor in the wave of deaths attributed to covid in the Spring of 2020. This is also referred to as the iatrogenesis hypothesis.

Dr. Jonathan Engler looked at what had happened in Lombardy [298] Italy and concluded that:

> "many of the deaths which occurred in the aftermath of the cataclysmic changes to the delivery of healthcare — especially of the frail and elderly — might have been caused by policy, rather than virus."

With regard to the spread of SARS-CoV-2 virus he says (using the chart shown in Figure 35 to support his statement):

> "A virus doesn't spread across thousands of kilometres within days and peaks at the same time."

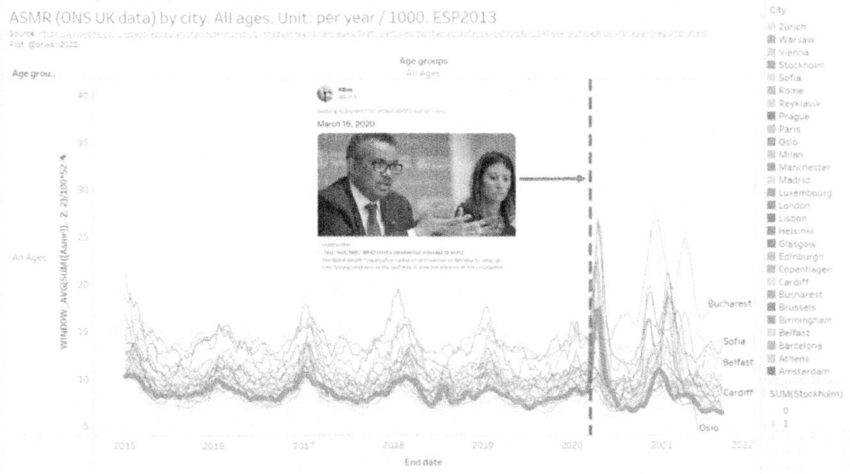

Figure 35 Age standardised mortality per year

Anna Farrow made a similar convincing case that this happened in Canada [299] while @NellyTells reports it was happening in Spain [300]. This especially revealing account is from South Carolina [301].

Likewise, there has been a long-term concern that excessive use of Midazolam was a contributing factor in the UK and the Daily Mail [302] newspaper reported on it as long ago as July 2020.

9.1.1. NG163 Death protocol

More detailed evidence to support the iatrogenesis hypothesis for the UK (and elsewhere) has been provided in twitter threads by Jikkyleaks and this recent thread [303] is particularly revealing.

The most damning evidence can be found in the NICE Rapid Guideline (NG163) [304] (published 3 April 2020) that has since been deleted. However, it can be found via the wayback machine here [305]. Jikkyleaks refers to this document as the "death protocol":

In particular, Section 6.5 of NG163 seems to support Jikkyleaks' claim that, while many elderly Covid-19 patients only needed three antibiotic tablets and standard post-viral pneumonia care, UK GPs were instead "told to euthanise them - care of @NICEComms".

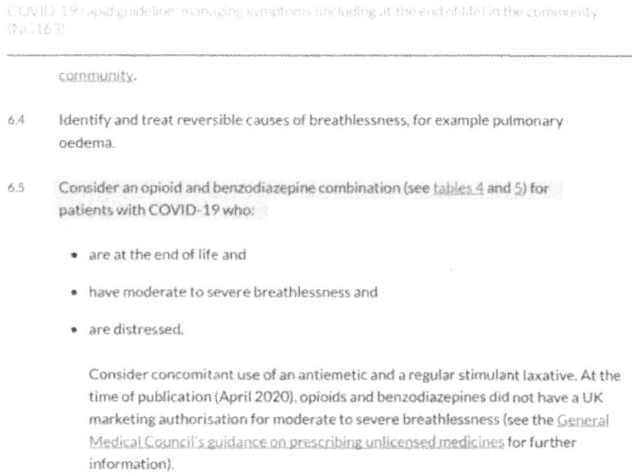

COVID-19 rapid guideline: managing symptoms (including at the end of life) in the community (NG163)

community.

6.4 Identify and treat reversible causes of breathlessness, for example pulmonary oedema.

6.5 Consider an opioid and benzodiazepine combination (see tables 4 and 5) for patients with COVID-19 who:

- are at the end of life and
- have moderate to severe breathlessness and
- are distressed.

Consider concomitant use of an antiemetic and a regular stimulant laxative. At the time of publication (April 2020), opioids and benzodiazepines did not have a UK marketing authorisation for moderate to severe breathlessness (see the General Medical Council's guidance on prescribing unlicensed medicines for further information).

Figure 36 NG163 death protocol

In 20 April 2020 in reaction to NG163 a rapid response letter [306] was sent by eminent experts in palliative care warning of the dangers of administering treatment more appropriate for end-of-life care to Covid-19 patients.

> "We are concerned that uncritical use of NG163 may create unintended risks for people with suspected or actual COVID-19 infection.
>
> The combination of opioid, benzodiazepine and/or neuroleptic is used in specialist palliative care settings for symptom control and for 'palliative sedation' to reduce agitation at the end of life. It takes great skill and experience to use palliative sedation proportionately so that extreme physical and existential distress are palliated, but death is not primarily accelerated. NG163 states: "Sedation and opioid use should not be withheld because of a fear of causing respiratory depression." If COVID-19 infection were uniformly fatal, this would be an acceptable statement.

But for people not previously known to be at the end of life, there is potential risk of unintended serious harm, if these medications are used incorrectly and without the benefit of specialist palliative care advice.

Another concern is that the recommended doses for morphine and midazolam are sometimes higher than current guidelines state for non-specialist use; and moreover there are inconsistencies between the maximum doses recommended by the oral or subcutaneous routes."

The role the UK Health Secretary, Matt Hancock (dubbed #MidazolamMatt), played in this has been very well documented [307] by @chrislittlewoo8.

This chilling video A Good Death? [308] by Jacqui Deevoy interviews family of those deceased in the UK and exposes the DNR scandal back in December 2021.

The fact that NICE deleted the guidelines - and that it can only be found with difficulty on the wayback machine is revealing.

9.1.2. Linking opioids to excess mortality

Figure 37 show the very close correlation between the Midazolam doses and excess mortality rate as reported by USMortality [309] in this tweet [310].

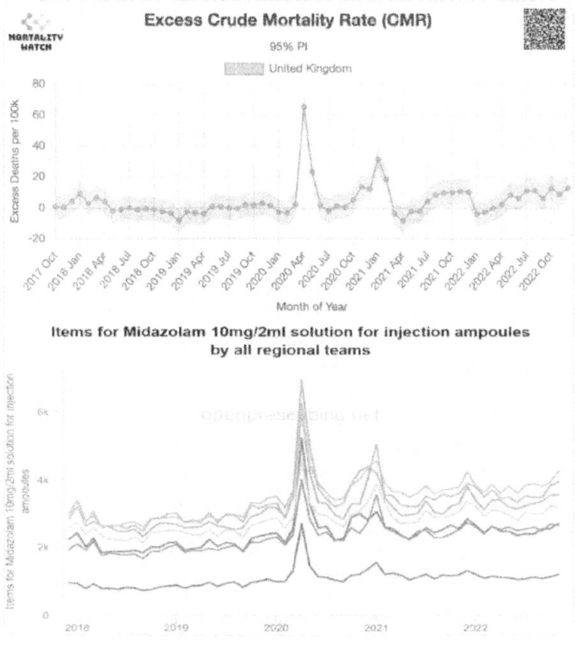

Figure 37 Midazolam and excess mortality

9.2. Covid-19 deaths exaggerated by re-attribution.

Figure 38 shows negative excess non-Covid respiratory deaths prepared by Joel Smalley suggesting many Covid-19 deaths were simply incidental because we were missing deaths from other causes. When Covid-19 deaths started falling those deaths started to reappear.

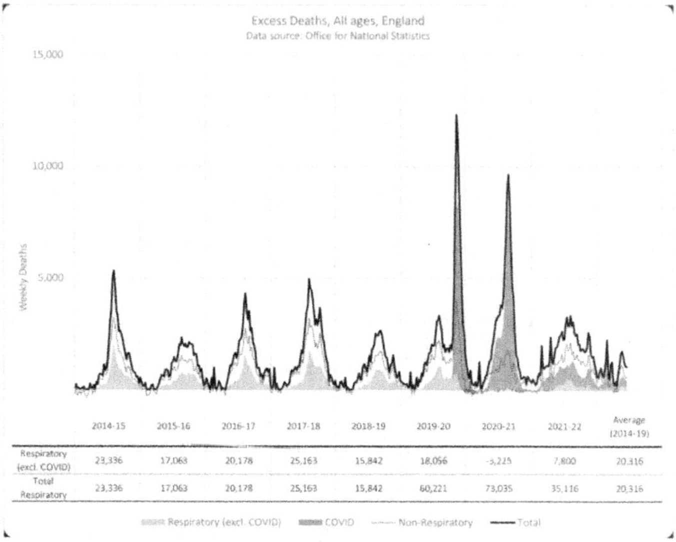

	2014-15	2015-16	2016-17	2017-18	2018-19	2019-20	2020-21	2021-22	Average (2014-19)
Respiratory (excl. COVID)	23,336	17,063	20,178	25,163	15,842	18,056	-3,225	7,800	20,316
Total Respiratory	23,336	17,063	20,178	25,163	15,842	60,221	73,035	35,116	20,316

Figure 38 Covid-19 deaths replacing other non-covid causes of death and deaths typically caused by other respiratory conditions

9.3. What really caused the surge in Covid-19 deaths in early 2020?

February 2023

Will Jones has published an interesting article [311] in the Daily Sceptic that strongly challenges the iatrogenesis hypothesis. This is the hypothesis that deadly health policies were a major factor in the wave of deaths attributed to Covid-19 in the Spring of 2020.

Jones's article provides some interesting data. We believe he is correct that there ***is*** something special about SARS-CoV-2 and that there is no evidence that non pharmaceutical interventions (NPIs) like lockdowns and contact tracing had any significant impact on death rates. However, contrary to what he asserts, neither of these invalidates the iatrogenesis hypothesis, and nor does his argument that Germany and Sweden (who he says had similar health policies to the UK, USA and Italy) did not get excess deaths at the same time. The case for the iatrogenesis hypothesis in the UK (and probably also USA and Italy) is not just the incorrect use of ventilators (which was common across all these countries) but specifically the inappropriate use of life-ending drugs and denial of potentially life-saving antibiotics, as well as "softer" issues such as denial of social care, relative visits and the social network which acts as the life-support system for the frail elderly.

Also, note that "lockdown stringency" does not necessarily reflect the level of dystopia within the health and social care system, specifically of the elderly; in terms of the early deaths, and hence the imputed case fatality rates, it is to this demographic we must look. Whether schools closed in March/April 2020 or whether football matches were banned and so on, has little to no bearing on elderly care.

Critically, Will also presents a set of graphs, Figure 39, that he believes destroys Engler's arguments. But, contrary to his assertions, these graphs may support the iatrogenesis hypothesis. Specifically, Will presents a set of graphs (Covid-19 hospitalisations, deaths etc) that he claims all follow the same pattern:

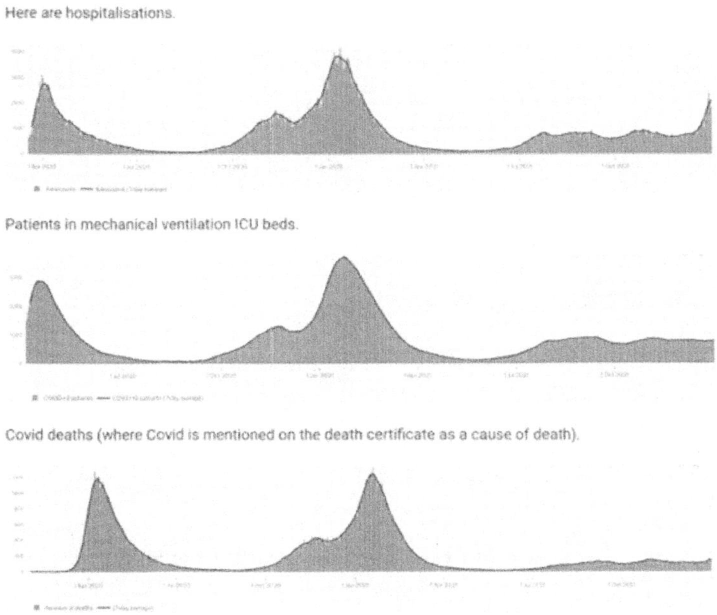

Figure 39 UK Covid-19 hospitalisations, ICU admissions and deaths

He includes, in Figure 40, the excess deaths (as reported from the Our World in Data website) and he concludes:

> "The close correspondence between these graphs is I'm sure obvious to anyone. The significance of that correspondence is that these are all showing different aspects of the same phenomenon, namely a viral outbreak that is causing a closely correlated rise in symptoms, PCR positives, LFT positives, variant genome detection, hospitalisations, ICU admissions, antibodies and deaths. No other cause for this multifactorial phenomenon is plausible. Thus, we must conclude that excess deaths during the pandemic are to a large extent explained by the effects of the virus that is causing all these things."

But there are two obvious problems with this conclusion. The first is that the excess mortality graph is *not* like the others. There is clearly a much higher (and, because of its extreme and vertical nature, a very unnatural) peak at the start of the pandemic than appears in the other graphs. This peak supports Jonathan Engler's hypothesis. The second problem (which is one we have pointed out many times) is that the data showing Covid-19 cases, hospitalisations and deaths etc from the Government's Covid-19 dashboard are completely inconsistent with the NHS dashboard [312] of Covid-19 emergency triage calls, as shown in Figure 41 (this dashboard was withdrawn in July 2022).

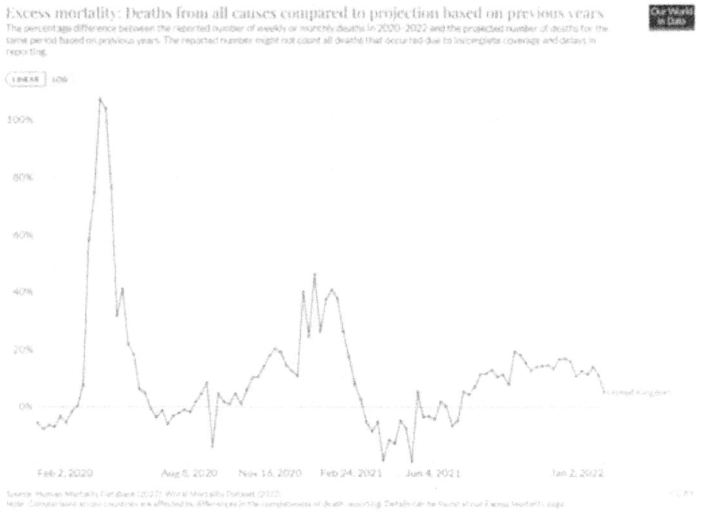

Figure 40 Excess mortality deaths from all causes

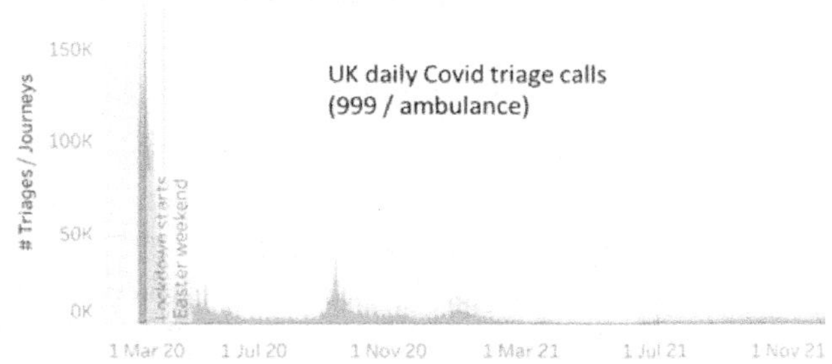

Figure 41 UK daily Covid-19 triage calls

This analysis [313] carried out by Joel Smally where he also concluded the pandemic was faked, where he said:

> "It would seem that there was only a COVID-19 pandemic in countries that were rich enough for their government's ill-conceived interventions to have a material impact on mortality and to shun the cheapest, safest and most widely available early treatments.
>
> Every single policy not only failed to mitigate death from the virus but evidently made the situation worse. All social distancing policies, zealous testing and, worst of all, the subjection of populations to participate in a mass medical experiment without proper consent, resulted in *increased* mortality.
>
> Is it only with the benefit of hindsight that we now know this? Absolutely not. The evidence was clear within weeks of every intervention, hampered only by the untimely provision of the necessary data by the public "authorities" and the illegitimate censorship of "misinformation" by the mainstream media."

9.4. In defence of alternative explanations for excess deaths

Other than a novel deadly virus spreading from Wuhan (1 March 2023)

The central thesis advanced in the Will Jones article [314] discussed in the previous section is that "the main thing driving excess deaths over the last three years... is the new SARS-like virus....".

We are hereinafter referring to this as "the default hypothesis" because it has somehow become widely accepted, though we would argue that this owes more to promulgation of state-sponsored propaganda than to rational analysis.

We believe that an alternative hypothesis—that excess deaths were primarily driven by changes to healthcare and other policies—cannot and should not be dismissed by 'sceptics'.

Overall, the central criticism of our alternative hypothesis appears to be founded in the following reformulation of the core message of the article: "we all know that it's the spreading virus which has driven excess deaths, and it might be reputationally harmful to the sceptical movement to challenge it".

Forgive us if we ignore such an exhortation. It is somewhat ironic that the statement "we all know that" expounds the overconfidence that has got the world into the mess it is now in. Likewise, the explicit call for consensus is paying an excessive heed to the risk of reputational harm to the 'movement', when sceptics should be speaking out against unwarranted assumptions and claims, whatever the sources. After all, we seek the same thing: truth.

Jones' article suggests that it is a given that excess deaths are caused by the novel virus, and that this must be the default assumption. Furthermore, the article implies that for any alternative hypothesis to displace this default explanation it must be unassailable in all its aspects, and that even a single apparent inconsistency demolishes it. This is rhetorical favoritism and assumes falsification is a one-way street.

Notwithstanding that this is not actually how scientific enquiry ought to be conducted, it belies the substantial holes in the hypothesis he advocates. Some of these holes in the

'Covid-19 is novel and deadly' hypothesis are helpfully revisited by Jones in an article [315] published a few days later, which can be summarized thus:

> "Look, I know there are all those anomalies in the default hypothesis which cannot be explained, but these do not have to be explained because this is what we all know actually happened."

We and a growing number of others [316] are perplexed at the official, default narrative (in relation to the main cause of deaths). We believe that the many and varied possible factors contributing to excess deaths, from 2020 onwards, should be subject to continued forensic examination. This viewpoint has emerged as a consequence of the fact that we regard Jones' default hypothesis of events as implausible.

To summarize, the default hypothesis (and to be fair it does not belong to Jones given that it is shared by many "thought leaders" on both sides of the Covid-19 debate), is that a deadly and novel virus spread from Wuhan for a few months before the start of 2020, and then spread throughout the globe. It then transformed itself in different places, sometimes continents or countries apart, and each outbreak occurred, with synchronicity, in early spring 2020. In all of these geographically separate locations plague-like vertiginous spikes in death rates manifested, with an intensity and duration that had never before seen before with any respiratory virus. Additionally, this only happened in particular locations in Spring 2020, the most important in relation to the global propagation of the "pandemic narrative" outside of China being Lombardy, Italy, and New York. It only lasted a few weeks, leaving neighbouring locations almost completely untouched. After this novel outbreak pattern, the virus returned in late 2020 and beyond, taking forms inconsistent with this initial outbreak.

What happened in Bergamo, other parts of Lombardy and parts of New York City in March and April 2020 was quite extraordinary and, critically, played a crucial role in moulding the pandemic response in the highly influential United Kingdom, and then globally. As described here [317], in Bergamo deaths increased 8-10 fold in some areas. Similar carnage was seen in New York [318]. Sudden sharp spikes in deaths, which also happened to coincide with the institution of special measures, and the fomenting of panic and fear, were observed. It is impossible to overstate the unusual nature of these peaks. Excess deaths of 800 to 1000% have never been seen before with a respiratory virus and are totally incompatible with the qualities of a "novel" coronavirus which is supposed to have been quietly spreading for many months beforehand.

Figure 42 shows percentage excess deaths in Bergamo since 2014 reveals the extraordinary nature of what happened.

In the French heatwave of 2003 [319] a mere 80% increase in deaths for a short period was regarded as a national scandal, having been shown to be caused largely by neglect of the elderly and a lack of basic care. This illustrates (1) how completely off-the-scale an 800-1000% increase is and (2) that short-term changes in basic care provision have the potential to cause dramatic spikes in deaths.

As can be seen from Figure 43, the worst winter flu seasons saw excess death rates spike at only around 20% in France, making the 80% spike from the August 2003 heatwave stand out starkly.

Yet in percentage terms, the excess death spikes in Lombardy in March 2020 reached levels 10 times those seen in this heatwave, and 50 times those generally seen in the French winter flu season. Likewise, events in New York City in Spring 2020 also look extraordinary, as shown in Figure 44.

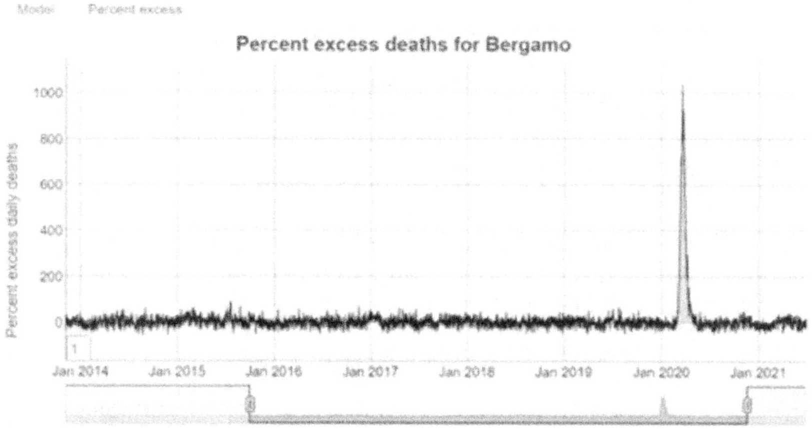

Figure 42 Percentage excess deaths Bergamo, Italy

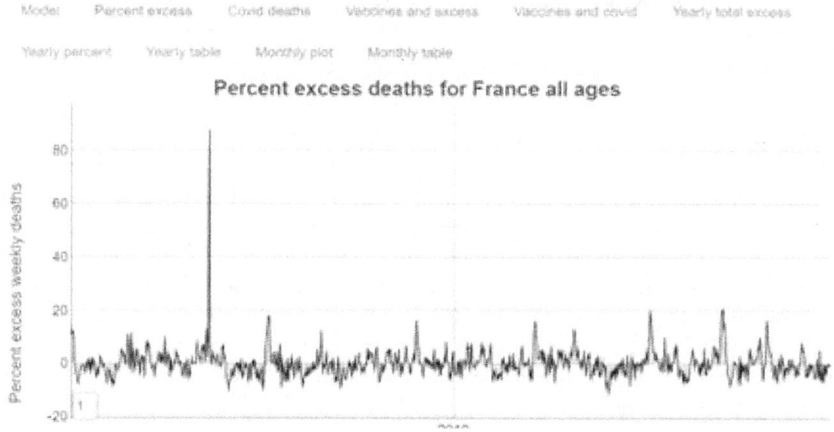

Figure 43 Percentage excess deaths, France

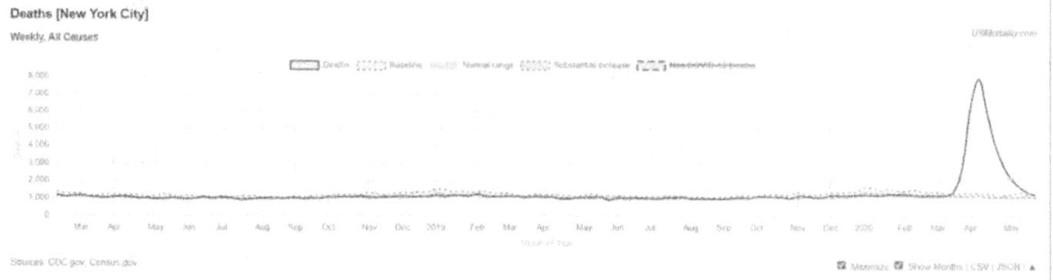

Figure 44 Deaths New York City

Raw weekly death counts in NYC are generally around 1000-1100 and show remarkable stability. In week 15 of 2020, 7,862 people died—an increase in excess of 700% over an average week, not dissimilar to that seen in Bergamo. Put differently, week 15 in April 2020 saw the equivalent of around 7 weeks of average mortality.

It is now generally accepted that whatever "the virus" is, it had an infection fatality rate (IFR) in the same ballpark as a bad flu season [320]. Even this is likely overstated as (1) the denominator underestimates community spread (2) the numerator will include many inappropriately treated people, as well as deaths misattributed to Covid-19.

So, in terms of pathogenicity, it wasn't particularly distinctive compared to other respiratory viruses we regularly see, and indeed, as Jones admits, the evidence for global prior spread months before the emergency is difficult to counter. Yet, consistent with such a low IFR, this prior spread saw zero noticeable excess deaths, although clearly some over-attribution started a few weeks before the emergency, as several places were recording covid-related cases, at low levels, without noticeable excess deaths. Jones seems to think that the finding of *any* excess death prior to lockdown is a "gotcha", falsifying the alternative hypothesis. However, this logic assumes that none of the fear and panic building in society and reported by the media is capable of inducing dysfunction in health or social care provision. We say that this dysfunction is a plausible explanation for at least some additional mortality before the governments formalized their response into legal restrictions or official policy.

One of the central planks of the default hypothesis is that there is no relationship between policy interventions and mortality. However, this shows a misunderstanding of the alternative hypothesis. Under the alternative hypothesis it is necessary to examine policy and care within the at-risk demographic in which almost all deaths occurred—the elderly and otherwise frail. And, when looking at explanations for mortality within this population, it is far more important to look at how they were treated compared to the wider population. Lockdown measures such as closing schools, parks, gyms, preventing indoor dining and so on may have correlated with the degree of mistreatment of the elderly, but not necessarily so, and those measures in and of themselves would not have been sufficient to contribute to the magnitude and pattern of mortality in Spring 2020.

Jones attaches some importance to the furin cleavage site (FCS) in support of the unusual nature of the virus, stating that "this essentially makes it like SARS-1 but with aerosol transmission, and so far, more transmissible". We are not aware of any evidence that it is the FCS itself which makes the virus aerosolized (and were in any case under the impression that SARS-1 was generally assumed to be aerosolized [321]). Aerosolized transmission appears to be a property shared by mucosal respiratory viruses in general, which includes SARS-1 and other coronaviruses and influenza. Droplet and fomite transmission was always an outlier hypothesis. Moreover, to explain the extent of the mortality spikes observed, the default hypothesis requires that the virus is able to spread between people at rates that have never been seen before, that it acquires this remarkable ability suddenly when it didn't have it before, then loses it again within a few weeks, and finally, it does so independently and near-synchronously at locations thousands of miles apart. However, if Jones is claiming (as he seems to be) that this property is a result of the FCS, nobody has argued that the FCS is something which came and went in this fashion in early 2020.

Furthermore, if the FCS enables entry into cells (as has been assumed by those who purport to understand such things), then it surely ought to be more virulent than SARS-1, as it presumably allows for faster spread within the airways themselves. Again, if this is the case, how did such a novel and deadly virus spread so far and wide and over months globally without being noticed before?

Clare Craig has argued (see here [322] and here [323]) that the surges occur not because of the virus per se, but because of a dramatic change in susceptibility to the virus—a so-called "seasonal trigger". It is true that host susceptibility to respiratory viruses is poorly understood, but there are many examples of neighbouring locations that experienced vastly differing mortality outcomes despite sharing the same climate. So, either the virus surge was highly geographically selective (unlikely), or another hypothesis explains the variation in outcomes and the excess death spikes.

In his second article [315], Jones attempts to explain "why, if it was in countries all round the world that winter, the explosive outbreaks only began in February and March 2020". This is, of course, the very question we are asking. He says that "this is because the virus's journey from first emergence in autumn 2019 to explosive outbreaks in early 2020 occurred in a slower and more staggered way than we might expect from a simple understanding of viruses. This is not because the virus wasn't present in countries prior to causing explosive outbreaks there—that's the simplistic assumption that is contradicted by the data—but because the virus doesn't always cause explosive outbreaks when it is present."

This appears to be a mere restatement, without explanation, of the core problem in his thesis—the implausibility in the way in which the qualities necessary to explain the mortality spikes appear to come and go. He gives the impression of thinking there must be a single explanation (the virus) for all observed outcomes, if only people would look hard enough to find that explanation (the virus). This assertion that absence of evidence is not evidence of absence cannot be falsified but given it can be applied to any causal assertion it fails to discriminate between plausible and implausible explanations.

Instead, we look to Occam's razor when evaluating whether the evidence at hand supports one hypothesis over others. All other things being equal, the simplest hypothesis with the fewest parameters that are consistent with the evidence should be preferred.

Whilst we accept that there are also unanswered questions in the alternative hypothesis, we would argue that it is more consistent with Occam's razor. The default hypothesis involves a myriad of assumptions about dramatic changes in viral behaviour in terms of pathogenicity and transmissibility that have never been seen before in any respiratory viral outbreak, and rests on new, unevidenced, assumptions about the way viruses evolve.

Viruses and society exist in a kind of adaptive symbiosis, and one affects the other via complex and poorly understood interactions that evolve over time. Thus, when a viral infection spreads through a population, which itself responds by suddenly and radically adapting its behaviour, the effects of the virus become difficult to extricate from the effects of the societal response. However, if there is little evidence of viral pathogenicity before the behavioural change in the society, one must consider the possibility that at least some of the subsequent morbidity is attributable to those changed behaviours.

In respect of the alternative hypothesis, it is obvious that the resources provided for, and the management of health and social care services differ significantly geographically, as do the underlying political and societal structures controlling them. Hence, the way each society or location responds to change will differ. There are also historical precedents for such changes, especially if precipitous, to be extremely harmful, and that some societies may be more vulnerable to such changes than others. So, it is not a huge stretch to conclude that it is possible that observed variation in outcomes is explained by variations in societal responses.

There are, in fact, numerous examples of responses that undoubtedly had the potential to elevate mortality. The list includes: medical staff absences while "testing positive", postponement of surgery and treatments, blanket do not resuscitate (DNR) orders, policies restricting the use of antibiotics, the emptying out of ICUs, the effects of fear on citizens' health directly or on the way in which healthcare workers responded, relocation of frail elderly patients and the substitution of normal care pathways with end-of-life treatments.

It must be emphasized that such policies will have adversely affected the outcome of both non-covid and Covid-19 patients. In respect of the latter, even those classified as ill with Covid-19 symptoms (i.e. respiratory) would have been affected. This is contrary to an assumption implied by the default hypothesis—that just because someone dies "from Covid-19" their death was somehow unavoidable. The evidence of inappropriate treatment suggests otherwise.

Jones has implied [324] that attributing all excess deaths to this societal response is an ABC ("Anything But Covid-19") position. But this mischaracterizes the alternative hypothesis as one that claims that coronavirus infections do not lead to any deaths. The argument being made does not hinge on explaining individual deaths. Rather, it revolves around explaining societal mortality in excess of that typically reported. Coronaviruses have long been implicated as a cause of cases of severe respiratory illness that leads to deaths (in the frail) prior to 2020, even though routine testing for them was not previously performed. Hence these deaths were rarely directly attributed to these viral infections. The common cold might be the ultimate cause of death in a frail elderly person dying of cancer or heart disease, but this would not be recorded as the primary cause of death. There is no reason to assume that coronaviruses ceased to be so potentially lethal for certain vulnerable people in Spring 2020.

Moreover, given that the number of people diagnosed with Covid-19 was substantially bolstered by over-attribution, via false positive Covid-19 tests and changes in death certification, it is plausible that a coronavirus was being misattributed as the direct cause of deaths when it was not.

It must be made clear that amongst the many things that we and other sceptics are *not* saying are that "viruses don't exist", "nobody has ever isolated this virus" or that "coronaviruses including SARS-CoV-2 don't ever kill people". We are also not making any comments here about the Covid-19 vaccines. In fact, our commentary is restricted to consideration of the events in early 2020 and no later. It is only by examining what happened when the emergency was imposed on a previously stable societal situation that reliable conclusions can be drawn about the matter at hand. Later, prolonged healthcare disruptions, vaccinations, "variants" and reïnfections (inter alia) dramatically complicate the picture, such that, whilst those periods are obviously important, they cannot provide much information about the origin of the pandemic narrative.

What we are imploring people to consider is this: given that the events of Spring 2020 which occurred in a few key geographically separate locations informed the extremely harmful global response, is the default narrative and hypothesis plausible, or should alternative hypotheses be tested?

If Jones accepts (as he surely must) that there has been:

> (1) some inappropriate treatment of persons considered (rightly or wrongly) to be "Covid-19 patients", and that this caused some deaths which would not otherwise have happened; and
>
> (2) some additional mortality consequent to policies affecting the health of individuals including their healthcare, but not regarded as "involving Covid-19"

... then it must surely also be accepted that at least some of the excess deaths observed would not have happened but for these factors.

Critically however, since we do not yet know what the quantum of these effects is, how can it be ruled out that together they account for all or nearly all of any excess deaths observed?

In conclusion, we should make it clear that we are not here taking Jones' approach in insisting that we must be correct–to do so would be unscientific. Rather, we are asserting that there are sufficient holes in the default narrative, in the form of contradictory evidence, that another explanation that may account for all or most of the excess deaths must be investigated and tested. This alternative hypothesis warrants sober and diligent assessment, without being dismissed as fanciful or subject to demands for consensus.

Chapter 10. A regulatory win, but bad news and bad data continue

10.1. Scottish cardiac ambulance data

Shows worrying increase in incidents (18 January 2023)

In early 2021 we wrote about the stark difference in trends between the 'official' UK Government data on covid case numbers and the number of 999 and ambulance calls for covid triage (here [325]).

In our view the ambulance data were a far more reliable indicator of covid illness than the 'case' numbers and showed that, while there was a genuine peak in March 2020, there were only small seasonal increases thereafter. This contrasted to the official claims that, for example, during the winter of 2020-21 the number of case numbers were five times higher than the March 2020 peak.

Consequently, we were intrigued this week when David Scott of UK Column alerted us to some very interesting data provided by Public Health Scotland on the number of cardiovascular incidents involving the ambulance service. The data are available here [326].

While it is possible to search by different reporting regions, we will just comment on the total for all reporting regions combined. Overall, since mid-August 2020 there has been a significant weekly increase in cardiovascular incidents in Scotland (averaging about 30% higher than the corresponding period in 2018-19), with especially large peaks between May-Sept 2021 (over 60% higher than the corresponding period in 2018-19). All of the charts can be seen in our article [327].

But the differences in age group patterns are interesting. For example, we directly compare the youngest age group (11-44) with one of the oldest age groups (75-84) on the same axis, as shown in Figure 45. Note that:

- The percentage increases in the young age group have been consistently higher than the older age group.
- In the young age group the average weekly increase peaked around July 2021 (83%) but has been consistently high since then (average weekly 40% higher) and never below 14% higher.
- In the older age group, the first peak was in April 2021 (34%), highest peak July 2021 (52% increase). Several below 0% since (averaging 16%).

So, in summary it seems:

1. The youngest have been proportionally worst affected with serious increased cardiac incidents.

2. There is some evidence of peaks in serious cardiac incidents occurring shortly after vaccination peaks in each of the different age groups.

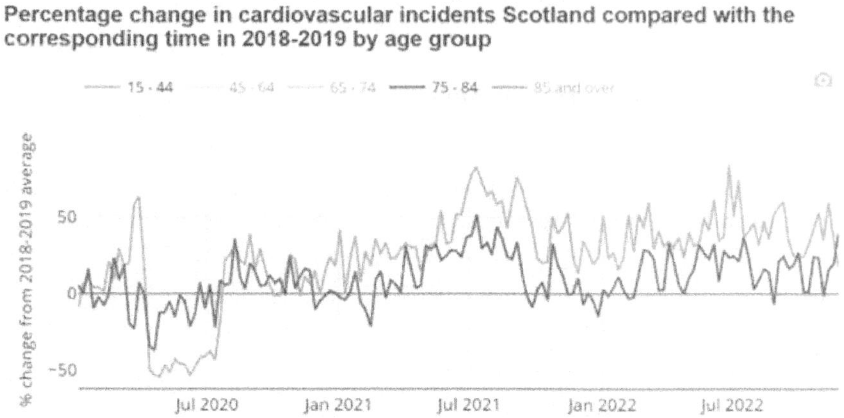

Figure 45 Percentage change compare young and old age groups

In case anybody suspects that the differences and large fluctuations are due to chance because of low incident numbers it is important to note the weekly numbers provided since 2020. The oldest age group has the lowest weekly number (averaging around 130 since start of 2021) while the 45-64 age group has the highest weekly number (averaging around 410 since start of 2021). These numbers are not small enough to have created the different patterns by chance.

10.2. UK Statistics Regulator agrees with us

We all should ignore claims of vaccine safety from the ONS (20 January 2023)

On 11 November 2022 we wrote a formal letter [328] of complaint to the Statistics Regulator about the Office for National Statistics (ONS) data on vaccine mortality. We said it was not fit for purpose:

Note that we concluded by saying:

> "The fact that these data are being used as continued justification for the efficacy and safety of the covid vaccines is therefore now a matter of national concern and scandal … In the meantime, we call for
>
> 1. the public withdrawal of the ONS dataset and
>
> 2. the retraction of any claims made by others that are based upon it."

We have now received the formal response [329] and it is on the Regulator's website (full pdf here [330]).

While there are aspects of the response that we are unhappy with, the crucial point is that they have completely accepted our main recommendation because they say:

> "Overall, then, our view is that the Deaths by Vaccination Status publication does not provide information on vaccine effectiveness or vaccine safety, and should not be used in this way."

Many researchers and news organisations have made claims of vaccine efficacy and safety based on the ONS reports. We therefore now call on all those who have made such claims to publicly retract them.

It is also important to note that the Regulator agreed with our conclusions that the ONS population sample was biased - with those excluded much more likely to be unvaccinated.

> "We consider that it is therefore likely that the sample used in the Deaths by Vaccination Status publication is not representative of the general population. Those who are missing are, we think, more likely to be younger and unvaccinated."

We therefore call on all of those - including especially the BBC - who have used the ludicrously low estimates of unvaccinated from the ONS [331] to publicly withdraw all material based on these estimates, as they have been deliberately used to represent the unvaccinated as a tiny fringe minority. The most egregious case of this was the BBC TV programme – 'Unvaccinated' - fronted by Professor Hannah Fry that reused the ONS claim that eight percent of the population remained unvaccinated:

> "In this timely, eye-opening investigation commissioned by BBC Factual for BBC Two and BBC iPlayer, due to air on Wednesday 20 July at 9pm, Professor Hannah Fry seeks to understand **why eight percent of the population** remain unvaccinated against Covid-19."

The original article containing the above quote can be found on the wayback machine here [332]. By 8 July 2022 the BBC saw fit to perform an Orwellian edit the page [333] changing the text to:

> "In this timely, eye-opening investigation commissioned by BBC Factual for BBC Two and BBC iPlayer, due to air on Wednesday 20 July at 9pm, Professor Hannah Fry seeks to understand **why a portion of the population** remain unvaccinated against Covid-19."

The not-so-good news is that, as expected the Regulator has gone to extreme lengths to defend the integrity of the ONS. In particular, they are putting forward the 'healthy vaccinee effect' which we have previously dealt with [334] and which we will be further dismantling in the next few weeks.

Our analysis of the most recent ONS report on deaths by vaccination status is here [335]. That report was published in July 2022 with the most recent data up to May 2022. Despite promises to do so, the ONS had not provided any updates to it since.

10.3. How to create the illusion your vaccine is 90% effective

3 February 2023

A major study claimed the covid vaccines are over 90% effective. But when you look at the details of the study you find that a whopping 37.2% of all vaccinated participants who were tested within 14 days of the first dose were confirmed as covid cases. None of these 'cases' were counted in the efficacy calculation. Also, out of the subset of 1,482 participants with confirmed symptomatic covid, that were part of the study, not a single one died, despite 812 of these being unvaccinated.

Deception is now endemic, and this article describes the 'how to guide' on manufacturing high efficacy illusions. Here we outline an easy to follow five step fool proof method to ensure a vaccine will be accepted as highly effective and look at a specific research paper to illustrate how this is done.

10.3.1. Step 1: Suppress legitimate criticism

We have reported the statistical tricks and biases commonly used in studies of vaccine efficacy many times. These tricks inevitably lead to exaggerated claims ("95% safe and effective") that are echoed throughout the mainstream media and are routinely used by censorship units like *Full Fact* as 'proof' to close down debate. We have also shown how, even when the flaws and biases committed by these studies are meticulously laid out in letters to journal editors, they refuse to even publish these letters, let alone retract the studies. A good example is our recent experience with Lancet [337] and its published study that supposedly 'confirmed' the 95% efficacy of the Pfizer vaccine. The same happened with the New England Journal of Medicine where another study reached the same 95% efficacy conclusion - they refused to publish this response by Mark Reeder [338]). These widely publicised studies essentially 'sealed the deal' for the efficacy of the Pfizer vaccination in the eyes of the public.

10.3.2. Step 2: Publish in a (bought and sold?) 'reputable' journal

Nothing has changed. Since then, there have been many even more fundamentally flawed studies that make similarly exaggerated claims. However, this study [339] of 109,865 healthcare workers in the 20 weeks from December 28, 2020, through May 19, 2021 (reported in 'Effectiveness of mRNA Covid-19 Vaccine among U.S. Health Care Personnel') is one of the most startling examples yet.

The study looked at both Pfizer's BNT162b2 and Moderna's mRNA-1273 and concluded the following:

> "The BNT162b2 and mRNA-1273 vaccines were highly effective under real-world conditions …."

In fact, for 'any' of the vaccines the effectiveness of 'complete vaccination' was stated to be 90.4% (with Moderna coming in at a whopping 96.3% and Pfizer at 88.8%). This information is all provided in their Table 3.

But before we look at the revealing information provided in the table, it is important to understand what kind of study this was. Most people assume that if you want to evaluate the efficacy of a vaccine in an observational study you simply compare the outcomes (e.g. infections, hospitalisations, deaths) of those in a large cohort of vaccinated people with those in a large cohort of unvaccinated people and then adjust for any known confounders. But that is not what was done here. This was a so-called "test-negative case–control study".

What they did was look at a set of people who tested positive for covid at some time during the 19 weeks of the study - they selected 1,472 out of the 8,365 testing positive (so this would contain a mixture of vaccinated and unvaccinated). These are the 'case participants' in their table. Then they try to find a set of 'matching' people who only ever tested negative during the 19 weeks. Again, this would contain a mixture of vaccinated and unvaccinated. These are the 'control participants'.

10.3.3. Step 3: Ignore infected cases that are vaccinated

The main trick to getting to the high efficacy figures is *to completely ignore vaccinated people who get infected within the first 14 days after their first dose* - they are not even counted as 'partially vaccinated' since that only applies to people post 14 days of their first dose and pre 7 days of a second dose.

So, imagine the most extreme case in which ***every*** vaccinated person gets covid within the first two weeks of their first dose. Then, assuming (as is likely) that none get infected a second time within the 19 weeks, according to the study definition no vaccinated people ever got covid over the whole period of the study.

If only one person in the unvaccinated comparative cohort had got covid, over the same period, the vaccine efficacy (defined as one minus the proportion of vaccinated infected divided by the proportion of unvaccinated infected times 100) will be reported as 100%.

Now, while it is certainly not the case that all the vaccinated here got covid within the first 14 days it seems that quite a lot of them did. A total 353 out of 948 (37.2%) who were tested within 13 days of their first dose were positive (the percentage is even higher, 40%, for those tested within the first 10 days). Does that sound like a vaccine that is effective in anything other than giving people covid?

10.3.4. Step 4: Don't look for covid if you don't want to find it

But the paper states "During the study period of December 28, 2020, through May 19, 2021, a total of 109,865 health care personnel were tested across the participating sites; of these persons, 8365 (7.6%) tested positive for SARS-CoV-2." So, over the whole 19-week period 7.6% of that population got Covid-19. That means (crudely) on average in any 2-week period the infection rate was about 0.8%. Yet the infection rate for people being tested within 2 weeks of their first jab was 37.2%!

Unfortunately, the study report provides no information whatsoever on how frequently people were tested. In theory if only people with Covid-19 symptoms got tested then having a high proportion of those being confirmed positive would not be surprising (if the test was accurate). But, as these were all healthcare workers, it's likely they were tested very frequently, and we know that during the first two weeks after vaccination it was routine to get tested. If people were tested every two weeks, then we could reasonably conclude the vaccinated were getting infected – within two weeks of their first jab – at a rate that was almost 50 times greater than the general rate for this population.

So, if you don't look for Covid-19, by not testing for it, or by ignoring the test results you won't find it.

10.3.5. Step 5: Ignore outcomes that make your vaccine look ineffective

And here's another nugget from the study: of the total of 1482 participants with a positive test and at least one Covid-19–like symptom *there was a grand total of zero deaths*: an infection fatality rate (IFR) of 0%. And 812 of those were unvaccinated. Bear in mind that this when covid was supposed to have been rampaging globally and causing widespread death. And of course, *that nugget somehow never got mentioned in the abstract, mains results, conclusions, or discussion.* It only appeared in the detailed results section (along with the fact that only 2% were hospitalised):

> "Only 2% of case participants were hospitalised during their illness; 1% of control participants were hospitalised during a non–Covid-19–related illness. No deaths were reported among the participants included in this study."

10.3.6. Why all observational studies (and many RCTs) of vaccine effectiveness and safety exaggerate vaccine effectiveness claims

All studies on vaccine effectiveness suffer from one or more (often most or even all) of the following systematic biases:

- ***Misclassificaton***: Participants who got a PCR positive test within 14 days of first vaccination (resp. second, third etc) are either classified as unvaccinated (resp. 1-dosed, 2-dosed etc) or simply not counted. Yet in many studies there are especially high infection rates for the vaccinated during this period. As explained here this would result in high efficacy rates even for a placebo vaccine.

- ***Delayed reporting*** If reporting of covid cases is delayed (e.g. by a week or two) during vaccine rollout then this results in exactly the same illusion/exaggeration of efficacy as misclassification.

- ***Illegitimate comparisons***: Efficacy assessed by comparing the never vaccinated only with the 'fully vaccinated' (based on whatever the definition of fully vaccinated was at time of study, e.g. at least two weeks after second dose, third dose etc).

- ***Different testing protocols between vaccinated and unvaccinated***: People who were unvaccinated were generally required to get tested far more frequently than the vaccinated even if they were asymptomatic. [337]. Hence, Covid-19 positives were more likely to be found in the unvaccinated irrespective of the true difference in susceptibility between groups.

- ***Survivor/selection bias***: People who were symptomatic or PCR positive when called for vaccination were recommended to wait until they were PCR negative before being vaccinated; this means that all such people had natural immunity when they did get vaccinated and hence were less likely to subsequently get covid.

- ***Study took place during period of naturally falling infection rate***: Timing of study coincided with period when infection rates were decreasing: This would be certain to create a statistical illusion of efficacy.

- ***Vaguely defined outcomes***: By not being explicit about the outcomes and end dates for the study, many studies can simply choose which outcome makes the 'best case' for the vaccine. So, in the above example, only in the detailed results do we find there were no deaths (in either the unvaccinated or unvaccinated) and almost no hospitalisations); hence the impact of the vaccine on these key outcomes were conveniently ignored.

10.4. The latest ONS data on deaths by covid vaccination status

23 February 2023

10.4.1. The saga continues

After a 7 month delay - the same (and worse) systemic problems and multiple flaws:

- None of the core limitations and flaws of the previous report have been resolved.
- The ONS appear to have ignored the UK statistics regulator who required them 'to address some of the sampling issues present in the first six iterations of the publication'.
- The higher non-covid mortality rates in the unvaccinated confirm there are biases/confounders still not adjusted for.
- There is still gross underestimation of the proportion of unvaccinated in the population. This artificially inflates mortality rates of unvaccinated and reduces rates of vaccinated.
- Use of new census data means the data in previous reports has changed significantly but seems no more reliable.
- The data for months Jan-March 2021 have been removed. These were the months that especially exposed misclassification of deaths shortly after vaccination.
- There are numerous errors in the data and key data are missing or difficult to analyse.
- Even if we were to trust their data, the evidence actually points to safety risks especially in the younger age groups.
- Ultimately, we don't think we can trust any public health statistics produced by the ONS. Given this the regulator has failed to maintain the public's trust in the ONS or government policies based on the data.

We have reported extensively on the problems with the ONS reports on deaths by vaccination status. We complained to the Statistics Regulator about the July 2022 reports, and he agreed with our recommendation to ignore any claims of vaccine safety or efficacy based on the data and also that the ONS underestimates the true population proportion unvaccinated.

After a 7-month delay since the previous update on 21 Feb 2023 the ONS finally released [340] a new version with data up to Dec 2022. The previous version (released July 2022) had data up to May 2022. So, there was great anticipation that the ONS would in the time available resolve the issues with their dataset and settle open questions about vaccine efficacy and safety. Unfortunately, this opportunity was missed.

To show how seriously they took their task, despite all that time they had to get it right, a corrected version was issued 24 hours later after many people pointed out errors (more of that below - in fact they only fixed some errors on month labels).

Inevitably, as in the previous report, the 'headline' figures are that the all-cause mortality rate - measured here by the age-standardised mortality rate (ASMR) - has been consistently lower among the vaccinated than the unvaccinated (although the difference is narrowing). If the data were accurate and reliable then, as we have always argued, the all-cause mortality rate is, indeed, the most objective measure of vaccine safety and efficacy. But, as in the previous version, it is easily shown that there are systemic flaws and biases in this latest version which make the stated ASMR figures meaningless.

Of course, this did not stop inevitable mainstream media publishing of predictable pre-prepared stories ridiculing 'anti-vaxx myths' [341] claiming the data proved that death rates were lower among the vaccinated. For example, The Daily Mail headline on 21 Feb 2023 was:

> "Death rates are NOT higher among Covid-vaccinated Brits, according to official stats debunking major anti-vacc myth"

A very quick look through the data reveals some obvious concerning changes from the previous version, namely:

- Data for those under 18 have been removed.
- Data for Jan-March 2021 has vanished.
- There are many changes to the raw data for April 2021-May 2022 between latest version and previous versions.

10.4.2. What the 'sceptical' papers say on ASMRs

There has been an enormous volume of discussion and analysis already about the data. We have not done any detailed analysis of it yet - for reasons partly explained here [342].

However, here we provide a round-up of the analyses already done by other sceptical writers and offer our brief comments on some of these analyses.

First, before going through these, it is important to note that (for reasons explained here [343]) the age standardised mortality rate (ASMR) is a terrible metric for assessing vaccination safety (also it cannot be reproduced by the data provided). While it accounts for age-confounding, it obscures the information needed to determine risk/benefit for different specific age groups.

By looking at raw mortality rates within each age category there is no need for the complex, obfuscated ASMR. The ONS ***do*** provide age categorised breakdown:

18-39, 40-49, 50-59, 60-69, 70-79, 80-89, 90+

(Although the 18-39 category is rather 'coarse' and, unlike previous versions, those aged under 18 are no longer included so we have less information than before).

Tore Aarhus Gulbrandsen [344] has produced the relevant all-cause mortality graphs for each of the age groups (note the ONS uses person years rather than number of people). As in previous ONS releases, there are wild fluctuations in mortality rates for the different categories of vaccinated. But in no age group is there any strong evidence of reduced all-cause mortality for the vaccinated.

The ONS summary data was trumpeted by the mainstream media and those continuing to push the 'safe and effective' vaccine narrative, since it shows the ASMR for the unvaccinated higher than that of the ever vaccinated. But a deeper look into the data reveals the key problems with this. Our full article [345] of 23 Feb 2023 included a chart which showed that the ASMRs reported by ONS changed dramatically for the unvaccinated between releases. The Jan-March 2021 data have been removed (the ONS says this is because they are using the new 2021 census which only includes people alive after March 2021), so it is important to remind people of what the previous report's data said about *non-covid* mortality.

There was a sharp peak in unvaccinated non-covid mortality in Jan-March 2021 (which was when the vaccine was rolled out). As we explained in detail [346], this must have been the result of misclassifying those dying shortly after vaccination as unvaccinated. But the fact that there was a continued (albeit decreasing) difference proves there was systemic bias/confounding of the data through one or more of:

- misclassification of vaccinated deaths as unvaccinated
- underestimating the population proportion of unvaccinated
- 'healthy vaccinee effect'

This bias influenced all of the mortality rates, but the ONS did not adjust for it at the time. They were however keen to assume a healthy vaccinee bias but presented no evidence to support this lazy assumption.

How did mortality change in the latest release? As shown by USMortality [347] there is still a significantly higher non-covid mortality rate in the 'unvaccinated' and so clearly the systemic problems have NOT been fixed in latest version. They have got worse.

10.4.3. Denominators

What about the critical problem with underestimation of the proportion of unvaccinated? Unfortunately, again, this problem has not been resolved even with the new census data. Clare Craig and Igor Chudov [348] have both analysed this.

As Igor Chudov pointed out as an example, the March 2022 ONS estimate for the 50-59 age group is that there were just 6.19% in this age group unvaccinated, but according to the UKHSA Week 13 vaccine surveillance report [349], (Page 17) 87% of the 50-59 age group were vaccinated in March 2022. So UKHSA say 13% were unvaccinated (a figure we know to be much more accurate).

10.4.4. Miscategorisation

We also know that miscategorisation is still happening. Indeed Note 17 of the ONS spreadsheet asserts:

> "There were some people who were vaccinated but not included in the NIMS data as they died soon after vaccination. Of these, 1,029 linked to our 2021 Census linked dataset. We included the latest vaccination records for these people in our dataset. This data is provisional and extends up to the 1 November 2022. This will be updated in future releases."

This led to an interesting twitter exchange between colleague Josh Guetzkow and the head of mortality at the ONS Sarah Caul MBE (Member of the British Empire) of the ONS shown in Figure 46.

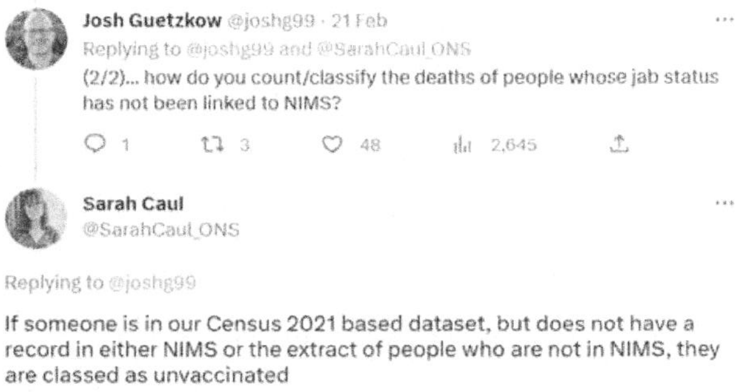

Figure 46 Anybody without a record in NIMS is assumed unvaccinated

10.4.5. Other issues with the ONS data

Joel Smalley has done an important analysis [350] that shows we consistently see elevated mortality rates for the vaccinated since the start of 2022 when Covid-19 represents less than 10% of deaths but the vaccinated disproportionally more of all deaths.

He showed that there are disproportionately more deaths in the ever-vaccinated population than one might expect from the percentage of the population vaccinated and Joel's analysis looks to be a powerful indictment of the vaccine's safety profile, but it is itself based on data we know we cannot fully trust.

Why can't we trust it? Because a cursory analysis of the death counts in the ONS dataset shows that the death counts from their Table 5 and Table 2 differ, as discussed in this twitter thread .

Dr Clare Craig asked the ONS about this discrepancy in death counts and explains [352] how deaths can occur amongst the population "ghosted" by the ONS. 'el gato malo' reaches the same conclusion as us about the data and highlights further concerns [353].

10.5. Postmodern science delivers immortality benefits

26 February 2023

In all of our deep dive reports we have compared ONS data against historical actuarial mortality rates. We believe that only by comparing with expectations can we determine if there is a pandemic and whether the vaccines are putting a dent in it, or indeed adding to the mortality burden.

Comparing mortality rates 'within' the ONS data set doesn't tell you whether the data as a whole stands up to scrutiny. For that we need to test against historical data and previous reports.

We pointed out that the ASMRs (Age Standardised Mortality Rates) reported for Feb-May 2022 were significantly lower than historical rates from 2016, for younger age groups (59 and below), giving rise to what we dubbed the '**dead presumed missing**' phenomena. We suggested that this can be explained by deaths that are missing from their dataset. Comparing the ASMRs in the latest ONS release reveals this same problem, (all the detailed tables and graphs from our analysis can be found in the full article [354]. The mortality risk of people in the ONS dataset remains significantly different from the general population and we can see there are huge changes in the reported mortality rates between this ONS report and the last one, with percentage changes in mortality ranging from -31% to +38%. Why these dramatic changes?

Between the old and new ONS reports the mortality rates changed significantly, with the mortality of unvaccinated and vaccinated older groups now exhibiting lower mortality figures, dropping by between -6% to -31%. How can this be? In contrast, for the unvaccinated younger age groups the mortality increased by between 23% and 38% between ONS reports. Odd. This is a massive change that cannot be explained. You'd think they would have checked for stability but obviously they are churning out garbage.

So, comparing across ONS reports shows dramatic changes that cannot be explained.

But much more significant than this is the fact that the mortality rates are crazily different from those from 2016. How crazy? Now you'd think in this age of real time big data we'd have the 2016 mortality rates at our fingertips but guess what - all we could find was a grainy image on an ONS web site. From this we produced rough estimates of the mortality burden by age group and compared them against the latest ONS mortality figures.

There was clearly something very wrong with this data. The most obvious thing is that, across all age groups, the all-cause mortality rate is significantly LESS from February 2022 than one would expect, compared to 2016, for BOTH the vaccinated and unvaccinated. And this occurs at a time when excess deaths in the UK are starting to increase and the covid case rate has plummeted,

So, more people are dying but in the ONS data set people are living longer!

There are a few things we can conclude from this. Either deaths are not being recorded in the ONS data set, and they don't bother to check (maybe they are with the coroners' courts or 'in the post'), or, if the data are correct then the vaccines are so good, they are improving mortality for everyone, whether you take them or not. Maybe all of that 'vaccine shedding' is a good thing after all? And with more of the vaccines, we will achieve immortality!

It seems to us that detailed blow-by-blow take downs of ONS are pretty laboured and this is the simplest and most obvious way of showing how useless the ONS data are. You don't really need any more than this to win the argument. It's clearly not representative of anything. It's postmodern science.

10.6. Summary remarks on new ONS data release

To date we have produced three exhaustive analyses of the ONS data, each of which has consumed a massive amount of time and effort. Recall that this data was said to be the gold standard produced by the best, most reliable official statistics department in the world.

Each time we looked at their data we, and many others, have discovered a litany of biases, errors, oddities, missing data, inconsistencies, contradictions and under/overestimates. The ONS have either ignored our analyses or made lazy off hand assumptions that they believe explains these issues. None of the issues we have identified have been addressed and none of their assumptions justified.

We had, perhaps naïvely, hoped that the ONS would have responded to the criticism from the UK statistics regulator and 'upped their game', but clearly, they have treated us, and the regulator, with contempt. Far from resolving all of the issues this report was replete with the same errors, was obviously hastily put together and even had to be fixed and updated within hours of release. More importantly all of the original issues and biases remain unaddressed. These events raise many legitimate questions:

- If the regulator doesn't require the ONS to produce accurate or useful information about vaccine safety and efficacy, what is the ONS for? What are we paying our taxes for?
- If the regulator can be ignored, where the official statistics produced by the system are as bent before and after regulatory intervention, why do we need a regulator at all? Why are we paying for this?
- Why should we accept anything the UK government has historically claimed about the covid vaccines based on this data? Why should we accept any of their public health claims in the future?

Chapter 11. The vanishing flu

11.1. Playing hide and seek with the flu

4 March 2023

We know the flu virtually disappeared globally after spring 2020 and in 2021 don't we? Here's the BBC [355] confirming it. It was 'out competed' by SARS-CoV-2 and then it came back with a vengeance. We are told this is a fact.

But what if the central underpinning 'fact' here is wrong and, like a child hiding behind a curtain during a game of hide and seek who forgets their feet are visible, the flu didn't disappear at all but was just poorly hidden. Or we didn't try hard enough to find it and didn't spot the kids' feet poking out from underneath the curtain.

Some have tried hard to find it. Eugyppius [356] had a good look at German data and couldn't. So, it wasn't hiding in Germany. If not there, then where?

Well, it is actually very easy to find out what countries experienced flu and which didn't from the WHO itself, by accessing the Influenza Laboratory Surveillance Information database [357].

As the charts in the original article version of this section [358] showed, it was hiding in France in 2020 and 2021 and also on Finland, India and Nepal. If we look further afield to countries neighbouring India and Nepal, such as Bangladesh and Pakistan we find that flu was present in winter 2021 and 2022, despite sharing land borders with countries where flu had disappeared. So, India and Nepal have no flu but neighbouring counties report cases beyond spring 2020 and into 2021. But how could the flu only spread within these countries and not cross the border into the immediate neighbours? Is it a religious thing - does Covid-19 only drive out flu in non-predominately Muslim countries in the Himalayan region?

And what about countries further afield, in the Caribbean specifically Haiti and the Dominican Republic? Haiti is on an island, and it shares this island with the Dominican Republic. There is flu in Haiti but no flu in the Dominican Republic.

So, here we have two neighbouring countries separated from the rest of the world, sharing the same island but where the flu virus doesn't circulate on one side of the border but does on the other. And what is even odder it appears to be happy spreading in the predominantly Muslim countries neighbouring India but not in India itself, or neighbouring Nepal.

This is all very odd. It appears the flu was considered gone, but only because no one was doing much seeking, and assumed, because they couldn't find it, it must have disappeared. But anyone spending 20 mins searching the online WHO flu database will find the flu's 'shoes poking out beneath the curtain'.

Either that or all we really need to prevent circulation of these pesky viruses is to do the opposite of what the globalists want. Every household simply needs to install its own international border post and sing a self-composed national anthem. Obvious really - if borders can stop the flu, they should have stopped Covid-19.

If border closures stopped viruses in their tracks, then the USSR and Eastern bloc countries should have stopped or significantly altered the circulation of flu in the northern hemisphere between the raising of the iron curtain and the fall of the Soviet empire.

Similarly North Korea should have a completely different variety and pattern of viral infections compared to elsewhere.

This section is based on a fuller article with relevant screenshots, charts, tables and figures here [358].

11.2. Peek-a-Boo Flu

1 April 2023

Is viral interference between SARS-CoV-2 and the flu a myth? And if we don't believe the PCR test can diagnose the presence of SARS-CoV-2 why should we trust it to diagnose the absence of influenza?

We found that flu had not actually disappeared but had been playing hide-and-seek and could be found hiding in the Hindu-Kush or sunning itself in Haiti. It clearly wasn't hanging around to witness the craziness of the West's response to the new 'novel and deadly' interloper.

Here we examine another part of the puzzle - the near-universal acceptance of the explanation for the disappearance of the flu: that it was out-competed by SARS-CoV-2 from Spring 2020 and failed to return until the end of 2021, just after the arrival of the SARS-CoV-2 Omicron variant. It reappeared just as quickly as it disappeared. And it did so globally and with a high degree of synchronicity across multiple countries.

Based on published empirical evidence we think that the explanation that flu disappeared because of competition from SARS-CoV-2 is wrong and, given this fact, we need to look elsewhere for an explanation for flu's disappearance.

This section is based on a fuller article with relevant screenshots, charts, tables and figures here [360].

11.2.1. Viral Interference

The disappearance of the flu supposedly rests on a well-accepted theory, called viral interference, whereby the circulation patterns of flu, and other viruses, fluctuate and change from year to year and hemisphere to hemisphere. Under this theory we are told to accept that this is the single and only plausible explanation for what happened to flu and that, after many decades of absolute respiratory viral dominance by flu, SARS-CoV-2 was just too fit and potent a competitor for flu to win the fight to occupy people's respiratory systems. This relationship between flu and SARS-CoV-2 has been likened to a see-saw[360].

As a result, flu disappeared and only returned after the circulation of the SARS-CoV-2 Omicron variant. This did not just happen with flu but was reported to have occurred with rhinovirus and RSV [361], which also absconded with the flu but then returned.

The biological mechanisms for viral interference look plausible and have been around since the 1960s. A good review of the various interference mechanisms can be found here, along with a review of results from epidemiological, ex vivo and in vivo studies, which show that sequential or co-infection with one virus can interfere with, and reduce the propensity of, infection by another. It is posited that production of a strong immune response to the first virus prevents other viruses from setting in.

However, it should be noted that even if this phenomenon is accepted as credible (and we do question its evidential basis below), it is surely a huge stretch to suggest that something which appears to happen at an individual level can result in synchronized population-wide suppression of influenza globally, and it doesn't explain how it bounced back.

11.2.2. Empirical evidence for viral interference with SARS-CoV-2

What empirical evidence do we have that viral interference occurs between the flu, rhinoviruses (RV), respiratory syncytial virus (RSV) and SARS-CoV-2?

Piret and Boivin [362] report on two experiments involving sequential infection of flu and SARS-CoV-2 in Syrian hamsters and ferrets but concluded that there was no detectable sign of viral interference. They concluded:

> "......previous infection with SARS-CoV-2 did not affect pH1N1 load in the lungs compared with a single infection.......further studies are needed to clarify the interactions between SARS-CoV-2 and influenza viruses."

Fage et al [363] looked at the replication kinetics and interactions between SARS-CoV-2, A(H1N1) flu, and RSV and concluded that:

> "Our results showed that during simultaneous infection, SARS-CoV-2 interferes with RSV-A2 but not with A(H1N1)pdm09 replication. The prior infection of nasal HAE with SARS-CoV-2 reduces the replication kinetics of both respiratory viruses. SARS-CoV-2 replication is decreased by a prior infection with A(H1N1)pdm09 but not with RSV-A2."

Replication of influenza A was reduced in the presence of prior infection by SARS-CoV-2 and vice-versa. So, both viruses had some ability to interfere with each other but there is no evidence that it was predominately one way, favouring the dominance of SARS-CoV-2.

Essaidi-Laziosi et al [364] investigated dual infections involving SARS-CoV-2 with RV and Influenza A and B viruses (IAV and IBV), using reconstituted repository airway epithelial cells and stated that:

> "We found that SARS-CoV-2 replication was impaired by primary, but not secondary, rhino- and influenza virus infection. In contrast, SARS-CoV-2 had no effect on the replication of these seasonal respiratory viruses."

In the viral interference theory if SARS-CoV-2 was infected first and then followed by another, secondary, infectious agent, we would expect that the effect of primary infection by SARS-CoV-2 would *decrease* the presence of the secondary infection. However, Essaidi-Lazios's experimental results did not match these theoretical expectations.

To hammer the point home, they concluded (our emphasis):

> "While infecting first with RV, IAV and IBV and then 48 h later with SARS-CoV-2 led to reduced SARS-CoV-2 replication even when inoculated with 2 logs higher multiplicity of infection (approximate MOI 0.1 for SARS-CoV-2 versus 0.001-0.002 for seasonal viruses), **no such effect was seen when the order of infection was inverted**, even when the incubation time between the two infections was shortened (in order to establish a co-infection during the exponential phase of SARS-CoV-2 infection). Our results indicate that the sequence of infection events influences the fate of SARS-CoV-2 infection. Regardless the order of infections …, no adaptation was observed in SARS-CoV-2 after co-infection (data not shown)."

Bai et al [365] investigated coinfection between SARS-CoV-2 and found that preinfection with influenza A significantly promoted the infectivity of SARS-CoV-2, leading to more severe outcomes.

> "The upcoming flu season in the Northern Hemisphere merging with the current COVID-19 pandemic raises a potentially severe threat to public health. Through experimental coinfection with influenza A virus (IAV) and either pseudotyped or live SARS-CoV-2 virus, we found that IAV preinfection significantly promoted the infectivity of SARS-CoV-2 in a broad range of cell types. Remarkably, in vivo, increased SARS-CoV-2 viral load and more severe lung damage were observed in mice coinfected with IAV. Moreover, such enhancement of SARS-CoV-2 infectivity was not observed with several other respiratory viruses, likely due to a unique feature of IAV to elevate ACE2 expression. This study illustrates that IAV has a unique ability to aggravate SARS-CoV-2 infection, and thus, prevention of IAV infection is of great significance during the COVID-19 pandemic."

Finally, and perhaps most significantly, this Nature paper by Bai et al [366] found that coinfection with influenza A (IAV) actually enhances SARS-CoV-2 infectivity! They tested whether IAV infection could affect the subsequent SARS-CoV-2 infection in both cultured cells and mice, stating that:

> "…..we found that IAV preinfection significantly promoted the infectivity of SARS-CoV-2 in a broad range of cell types. Remarkably, in vivo, increased SARS-CoV-2 viral load and more severe lung damage were observed in mice coinfected with IAV. Moreover, such enhancement of SARS-CoV-2 infectivity was not observed with several other respiratory viruses, likely due to a unique feature of IAV to elevate ACE2 expression. This study illustrates that IAV has a unique ability to aggravate SARS-CoV-2 infection…."

So, is the theory that viral interference caused the eradication of the flu a myth?

11.2.3. Observational studies of viral interference with SARS-CoV-2

An observational study by Stowe et al [367] reported interactions between SARS-CoV-2 and influenza, and the impact of co-infection on disease severity. They used data for influenza and SARS-CoV-2 collected from England's national surveillance systems between 20 January 2020 and 25 April 2020.

In their paper they conclude two things:

- The risk of testing positive for SARS-CoV-2 was 58% lower among influenza-positive cases and
- Patients with a co-infection had a risk of death of 5.92 (95% confidence interval: 3.21–10.91) times greater than those with neither influenza nor SARS-CoV-2. The odds of ventilator use, or death and intensive care unit admission or death were greatest among coinfected patients.

So here we see lower co-infection rates, but significant numbers of co-infections were indeed discovered. However, the study sampled people who were tested for both influenza and SARS-CoV-2 within 7 days of each other, without recording the order of the tests, so we can conclude little about whether previous infection with SARS-CoV-2 prevented infection by flu.

It is notable that in Spring 2020 there was up to a 10-times higher risk of death in people with a SARS-CoV-2 co-infection with flu. And this correlated with ventilator use. However, with hindsight we now know that, as a matter of protocol rather than genuine health needs, many Covid-19 patients were unnecessarily put on ventilators leading to increased risk of their death.

Of course, tracking of both flu and SARS-CoV-2 was routinely performed worldwide by national health bodies. The independent [368] newspaper reported for Public Health England (PHE):

> "...of the 685,243 samples that have been reviewed at PHE's laboratories since the first week of January, not a single one has tested positive for influenza. In the week up to 31 December 2020, just one case of flu was confirmed by laboratory analysis."

Think about this. Nearly seven hundred thousand tests and they are all negative, except one. And that single positive was confirmed to be a true positive. So, there was not one single false positive test result. This is not possible for any test, as it implies a specificity of 100%, zero chance of cross contamination and perfect laboratory conditions, which we know cannot possibly be true.

Next, in October 2022 the CDC published a paper [369] on circulation of human coronaviruses (HCoVs) and found that the cold season had shifted in 2020 and they also reported evidence of coinfection of HCoVs and flu in data collected from 2014 until 2021. From this study it is clear that HCoVs can happily coinfect with flu and other coronaviruses, showing that people might carry a nexus of infections by a host of different viruses. Given that SARS-CoV-2 is simply another coronavirus there is no reason to suppose that it behaves any differently from the others.

Another study, published in Nature Communications, by Butler et al [370] used shotgun transcription to test for many kinds and strains of virus extant in the initial spring wave in New York City (NYC) in Spring 2020:

> "Among respiratory viruses discovered across all patients (COVID+ and COVID–), we found frequent Influenza A (23% of viral positive cases), rhinovirus A (16%), and human metapneumovirus (12%)."

So, during the NYC deadly Spring wave, when SARS-CoV-2 was rampant, over 23% of patients being admitted to hospital were found to have influenza A. Bearing in mind that in a typical peak flu season we might see 20-40% of ILIs testing positive for flu this shows that in March-May 2023 the flu season was in full swing in NYC despite a co-occurring peak in SARS-CoV-2 prevalence.

They also observed a coinfection rate of around 3% between SARS-CoV-2 and other viruses:

> "These data also enabled an examination of co-infection within COVID+ patients. Among qRT-PCR positive cases, only 7 (3.2%) harbored sequences mappable to other respiratory viruses. Among these, we found human coronaviruses 229E, NL63 and HKU1, influenza A, and human mastadenovirus and metapneumovirus."

Dao et al [371] conducted a meta-analysis of dozens of studies reporting rates of coinfection and found wide variability in rates in many studies, but some very high rates in some.

This Chinese paper by Yue et al [372] reports on 307 SARS-CoV-2 infected patients, finding significant levels of coinfection:

> "Unexpectedly, there were only 42.7% (131) of SARS-CoV-2 single positive patients. Most of the SARS-CoV-2 infected patients were also positive for influenza viruses, including influenza A (49.8%) and influenza B (7.5%), taking up 57.3% (176/307) in total. Notably, early patients with COVID-19 were almost all coinfected with influenza B virus while influenza A virus infection has become prominent in the co-infection patients since 28 January onwards, which indicated that the two types of influenza viruses appeared a competing relationship."

It should be noted that the rate of coinfection found in all of these studies will depend on the testing process and potential influence of testing protocols, procedures and the effect of quarantines, as described by us here [373]. Hence, we should not be surprised by such wide variability in these results.

11.2.4. The Twindemic

The return of flu was presaged by a sequence of significant events:

In August 2020 The New York Times warned of the possibility of an upcoming Twindemic [374] of flu and SARS-CoV-2.

The omicron variant of SARS-CoV-2 emerged in South Africa on 24 November 2021 and was said to have then spread [375] at an unprecedented rate thereafter.

Then in January 2022 something odd happened: Israel reported the first coinfections of flu and SARS-CoV-2, referred to as flurona [376]. The Washington Post [377] reported that flurona coinfections were increasing as omicron surged.

Given the omicron variant was said to be milder and had outcompeted all other SARS-CoV-2 variants prevailing beforehand, this was presented as the main reason for relaxing lockdowns and quarantines throughout the world. Omicron came just in time to enable flu to reappear and then for coinfection of flu and SARS-CoV-2 to become possible, whereas before it was considered impossible. And with amazing prescience the New York Times predicted that a twindemic was imminent at a time when co-infection was deemed highly improbable, because flu had disappeared.

11.2.5. PCR testing for influenza

We are all painfully aware of the inaccuracy of using PCR to test for SARS-CoV-2, and a useful review of SARS-CoV-2 PCR can be found in this Daily Beagle [378] article.

Another recent publication by Collateral Global [379] highlights the PCR scandal in the UK. Our interpretation of their conclusions is that PCR testing in the UK is not effectively regulated, and that PCR testing is effectively as opaque as a black box.

Much of the discussion in the Daily Beagle focused on cycle thresholds which might determine whether there is SARS-CoV-2 in the sample or not. But focusing on this alone side-step's questions of cross-reactivity, non-specificity, cross contamination or some outcome synergistic with high amplification. These are central to whether we can determine whether another pathogen (such as flu) might be the actual cause of a false positive test result for SARS-CoV-2.

This article noted that the possibility of cross reactivity with flus, other coronaviruses and bacterial contamination was actually the reality, and this reality was recognised as far back as 2020 (such as reported by the smoking man [380]). However, it appears that the magnitude of the problem was underappreciated and misunderstood at the time.

There is so much PCR kit heterogeneity that it can be difficult to know which PCR test kits can be trusted, and which cannot. Some PCR kits claim to be perfectly accurate, with no cross reactivity, such as GeneXpert [381], GenMark [382] and BioFire [383]. However, in June 2020 this Australian validation of the Beijing Genomics Institute (BGI) [384] test kit reveals a specificity of 97.5% at one laboratory. Also, this study [385] that appeared in the Journal of Clinical Virology looked at the accuracy of the Australian Diagnostics multiplex kit, which also tests for flus, and found a specificity of 92% (inevitably multiplex kits are more prone to producing at least one false positive because they are testing for more viruses).

We should be wary of taking PCR manufacturer data at face value when we know that viruses continually mutate and are a moving target. As they mutate the potential for cross reaction and non-specificity obviously increases and the test, invented at a particular point in time, inevitably become progressively less trustworthy. The central question about PCR is therefore this:

If we don't believe the PCR test can diagnose the presence of SARS-CoV-2. Why should we trust it to diagnose the absence of influenza?

Australia in 2020 is used by some as the basis to claim that SARS-CoV-2 PCR kits are perfect as they had a long stretch of 1:10K positivity off-season (private correspondence with Kevin McKernan). In response to an FOI request [386] the ONS deployed the same lazy logic with regards PCR testing in the UK:

> "We know the specificity of our test must be very close to 100% as the low number of positive tests in our study over the summer of 2020 means that specificity would be very high even if all positives were false."

The ONS are claiming that because the number of PCR positives were so low in the summer, when SARS-CoV-2 was not circulating, then the tests must therefore be perfectly specific. However, this claim only makes logical sense if the PCR tests undertaken were subject to challenge by other circulating viruses or bacteria that had the capacity to trigger a non-specific false positive result. In the absence of a competing challenge then a negative test result would be inevitable and proves nothing (Kevin McKernan on PANDATA PCR Smoke and Mirrors [387] twitter space 2nd April 2023 (from minute 37). Further, given that both SARS-CoV-2 and the flu have greater circulation during winter then the absence of both in summer would logically lead to a high rate of true negative PCR test results in summer.

To put it another way if SARS-CoV-2 PCR cross reacts with flu then when flu is present during the winter this will generate PCR false positives for SARS-CoV-2. If flu is absent in the summer but other non-seasonal pathogens or contaminants were circulating, that caused false positives, we would observe a high false positive rate during the summer season. The fact that we did not see high false positive rates during the summer logically means that the kits are predominately picking up flu in the winter when it is circulating. We could use similar arguments for cross reaction with other competing winter coronaviruses (which as far as we know continued to circulate and were unaffected by viral interference).

Back in December 2020 we raised the issue of the role of confirmatory testing being done in the summer but not in the winter flu season in the UK. By performing confirmatory testing [388] for SARS-CoV-2 during a period of low prevalence the false positive rate would depress case rates to make the PCR testing look accurate and, when confirmatory testing ceases, it will inflate the SARS-CoV-2 case rate.

In the early part of the pandemic doctors were incentivised to diagnose SARS-CoV-2, where the symptoms are indistinguishable from flu, for symptoms which would have hitherto been attributed to Influenza-like-illnesses (ILIs). That incentive was achieved by a combination of authoritative diktat by the WHO, who mandated that a respiratory death should be certificated as Covid-19 deaths on the flimsiest of grounds, and the all-pervasive fear caused by the ceaseless propaganda about a novel and deadly virus. And this despite the fact that the UKHSA (Health Security Agency) had ruled [389] that Covid-19 was not a High Consequence Infectious Disease.

In early 2020 we assume influenza and SARS-CoV-2 testing was performed by different PCR kits but by July 2020 the CDC [390] approved the first multiplex (multi-virus) kits under EUA to detect both influenzas and SARS-CoV-2. After their near universal global roll-out flu disappeared over winter 2020/21. This may be a coincidence.

It seems to us that single virus, rather than multi-virus test kits, which are sensitive and specific to a single organism, would surely reduce the risk of shared failure modes and common causes of error. Diverse types of PCR kits specialising in the diagnosis of separate and different viruses would reduce the risk of cross-contamination or confusion about whether a positive means a Covid-19 positive or an influenza positive or both.

Note that we have not discovered a smoking gun that exposes systemic problems with ALL multi-virus PCR kits. Some of the early PCR kits we know to be unreliable but after the CDC EUA approval of multi-viral kits many were declared to have perfect specificity. We have no idea how and why there was a step change in reliability for these kits, if indeed there was any real improvement. In any case, given the huge variety of kits available, of unknown provenance, we cannot simply assume perfection across the board.

The global downward trend in bacterial infections, as well as in virtually all other infections during spring 2020 was amply illustrated in a chart published by the BioFire syndromic trends [391] reporting system, showing the percentage detection rate of pathogens, in the USA, by BioFire clinical diagnostic systems (PCR), from 2019 through to 2021 (Figure 47). The reported rate of viral and bacterial pathogens detected at least halved after SARS-CoV-2 appears on the scene in the USA, UK and Europe in February 2020. This is also shown by the Seattle Flu Study [392].

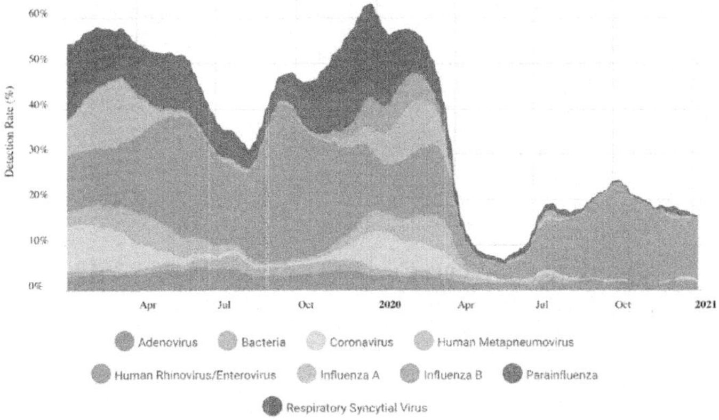

Figure 47 Percentage detection rate of pathogens, in the USA, by BioFire PCR, from 2019 to 2021

A drop in virtually all pathogens tracked by BioFire globally cannot be explained by viral or bacterial interference.

There are some potential failure modes worth investigating that might provide some insight into what is going on:

- Co-infection with both flu and SARS-CoV-2 may occur at the same time. Is a positive for SARS-CoV-2 somehow prioritised by the tests? Perhaps by SARS-CoV-2 masking the existence of flu or the tests showing this?
- Often when people think of PCR they think of a biological/chemical reaction without considering that it takes place within a wider system involving technology, people, procedures and policies. Each and all of these have a potential role to play in generating results and are thus potential sources of systematic or random error. One potential vulnerability is that PCR equipment uses proprietary software algorithms and are connected to the internet. Yet we do not know whether the software is independently audited. Likewise, we do not know whether the chain of custody for samples, or their reporting, is respected. It is therefore not inconceivable that these, and more, vulnerabilities exist in this wider system that might be exploitable.

Clearly, we are speculating here. But things do not add up, as shown in Figure 48 with data from CDC [394] and Our World in Data.

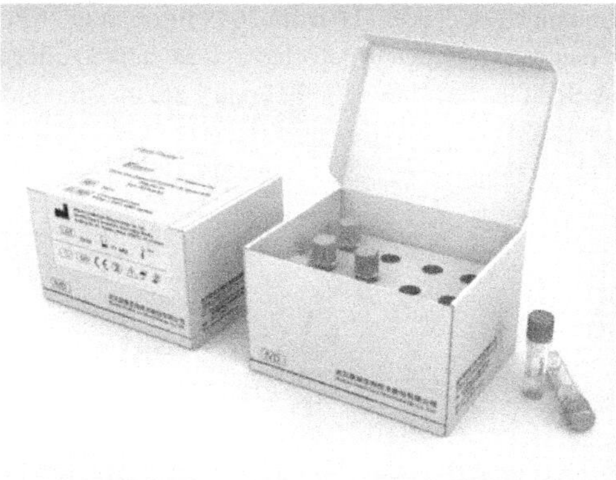

Year	Flu Cases	Covid Cases
2010-2011	21m	0
2011-2012	9m	0
2012-2013	34m	0
2013-2014	30m	0
2014-2015	30m	0
2015-2016	24m	0
2016-2017	29m	0
2017-2018	41m	0
2018-2019	29m	0
2019-2020	36m	0
2020-2021	0	57m

Figure 48 Flu versus Covid-19 cases in the USA 2010 to 2021

11.2.6. Discussion

In theory there is no difference between theory and practice,......while in practice there is.

Microbiology or virology theory is not our area of expertise hence we have not presented any arguments here rooted in theory. Instead, we have taken the sceptical option and asked - where is the empirical evidence? Anyone, no matter their credentials, can and should be able to ask this question.

We have found there is little empirical evidence that proves SARS-CoV-2 interferes with the flu in a dominant way. Therefore, there is no support for the widespread assumption that SARS-CoV-2 prevents flu's transmission or infection. This is one of the central planks of the Covid-19 crisis and it looks to be wrong.

Flu did not globally disappear since we know it was playing hide-and-seek in some far-flung places. If we accept flu was in circulation, then we must entertain the possibility of alternative explanations, not for the disappearance of flu, but for the disappearance of *positive* flu test results, especially false positive results.

Also, recall that flu disappeared simultaneously just as SARS-CoV-2 appeared simultaneously across the globe. The omicron variant of SARS-CoV-2 appeared at the end of 2021, and it did so in near synchronicity across the globe. Coincidentally flu then reappeared and did so simultaneously globally with no evidence of transmission from place to place. The sequence of these events does not concord with another central plank of virology - the idea of viral spread. A seasonal trigger is often touted as an explanation for the synchronous appearance of flu at the end of 2021, yet this does not explain the fact that flu had not disappeared from Haiti, Afghanistan, Pakistan, Bangladesh and Laos.

Despite the similarity of the symptoms of flu with those of SARS-CoV-2 it was, at least initially, the infection fatality rate for SARS-CoV-2 that differentiated it from the flu - its novelty was dependent on its perceived elevated lethality. However, over time the infection fatality rates for SARS-CoV-2 have converged on that for the flu and now the deadliness of one is indistinguishable from the other. Why then, three years later, do we consider SARS-CoV-2 to be more novel than flu or any other respiratory viral infection? Given that the symptoms of both overlap to an extent which makes each indistinguishable from the other based on clinical presentation, legitimate questions [394] have been raised as to the circumstances that led SARS-CoV-2 to be identified as a novel virus in the first place.

Given we cannot trust PCR tests for SARS-CoV-2, why should they be accepted as proof of the absence of flu? The evidence suggests that influenza and SARS-CoV-2 do not significantly interfere with each other, and given no false positives for flu were reported at all, how else can we explain the disappearance of flu except by changes in the PCR testing process? We know from the BioFire testing that all bacterial and viral pathogens except for SARS-CoV-2 decreased precipitously just when the pandemic was announced. This cannot be explained by viral or bacterial interference.

If flu has vanished there would surely be reduced evidence of zoonotic transmission of flu in animals, or from animals to humans via animal virus reservoirs (noted by "sl" [395]). Dogs, cats and other animals all get flu and coronaviruses, yet we have no evidence that flu has been displaced by SARS-CoV-2 in these various animal populations.

Of course, non-pharmaceutical interventions, such as masks and social distance are also touted as the reason for the disappearance of the flu but there is zero empirical or theoretical evidence to support this either. Indeed, if they worked for the flu why did they not work to prevent the transmission of SARS-CoV-2, given that the primary mechanism for both appears to be aerosol transmission?

The fact that flu did return and co-existed with SARS-CoV-2 during the twindemics of 2021/22 and 2022/23 should be the nail in the coffin for the idea that flu disappeared because of viral interference from a novel interloper.

These are no doubt controversial conclusions but, given the evidence, a reasonable question to ask is: Was Covid-19 disease actually entirely new, or is it simply caused by misattributing flu, or the myriad of other causes of respiratory illnesses, as SARS-CoV-2? Or is there some other unknown mechanism that generates one or the other or indeed both?

Chapter 12. The vanishing flu detection system

12.1. Sensors set to off

11 May 2023

Identification of any virus relies not only on the test itself but also on the protocols, procedures and the public health bureaucracy that govern when the test should be administered and how the test result is validated, interpreted and reported. So, a systematic assessment of the effects of seemingly unrelated policy decisions is needed to determine whether policies were enacted - wittingly or unwittingly - which brought about a particular result as a kind of 'spooky action at a distance' that caused flu to appear to vanish from some countries but not others.

Quarantines were promoted as measures to reduce the spread of SARS-CoV-2 and are claimed to have prevented the spread of flu. In this article, we investigate the possibility that what they actually did was dramatically reduce the chance of a positive flu test result. If you don't have a positive flu result, there is little possibility of being diagnosed with flu in the presence of an extremely contradictory explanation. Given that PCR tests for SARS-CoV-2 were mandated (when not enthusiastically and voluntarily performed by a populace terrified by propaganda) there was a very high chance of being diagnosed with Covid-19 instead of the flu.

This section is based on a fuller article with relevant screenshots here [396].

12.1.1. Algorithms and Policy

When examining the algorithms that govern the application of any tests we need to focus on the overall context, including:

- Pre-conditions exist that determine whether the test is encouraged or allowed to be done.
- Limitations on interpretation of the test result and whether it needs to be validated (i.e., confirmed by a repeat of the same or another type of test).
- Official information made available about the test performance specifications which influence the informativeness of the test result given the context of use.
- The probability of the patient having the virus given a positive or negative test result and how this might vary according to the background prevalence of infection.
- The cognitive dissonance at play when deciding what to do about test results for competing viruses (SARS-CoV-2 and flu)

So, a flu test result is only one part of the decision-making process that determines whether you have flu.

12.1.2. Influenza Testing Algorithms

Before we look at flu testing let's remind ourselves of the CDC protocols on SARS-CoV-2 testing and in particular testing in 'broad settings' [397]. Here the assumption is that testing takes place *en masse* with social distancing, masks, pre-screening, temperature checks and at special screening centres. Within these documents there is a huge amount of information on the context and conditions for testing - creating an impression of a wartime emergency, and thus reinforcing the view that SARS-CoV-2 is deadly.

But nowhere do these documents present an algorithm for deciding if a patient is infected with SARS-CoV-2. It's absent and entirely implicit. The idea that there is an outbreak is taken for granted. There is no recognition of any competing explanations for symptoms, such as other viruses, and because of this any reference to the possibility of false positives and negatives is entirely absent.

Ultimately, clinical judgement regarding Covid-19 is delegated from the physician to diagnosis based on PCR-test. Cultured samples aren't mentioned, and neither is confirmatory testing. In other words: "It's all about the test".

Now let's look at the CDC algorithms for the flu, the governing protocol for which is documented here [398] (10th August 2020). In the UK, annual flu numbers are estimated using modelling techniques, with the most important data used being those obtained from "sentinel testing" sites, which are specific GP surgeries who are asked to perform flu testing on anyone with symptoms suggestive of flu, for public health planning purposes. There is no easily accessible UK information equivalent to that issued by the CDC in the USA, but it can probably be assumed the general principles are the same.

In contrast to SARS-CoV-2, flu testing is remarkably straightforward but loaded with qualifying criteria that the physician is instructed to actively consider.

PCR is only recommended for symptomatic hospitalised patients but for symptomatic outpatients the rapid molecular assay test should be considered. Other, less reliable, tests, such as rapid antigen tests are only recommended if other tests are unavailable. Culturing of virus samples is only recommended for the purposes of confirmation. Furthermore, testing is recommended within 4 days of symptom onset, presumably because of the decay in the presence of live virus and the reduced capability of tests to detect virus in diminishingly small quantities.

It is fascinating to learn that flu testing is governed by a single question acting as a pre-condition to the testing process: Is flu in circulation in the community? When there is no epidemiological outbreak present this algorithm [399] is applied, but a completely different algorithm [400] applies when flu is acknowledged by the public health authorities to be in circulation. In the event of a positive test the clinician is asked to pause and consider if this is a false positive. Furthermore, they would need to justify any decision to support the positive result and diagnose flu with an assessment of whether there is evidence of an epidemiological link between this case and others (i.e., link to existing circulation in the community).

Likewise, the clinician would also have to consider the signs and symptoms of flu, but given these will heavily overlap with covid, which the authorities are proclaiming as an epidemic, it looks like the cards are stacked against them.

Finally, it calls for the clinician to initiate antiviral treatment as a consequence of the positive test result, thus incurring expense and potential waste.

The default here is that influenza is highly likely given the flu test result is positive. There is no call to reconsider the symptoms or to consider if there really is a genuine outbreak. Also, there is no call to consider expensive anti-viral treatment (whether or not there are incentives to use them depends on norms of practice in different locations). All in all, this is an easier call to make than diagnosing flu when it is 'not in circulation'.

There is an elegant logical circularity at play here that a doctor needs to consider. You need an outbreak and an epidemiological link to help justify a positive influenza test, but surely you only know there is an outbreak, and can determine an epidemiological link, if you and others, in coordination, have already accumulated enough positive test results. It's a chicken and egg situation. Who determines whether there is an outbreak? None of the CDC documents say. Clearly individual physicians do not have the authority to make such a decision themselves. A hospital's authorities could maybe do so after liaising with public health authorities, but at a national or international level such a decision would be in the hands of the centralized public health bureaucracy.

So, compared to SARS-CoV-2, diagnosing flu 'out of season' appears fraught with tricky clinical and bureaucratic questions.

12.1.3. Accuracy of flu testing

The controversy around the accuracy of the SARS-CoV-2 PCR test is well known, but there is much less discussion about the accuracy of the flu tests. The reported accuracies for the flu rapid molecular assay test are that they have a perfect specificity (!) and high sensitivity (between 90-95%). These are CDC numbers. Values from research papers can vary wildly, sometimes down to around 60%. Also, specificity numbers are usually not given but implicitly assumed to be 100% based on a very small number of challenge samples.

The one thing the CDC are very careful to advise about is the time from onset of symptoms to the application of the flu test, which they say should be less than four days. This is the time window for viral shedding. Any upper respiratory tract test will be more reliable the shorter the delay between symptoms and administration of the test. Waiting for longer than four days might lead to the test failing to detect live virus in someone who has suffered or is suffering flu.

The seminal paper on influenza and immunology was written by Nobel laureate Peter Doherty (Doherty et al. [401]) and appeared in nature in 2006, and states:

> "Influenza viruses grow rapidly in the human respiratory mucosa, allowing transmission to colleagues and family members via respiratory droplet inhalation (coughs and sneezes) even before the development of obvious symptoms."

Exposure to flu for the first time provokes a primary response by the immune system which reduces viral titres to zero within 10-12 days. So, someone young, who contracts flu for the first time in their lives, would largely clear the virus within 10 days. Someone older who has contracted flu more than once in their lives will enjoy a secondary immune response and will clear the virus within five days.

Liu et al [402] report that co-infection rates for flu and SARS-CoV-2 should be much higher than reported simply because of the shorter time window for incubation and viral shedding in flu compared to SARS-CoV-2:

> "Results from a meta-analysis of 54 related publications indicated an overall proportion of coinfection with influenza viruses in SARS-CoV-2-positive patients of 0.7%. An over 18-month period study with 17,011 adults with SARS-CoV-2 infection shows 1.3% of coinfection with influenza viruses. However, the actual coinfection rate may be much higher in that some coinfected patients may have undetectable influenza virus at the time SARS-CoV-2 infection is diagnosed. This happens because the mean incubation and viral shedding times of influenza viruses (2 and 3 days, respectively) are much shorter than those of SARS-CoV-2 (6 and 17 days, respectively)"

A positive flu test should only occur when there is enough flu virus to detect. For those who are older and have been pre-exposed to the flu this means the test needs to be applied after symptom onset, giving a target time window of 4 days. For younger people, previously unexposed to the flu, the target time window to apply the flu test would be, at most, 10 days. After that the chance of a positive would reduce substantially.

12.1.4. Quarantines and their effects

So, what could cause a delay in testing and a reduction in the chances of a test detecting a flu virus? Policy requirements for SARS-CoV-2 quarantines of course!

From Spring 2020 to end of 2021 the advice was that a person should not visit a GP or hospital if they had respiratory symptoms, on the assumption that these were diagnostic of SARS-CoV-2. For example, (as can be seen in the screenshots shown in the full article [396]):

> US Alaska state advice on Covid-19 was simply: "STAYE HOME IF YOU FEEL SICK"
>
> US Georgia state advice on Covid-19: "If you no symptoms but have contacted someone who tested SARS-CoV-2 positive you are required to quarantine for up to 14 days and only seek admission to hospital if a respiratory condition develops and then significantly deteriorates. You need a negative covid test to re-enter society, sourced from a centralised centre." Note that these centres only tested for SARS-CoV-2, hence flu was never tested for.

If symptoms were severe and someone was admitted to hospital a SARS-CoV-2 PCR test admission would have been performed immediately. People with symptoms would already have stayed at home, in quarantine, for a period up to two weeks from symptom onset. Thus, crucial time was lost from symptom onset to presentation to hospital or GPs, and this introduced a delay, supposedly to keep society safe.

So, most people with respiratory symptoms would have stayed away from all health services for much longer than four days.

After four days the accuracy of the flu test would have deteriorated significantly, and had they been tested for flu the test result would likely have been negative given it was done up to two weeks after symptoms started.

Likewise, the availability of flu tests was resource limited, yet Covid-19 tests were readily available. The effects of this on Covid-19 and flu rates were recognised in the UK national influenza report [403] which said:

> "Surveillance indicators suggest that COVID-19 activity at a national level has increased during week 51. There is currently limited testing for other respiratory viruses, however, laboratory indicators suggest that influenza activity is low."

It is inevitable that influenza activity will be low if there is limited testing for it!

In parallel with this, the ready availability of a mandated covid test, subject to excessively high cycle thresholds (or deliberate gene miscounting) would have increased the chances of a covid false positive test result.

Before the widespread adoption of multi-viral PCR test kits, which test for multiple viruses in parallel, most of the testing done in 2020 and 2021 would have involved sequentially testing people for different respiratory viruses. Here the decision to conduct a subsequent test would only be made following the obtaining of a negative previous test. This process efficiently minimises the amount of testing done and allows the physician to target the most likely pathogen. So, even if a physician was considering flu as a possibility, the SARS-CoV-2 PCR test would always have been the first test performed and given the high likelihood of a positive test result subsequent tests for flu would not have taken place. And as we say, if a flu test was performed it would likely show negative for flu even if that was the causative agent because of the time delay introduced by quarantine.

12.1.5. Cognitive dissonance

Even if the SARS-CoV-2 test was negative and the flu test was positive the flu test result would likely have been discounted as a false positive. Why? Because the CDC flowchart instructs the physician to suspect that it is!

The rationale would go something like this a) there is no outbreak of flu b) there is no epidemiological link to get the result accepted by health authorities c) Covid-19 disease is deadlier than the flu so a diagnostic misclassification would be risky and d) the antiviral treatments for flu do not apply to Covid-19.

If a flu test was done and it was positive the physician might have a conundrum if there was a positive SARS-CoV-2 test result for the same patient. How would this be resolved? There may be potential for cognitive dissonance here. Recall that all advice on Covid-19 diagnosis was to assume, even in the absence of a SARS-CoV-2 positive test, that the patient had been infected with SARS-CoV-2. With the weight of coercive pressure on the side of SARS-CoV-2 diagnosis, and with the incentives in place to diagnose SARS-CoV-2, it is inevitable that there was no logical reason for a physician to consider that a flu test result is anything other than a false positive. And even more so given they have been told that flu had disappeared and that there was a SARS-CoV-2 epidemic and 'flu had been driven out by SARS-CoV-2".

Imagine going to your boss admitting having done a flu test and presenting them with a positive when the WHO and every health authority in the world has said it has disappeared? It would be professional suicide.

A clinician's cognitive decision-making process can be simulated by a Bayesian model showing how all the above factors combine to drive a diagnostic decision that favours Covid-19 and suppresses any chance of a true positive for flu (see the appendix here [396]).

12.1.6. Changes to death certification helped vanish the flu

The WHO guidelines [404] on cause for death certification and coding essentially caused reporting of flu and other viral infections as causes of death to disappear:

> "A death due to COVID-19 is defined for surveillance purposes **as a death resulting from a clinically compatible illness**, in a probable or confirmed COVID-19 case, unless there is a clear alternative cause of death that cannot be related to COVID disease (e.g. trauma). There should be no period of complete recovery from COVID-19 between illness and death.
>
> A **death due to COVID-19 may not be attributed to another disease** (e.g. cancer) and should be counted independently of preexisting conditions that are suspected of triggering a severe course of COVID-19."

And with regard to the death coding (ICD-10):

> "COVID-19 is not considered as due to, or as an obvious consequence of, anything else in analogy to the coding rules applied for INFLUENZA. Further to this, there is no provision in the classification to link COVID-19 to other causes or modify its coding in any way."

And on the requirements of public health versus an accurate medical diagnosis:

> "...whether a sequence is listed as 'rejected' or 'accepted' may reflect **interests of importance for public health** rather than what is acceptable from a purely medical point of view. Therefore, **always apply these instructions, whether they can be considered medically correct or not**."

Given influenza is clinically compatible with Covid-19, but a doctor is prohibited from coding the cause of death as influenza then the death certificate will give the primary cause of death as Covid-19 even if the supposed underlying cause of death was influenza (or any other viral infection).

Reporting requirements were made clear at local levels, showing that the central instructions emanating from the WHO propagated throughout national healthcare systems within days of being released. The Covid-19 death certification protocol [405] for Cambridgeshire and Peterborough in the UK (which could be applied by video link!) Mere suspicion of Covid-19 as the cause of death was judged sufficient:

> "If a patient dies with clinically probable COVID-19 but the results of confirmatory swabs are not yet available, put cause of death as COVID-19 infection."

12.1.7. Discussion about the vanishing flu

Prior to 2020 some patients would have been picked up by sentinel testing [406] in outpatient settings or at GPs and would have been reported as a flu case if they tested positive simply because they would have been tested in time. But post spring 2020 until winter 2021 the chance of such a positive result from the medical system would have been vanishingly small even if testing was performed, which was extremely rare.

Also bear in mind the sheer hysteria around Covid-19 in 2020 and 2021 would have affected clinical decision making. Key variables would also have heavily influenced decision making, including unfounded assertions from governments and the mainstream media like:

- Symptoms previously associated with the flu were now firmly associated with SARS-CoV-2.
- Asymptomatic people were told to assume they had the SARS-CoV-2 virus.
- SARS-CoV-2 was recognised as more infectious and deadlier than the flu.

In conclusion, the delays built into the quarantine system may have created a substantially depressed likelihood of detecting and diagnosing flu, if someone was lucky enough to get a flu test. Similarly, there would have been a hugely increased chance of a positive being overridden by a Covid-19 false positive or being dismissed as a false positive anyway, given that an epidemic of SARS-CoV-2 had been declared and flu was said to have disappeared.

In any case there is ample evidence that WHO directed changes to national death certification systems essentially eradicated flu from death certificates and replaced it with Covid-19, whether there was a positive Covid-19 test result or not.

12.2. Finding the Flu is easy, just Google it!

26 May 2023

This section is based on a fuller article with relevant screenshots here [407].

The flu supposedly vanished during the SARS-Cov-2 pandemic, but internet searches for 'flu' continued as normal.

Detecting trends in searches for salient terms made on internet search engines, such as Google, has been touted as a way of better predicting and potentially managing events. One obvious application is to predict health emergencies, such as pandemics, in advance of, or as they occur. For instance, Sam Gilbert, an affiliated researcher, for the Bennet Institute of Public Policy [408] at Cambridge University describes various ways in which he helped UK SAGE (Scientific Advisory Group for Emergencies) use Covid-19 search data.

At a national level the use of search data is already used as a signal of flu trends. An example is the UK's flu-detector [409] system that tracked internet searches using Google Trends [410]. Other countries use similar systems too.

It is believed in public health circles that there is a well-established relationship that an increase in internet searches for keywords is a reliable indicator of some spreading disease or pathogen affecting the general public.

Given that official sources stated that the flu had vanished from many countries during their normal flu seasons in 2020/21 and 2021/22 we would expect that the frequency of internet searches by the general public would therefore have decreased significantly during those times. This is especially so given that the world was in SARS-CoV-2 panic mode and Covid-19 propaganda was in full swing. But is this the case?

Let's look at the Google Trends results for a number of countries, that the WHO reported, via their FluNet surveillance system [411], which had experienced no flu in 2020/21 and 2021/2022.

A self-explanatory red box is used to highlight areas of obvious difference between Google Trends and FluNet. In order, we will look at: UK, USA, Canada, Australia, New Zealand and Sweden as shown in Figure 49.

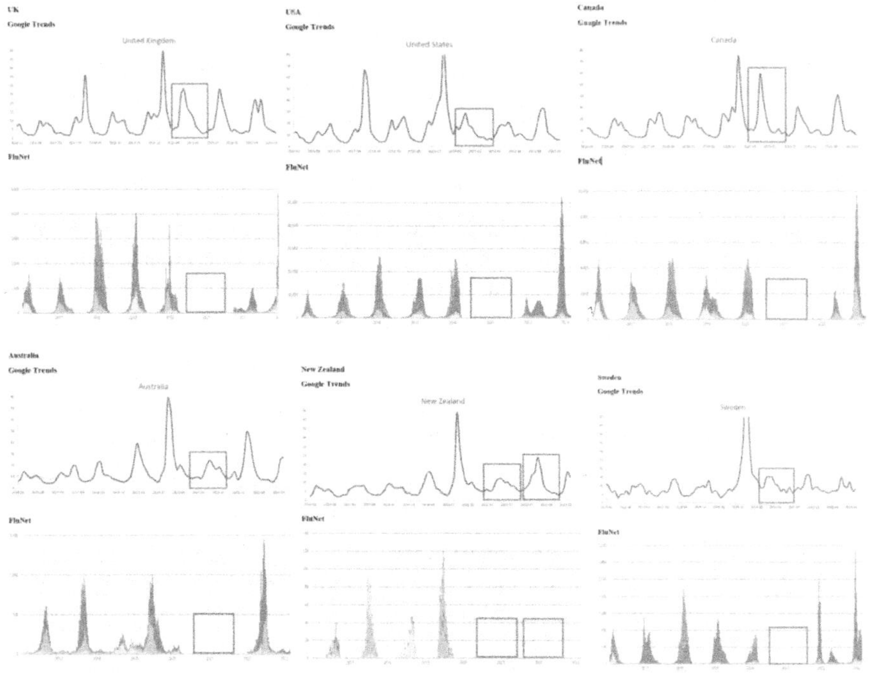

Figure 49 Google trends compared with FluNet surveillance system

Google search data for 'flu' shows that people were concerned enough to search for flu at the very time when flu had as reported by the WHO, scientists and national public health authorities, apparently vanished. And the public in each country performed these searches at the very time when the seasonal flu normally affects their country. This is clear across the globe, in northern hemisphere countries that experience summer flu seasons and in southern hemisphere countries with (their) winter flu seasons.

Some countries only 'missed' one flu season. Others missed two. Yet in all cases people in those countries searched for flu at the exact times when flu was expected.

Can the absence of flu from all of the above WHO FluNet charts be simply explained by a lack of reporting? Apart from New Zealand in 2023 (which is not red boxed) the answer to this question is a resounding no.

The WHO FluNet data is assumed to be 'ground truth' and relied upon as such. Many dozens of scientific research papers and hundreds of newspaper reports have asserted or reported that flu had vanished. Scientific and health policy making have subsequently mistakenly assumed the disappearance of flu as an unquestionable fact. For example, in virology an edifice has been built to prove the idea that viral interference between flu and SARS-CoV-2 is true and, in turn, this supports the notion that Covid-19 was both novel and deadly.

All of these major mistakes are now 'baked in' to the historical record. At best, the public health authorities may simply be wrong, or, at worst, this discovery suggests a scale of data manipulation that cannot be explained by simple human error.

If flu was in circulation, as these internet searches appear to suggest, does this mean that some or all of the respiratory infections and deaths that were originally attributed to SARS-CoV-2 may actually have been caused by flu?

The national and international health authorities have - wittingly or unwittingly - suffered a catastrophic failure in flu detection and reporting. Either that or Google's data cannot be trusted. We will leave it up to the reader to decide which of these options presents the most credible explanation.

12.3. Do Not Seek and Ye Shall Not Find

1 June 2023

This section is based on a fuller article with relevant screenshots, charts, tables and figures here [412].

Did flu surveillance and reporting systems (intentionally?) fail to detect flu?

In this section we look into flu surveillance systems and flu data reporting, mainly in the UK. A hodge podge of flu surveillance systems have consistently reported on flu prior to 2020 and continued to have some role to play post Spring 2020 until flu returned at the end of 2021. In the UK flu surveillance is done via clinical surveillance by primary care (based on networks of GPs), and the FluDetector and the FluSurvey systems.

Our investigations into flu surveillance use in the UK suggest they were either not picking up signals, that were in fact present, or were (intentionally?) deactivated for the duration of what would have been a normal flu season in 2020-2021.

We also looked at UK ONS data for influenza and pneumonia in 2020-2022. We discovered a reporting gap for flu in 2020 when all respiratory disease reporting switched to focus myopically on Covid-19. And then, in 2021 and 2022 the ONS re-started flu reporting and influenza and pneumonia deaths returned.

However, we discovered a hitherto much ignored source of government statistics: The UK NOMIS system. This showed that, for the whole of 2020, there is no significant change in the number of deaths caused by flu, compared with previous years, directly contradicting the ONS data. Likewise, the 2020 deaths recorded as caused by flu in the USA were also similar to that seen in previous years.

12.3.1. FluDetector

Credence has been given to the idea of tracking pandemics, such as the UK's flu-detector [413] system, which tracks internet searches using Google trends (note that this guidance document was withdrawn in October 2022, without explanation and replaced with new systems). The chart produced by UK the flu-detector [414] system from April 2017 to the present showed there was no flu signal in the winter of 2020-21. But it is important to realise that the output of the system isn't raw data but is rather modelled output that processes the data through a sophisticated machine learning system (a non-linear Gaussian process model).

We can easily verify this 'modelled' output against the raw data by turning to Google Trends for the ground truth on searches for "Flu". As we showed in our previous article (see Figure 49 above), there is a clear signal in winter 2020-21 showing that people were in fact searching for flu. Yet the UK surveillance system, that claims to use Google's own data as the basis for its calculations, has either not detected this Google signal, or somehow suppressed it. How can this difference be explained? Have the Gaussian process models simply failed and performed so catastrophically, or is there some fault in Google's search data archives?

Data from the UKHSA national weekly flu reports [415] confirm the NHS were recording people with cold/flu symptoms at the time they were searching for flu on Google. The peak for cold/flu of just over 20,000 online assessments in September 2020 (when flu was said to be absent) is even slightly higher than the peak for covid during the same period. Yet, despite this, the 'modelled' data from the flu surveillance system fails to pick up this signal.

So here we have independently checked the FluDetector system against that provided by UKHSA and Google itself, both of which report a signal for flu in 20/21, and yet FluDetector shows no signal for that season. It is hard to explain away this failure and the implications of this difference are potentially quite sinister. Were machine learning systems introduced to suppress the flu signal and help convince the world that flu had disappeared from the UK? Or is there some innocent explanation? Or is this story repeated in different countries which also used automated flu surveillance systems?

12.3.2. FluSurvey

The UK FluSurvey was originally conceived to survey a panel of self-selecting participants for signs and symptoms of influenza-like illnesses (ILIs). In March 2020 it was repurposed to cover both Covid-19 and flu symptoms, and the routine questionnaire was adapted to capture Covid-19 specific information.

In June 2020 the FluSurvey reported the 2019/20 provisional results [417] for flu, which only ran up to week 12 - the end of March 2020. The last 3 months' worth of data up until June 2020 are entirely missing. Note that all reports FluSurvey use links to archives of their website accessible using the web archive Wayback machine. By October 2020 this had not been updated [418] despite the survey continuing. However, 'health care seeking behaviour' reports were produced instead, and the symptoms fever, cough and loss of smell were tracked but not explicitly attributed to either flu or Covid-19.

This kind of reporting continued until January 2021 when the FluSurvey website announced [419] that they had decided back in November 2020, at the start of the normal UK flu season, to discontinue using FluSurvey to track both flu and Covid-19:

> "The 2020/21 flu season has now began, we are not reporting both influenza like illness (ILI) and Covid-19 related symptoms using this platform. Changes to how we report the data commenced on the 2nd of November, 2020."

In January 2021 they then helpfully updated the ILI incidence chart to include up to week 20 of 2020 (only half a year's data),

Fast forward to the next update of the website on November 30 2021, almost a full year later, and we find this statement [420] on the website:

> "The 2021/22 flu season has now begun, we continue to report both influenza like illness (ILI) and Covid-19 related symptoms through the surveillance system. Data represents UK residents who have registered to participate during the survey period."

So, they make a spontaneous decision to do an about turn and track both Covid-19 and flu together using FluSurvey at the end of 2021. And they state that they know the 2021/22 flu season has now begun! How do they know this when the chart previously reported in January 2021 had apparently not been updated at that time, in November 2021? And how do they know it would come back when flu had disappeared?

FluSurvey reports fed into the UKHSA national flu report for the first time from 8 October 2020. They did not explicitly appear in any national flu report before that date, including before the covid pandemic.

The UKHSA week 28 national flu report (15 July 2021) [421] contains the FluSurvey 'healthcare seeking behaviour' chart, show in Figure 50, can be found on page 32.

Notice that the rate of fever and coughs between weeks 37 of 2020 and week 3 of 2021 is consistently above 25 per 1,000 participants and peaks at 50 per 1,000 participants (right hand scale on chart). Also note that the ILI line in the chart is blank up to week 43 confirming the decision to not formally track ILIs as noted on the FluSurvey website and instead formally attribute cough and fever symptoms to Covid-19.

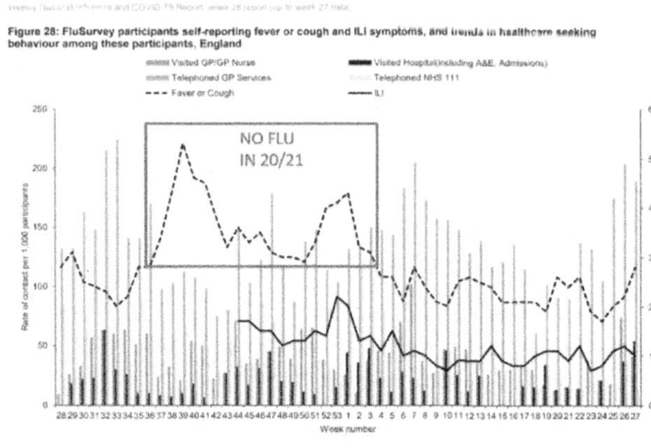

Figure 50 UK FluSurvey 'health care seeking behaviour' report from July 2021

The UKHSA week 4 national flu report (27 January 2022) [422] contains the FluSurvey 'healthcare seeking behaviour' chart, shown in Figure 51, which can be found on page 35. Here the rate of fever and coughs peaks at approximately 70 per 1,000 participants during the 2021/22 flu season, weeks 37 2021 to week 3 2022. Notice that throughout this period the ILI (black line) is charted and acknowledges the rate of ILIs.

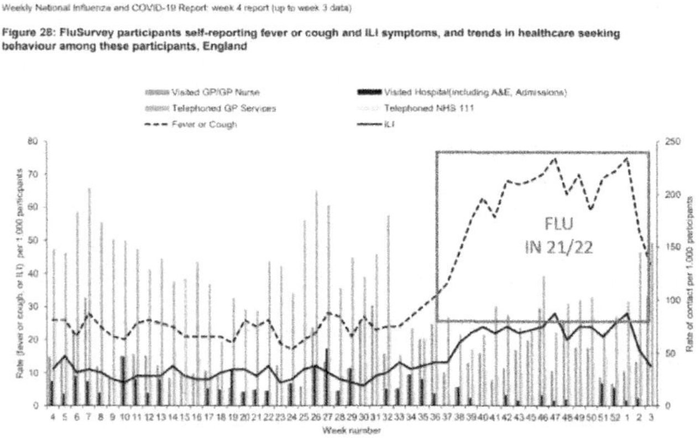

Figure 51 UK FluSurvey 'health care seeking behaviour' report from January 2022

The peaks marked in each of the above charts are remarkably similar. Given the purpose of the FluSurvey is to track flu symptoms, and fever and cough are a primary method for doing so, this surely suggests that there is evidence of a flu peak in 2020/21 when it was claimed to be absent. And at a time when FluSurvey decided to change its reporting standards (November 2020).

Let's review the sequence of events:

- FluSurvey tracked ILI incidence only until week 20 of 2020 and never updated this data.
- They decided to no longer track both flu and covid from November 2020 but only report this change in policy in January 2021.
- FluSurvey stated they (presciently) knew in January 2021 that the flu season had now begun and did so after witnessing the near eradication of flu from March 2020 to May 2020.
- Fever and cough symptoms were tracked and peak in a similar way and this continued, but tracking ILI incidence was abandoned, thus reducing the strength of the flu signal.

This surveillance data and timeline of reporting policy decisions is suspicious:

- Why decide to track both viruses March 2020 to November 2020 (outside of the normal flu season), then stop doing so without explanation?
- Why was ILI tracking abandoned when fever and cough symptoms were peaking in 2020/21?
- Why claim the 2020/21 flu season had begun and stop reporting flu and Covid-19 using the system?
- Why then switch back to reporting both viruses again in November 2021 and declare the flu season had begun with ZERO surveillance evidence flu had returned?

Even more damming is the evidence that in the UK Covid-19 test results were fast tracked and had to be reported [423] within 24 hours, whilst positive influenza tests were allowed to take up to 7 days. The Public Health England week 50 influenza and Covid-19 report (page 43) [424] makes clear that up to week 41 of 2020 all tests were SARS-CoV-2 only. Apparently, no testing for influenza was being done!

12.3.3. Anecdotal reports about flu testing

This self-explanatory comment [425] concerns flu testing in Germany:

> "I would like to contribute some information about what happened to the flu here in Germany.
>
> My sister-in-law Marianne is working as a receptionist in a so called Sentinel-Klinik in south-west of Baden-Württemberg. A sentinel-clinic is a clinic which reports regularly to Robert Koch Institut (RKI) which is the federal authority of health. There are some 200 sentinel-clinics in Germany. On basis of these reports number of flu-cases and flu-deaths is estimated by RKI. Which ends up in quite an exact estimation.
>
> Marianne told us in Winter 2020/21 "In former years when a patient was brought to us into our hospital who had respitorial problems we always did a test on influenza.

> And we all ways reported the result to RKI. This was obligatory. In this winter in case a patient arrives with respitorial problems we don't do any test on influenza. Not one!"
>
> In other words: All of the flu-deaths in Germany have been mislabeled into corona-deaths. These deaths were urgently needed in order to fabricate the "second wave" of which people had been frightened so much. Without this trick no "second wave" of corona would have appeared and vaccine rollout would have been hampered."

Australia did not experience flu or SARS-Cov-2 in 2020. This report [426] attributes the disappearance of flu in Australia to physical distancing and good hand hygiene.

There are obvious questions about whether NPIs can really explain the absence of flu in Australia given they weren't mandated in summer 2020 and were not stringently applied. Furthermore, they subsequently failed to prevent Covid-19. In the comments section of our substack Dr Emilie Larkin and Dr Irandani Anandi Ranasinghe-Markus also drew our attention to changes in testing policy involving drastically reduced flu testing.

Here is another report [427] highlighting the same issues from the WHO:

> "Sentinel surveillance for influenza stopped in early March and was redirected to the detection of SARS-CoV-2. Influenza surveillance has resumed for the 2020/21 season. One challenge for resuming influenza surveillance is getting access to representative samples from the hospital laboratories due to the externalization of SARS-CoV-2 testing."

Finally in this video interview [428] Lisa Brackenridge, former nurse, states that the normal flu screening was 'more or less abandoned' and whereas historically normally people would be given a flu screen, if they presented with respiratory symptoms, from January 2020 to January 2021 she only, say, five or six screens done over that whole period.

This evidence suggest testing resources were indeed diverted to SARS-CoV-2 testing from routine flu testing, and hence routine surveillance systems were dismantled.

12.3.4. Change in the gold standard

Some hospitals (see, for example the screenshot from Northwell Hospital in Figure 52) were not culturing flu viruses [429] in the same way as before, so the gold standard had changed just as the pandemic began, with a switch over the multiplex array PCR. The head of Northwell Health Laboratory said in a call [430] to the CDC that they were prioritising testing for SARS-CoV-2. It is conceivable that this change may have occurred globally.

Three days earlier the streptococcus pneumoniae antigen, serum test was withdrawn and replaced with a urine test (for a respiratory pathogen!)

12.3.5. ONS and FOI responses

The UK ONS report mortality statistics for each year. The statistics for England and Wales are available for download here [431]. The 2020 dataset [432] contains information that excludes any report on influenza and pneumonia deaths, and instead is wholly focused on deaths 'involving' Covid-19. In contrast the 2021 dataset [433] does contain data on influenza and pneumonia deaths, starting on January 8th 2021.

Unlike the 2021 dataset, the section "Weekly figures by cause" is not present in the 2020 dataset. The ONS do not provide weekly figures by cause data for anything other than Covid-19 before 2021.

In 2020 all Covid-19 deaths are categorised as 'involving' Covid-19 (codes U07.1, U07.2, U09.9, U10.9) rather than due to Covid-19 (codes U07.1, U07.2, U10.9) and in 2021 Covid-19 and pneumonia & flu deaths are categorised as 'involving' (J09-J18) and 'due to' (J09-J18). So, in 2020 official ONS statistics any reporting of flu deaths was completely abandoned in favour of Covid-19 reports.

☐NEW TEST ☒TEST CHANGE
NOTIFICATION DATE: MARCH 5,2020
EFFECTIVE DATE: Immediately

Viral Respiratory Culture (V VCR)

Effective immediately, in order to prevent inadvertent culture of SARS-CoV-2, the cause of COVID-19, the Viral Respiratory Culture (V VCR) test will become nonorderable. The alternative test is the (V RVP RAP). If a Viral Respiratory Culture is ordered this test will be cancelled and the alternative Respiratory Viral/Bacti Detection by NAT (V RVP RAP) test will be added on.

Test Requirement/Parameter	New Test Order V RVP RAP	Previous Test Order V VCR
Method:	Multiplex Amplified nucleic acid test PCR	Viral Culture
Sample	Collect specimen using a flexible shaft nasopharyngeal flocked swab. Dacron, rayon, or nylon swabs with plastic or wire shafts is also acceptable. **(Calcium alginate, charcoal, or cotton tipped swab with wooden or metal shaft are not acceptable.)** Place the swab into a tube containing 2 to 3 mL of viral transport medium (M4 or UTM) close tightly. Indicate source	Same collection

Figure 52 Northwell hospital stop culturing flu virus

An official response to an FOI request [434] for deaths from influenza January - April 2020 stated there were 2,287 recorded deaths, in England, caused by influenza and pneumonia in March alone, and up until May 2020 there were 31,315 deaths from 'respiratory disease' as the underlying cause of death:

> "We publish a dataset for deaths registered weekly in England and Wales [435], which includes figures for deaths by all respiratory diseases and the coronavirus (COVID-19). In this publication, influenza deaths are not shown separately, instead they are included in respiratory deaths (ICD Code J00 - J99). The totals shown in this dataset are for underlying cause only. As at 1 May 2020 (latest available data), **the total number of deaths where respiratory disease was the underlying cause of death, in England and Wales for 2020, was recorded as 31,315 deaths.**

The accompanying bulletin [436] for deaths registered weekly in England and Wales reports the number of deaths involving influenza and pneumonia (where COVID-19 was not also on the death certificate) in Figure 1. Additionally, the bulletin reports the total deaths involving influenza and pneumonia (but not COVID-19), in England and Wales for 2020, as at 1 May (latest available data) is 44,240 deaths. This total includes all deaths where influenza and pneumonia were mentioned somewhere on the death certificate and COVID-19 was not mentioned.

On 16 April we published analysis into "Deaths involving COVID-19, England and Wales: deaths occurring in March 2020", [437] which provides further detail into underlying causes, however, please note that the analysis presented is for England and Wales. This shows the breakdown of COVID-19 deaths with an underlying cause of Influenza and pneumonia. Table 1 of the data tables [438] accompanying this publication also provides a breakdown of underlying cause for all deaths for March. **There were 2,287 recorded deaths, in England, caused by influenza and pneumonia**."

Hence, flu deaths have been included in a catch-all category with ICD code J00-J99 for respiratory deaths up until May 2020, but we have specific influenza death data only for the single month of March 2020, when the pandemic started.

The ONS 2020 mortality report [439] makes no mention of reported flu deaths in 2020 giving the impression flu was absent, but when we examine the ONS reports for deaths caused by pneumonia & flu in 2021 and 2022 there were 16,079 and 20,008 reported respectively, so for all years apart from 2020 they are happy to provide accurate flu data.

AlternativeNarrative noticed that the ONS report [440] on deaths registered weekly in England and Wales, from January 2021 reported these flu deaths:

> "Of the 8,433 deaths involving COVID-19 in Week 4 in England and Wales, 7,610 had this recorded as the underlying cause of death (90.2%).
>
> Of the 5,719 deaths that involved Influenza and Pneumonia, 298 had this recorded as the underlying cause of death (5.2%)."

12.3.6. NOMIS and WONDER mortality statistics

Of course, absence of evidence is not evidence of absence - can we find evidence for flu from other data sources? Luckily, we can.

Data for pneumonia and flu deaths can be extracted from the UK NOMIS (official census and labour market statistics) [441] system. However, this only provides yearly totals rather than weekly figures. The coding system used shows deaths 'due to influenzas or pneumonia' rather than 'involving' (codes J09-J18). When we queried this system, we were quite shocked to find that it returns influenza and pneumonia deaths for 2020, and these are reported at a rate consistent with previous years (the data for 2021 is flagged as provisional in the system). See Figure 53.

So why does the NOMIS system list flu deaths in 2020 but the ONS reports do not in 2020? Perhaps they never got the memo? Why did the ONS only release flu data in response to an

FOI request? The FOI request stated there were 2,287 deaths in England in March alone, at a time there was supposed to be little to no flu. At the same time the 3,234 Covid-19 deaths was taken to be a sign of a pandemic caused by a novel and deadly virus.

The presence of flu deaths in 2020 in the UK is repeated elsewhere. In the USA influenza and pneumonia numbers are similar in 2020 to previous years, as reported in the CDC WONDER system [442], with 53,544 deaths in 2020 compared to between approximately 50-60k deaths in each year from 2015 to 2019.

Mortality statistics - underlying cause, sex and age

ONS Crown Copyright Reserved [from Nomis on 3 May 2023]

area type	countries	
area name	England and Wales	
gender	Total	
age	total (all ages)	
measure	Deaths	
Date	**A00-R99,U00-Y89 All causes, all ages**	**J09-J18 Influenza and pneumonia**
2018	540,265	29,451
2019	529,553	26,342
2020	607,099	20,130
2021	585,484	16,232

Figure 53 UK NOMIS mortality statistics for influenza and pneumonia

Routine mortality reporting by the ONS switched to Covid-19 in 2020 and flu is only included in surveillance reports from 2021, thus giving the impression flu had disappeared.

The NOMIS system shows for whole of 2020 that there was no significant change in the number of deaths caused by flu and pneumonia (20,130), compared to previous years, directly contradicting the ONS, which deliberately published no comprehensive data on flu.

In the USA the CDC also report flu deaths in 2020 at levels consistent with historical patterns where we can interpret an influenza death is simply a flu-positive pneumonia death.

Despite these facts the WHO's international flu surveillance system, FluNet, shows no significant flu for 2020/21 in either the UK or USA.

Chapter 13. The fightback against vaccine hesitancy relied on dodgy data

13.1. Claims the unvaccinated were at higher risk were wrong

They were based on deliberately murky record keeping (7 March 2023)

13.1.1. Switching narrative to counter vaccine 'hesitancy'

By late 2021 it was already clear in the UK that the covid vaccines did not stop infection or transmission. And there were also already plenty of concerning safety signals. So, even though the "vaccine pass" was then required in the UK to participate in daily life, 'vaccine hesitancy' was on the increase.

Given this increasing resistance against the vaccine programme, the official messaging was changed from "vaccines stop you getting covid" to "vaccines stop you being hospitalised and dying from covid".

To push this new narrative the Government started pumping out 'data' to support the claim that almost all of those ill in hospital with covid were unvaccinated. Figure 54 shows an NHS text that was sent to everybody registered with a GP in the UK in November 2021

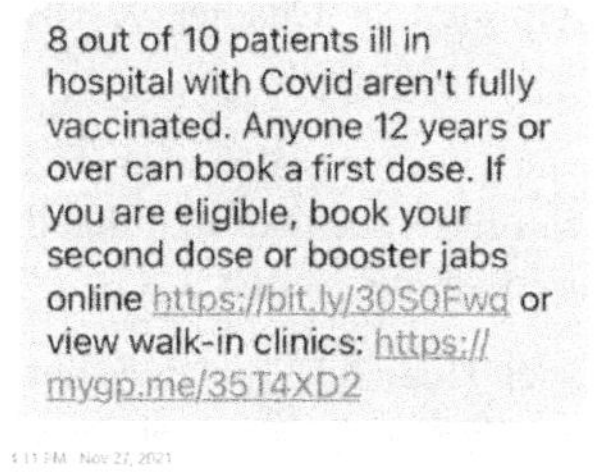

Figure 54 NHS text message booster invitation

At the time the text was sent out, "fully vaccinated" in the UK was defined as: "at least 14 days since 3rd jab" or "between at least 14 days and less than 6 months of 2nd jab". So, the official figure of 8 out of 10 "not fully vaccinated" might have been right but was totally misleading since almost ALL of those who were vaccinated (i.e., had at least one jab) at that time were "not fully vaccinated".

This creates a false semantic equivalence between 'unvaccinated' and 'not fully vaccinated'.

Many media sources, including the BBC [443], pushed the 80% unvaccinated claim without even mentioning the 'fully vaccinated' criteria (screenshots for all of the following media claims are on the full version of this article [444]). For example:

> 17 Dec 2021. BBC Headline: "Covid: Addenbrooke's boss says 80% of virus patients are unvaccinated"

1 Nov 2021. Independent Headline: "Unvaccinated Britons 32 times more likely to die with Covid" (note the use of "with" rather than "of").

6 July 2021: Guardian Headline: "99.2% of US Covid deaths in June were unvaccinated, says Fauci"

15 Dec 2021: Bloomberg UK News Headline: "Unvaccinated Covid Patients Push Hospital Systems past the Brink"

With respect to patients in ICU claims [445] that high proportions of those with covid were unvaccinated were widely cited - and never challenged - in the mainstream media:

29 July 2021 ABC News headline: "Vast majority of ICU patients with COVID-19 are unvaccinated, ABC News survey finds"

CTV News: "Inside an ICU where 70 per cent of COVID-19 patients are unvaccinated"

9 Sept 2021: NHS Bart Health Headline: "Almost 90% of patients admitted to Intensive Care Units in North East London are not fully vaccinated"

A particularly serious example was the ludicrous claim made in the BBC documentary 'Unvaccinated' [446] by Dr Mehool Patel (Consultant, University Hospital Lewisham) that we covered in detail in Chapter 7. He claimed that 20 out of 21 patients admitted to intensive care were unvaccinated (95%) and that 7 out of 7 (100%) who did not survive were unvaccinated. Yet, as we reported in Chapter 7, BBC's Complaints Director Jeremy Hayes conceded:

> "I have approached the programme makers for information about the data which were quoted by Dr Patel. I have been advised that the figures were compiled by Dr Patel himself for the purposes of research.
>
> "Lewisham and Greenwich Hospital Trust does not record the vaccination status of patients in ICU so Dr Patel's figures cannot independently be verified."

13.1.2. Deliberately murky record keeping used to manipulate data

But the scam was based on something even more ludicrous than classifying "not fully vaccinated" as "unvaccinated".

As a result of Freedom of Information Requests sent to some individual NHS trusts we now know that some hospitals were using the NIMS system to classify vaccine status of patients while others were using their own systems. This meant that, in many cases even if a patient had a vaccination record in NIMS, if the patient was not vaccinated in that particular hospital/Trust they were recorded as unvaccinated. Some hospitals were using a mixture of both systems (NIMS where a death was recorded and an internal system where a covid case was recorded). For those relying on NIMS, since it was not operational until June 2021, all deaths within the hospital would have had an unknown vaccination status between Jan-June 2021. The problem is that some hospitals were classifying "unknown" as "unvaccinated".

So, deliberately murky record keeping was used to manipulate the data.

To see the implications of this, Figure 55. shows the data on hospital deaths (all deaths, not just covid) from the start of the vaccine programme until the end of 2021 from an undisclosed NHS trust who responded to an FOI request.

		Vaccination Status			
Year	Financial Week	Single vaccinated	Double vaccinated	Triple vaccinated	Not vaccinated
	18/01/2021				14
	25/01/2021				68
	01/02/2021				41
	08/02/2021				42
	15/02/2021				46
2020/21	22/02/2021				36
	01/03/2021				31
	08/03/2021				38
	15/03/2021				18
	22/03/2021				27
	29/03/2021				35
	05/04/2021				3
	12/04/2021				36
	19/04/2021				28
	26/04/2021				42
	03/05/2021				31
	10/05/2021				32
	17/05/2021				40
	24/05/2021				32
	31/05/2021				39
	07/06/2021				30
	14/06/2021				33
	21/06/2021		11		20
	28/06/2021	3	16		8
	05/07/2021	4	30		10
	12/07/2021	2	21		18
	19/07/2021		24		9
	26/07/2021	1	36		10
	02/08/2021	2	25		16
	09/08/2021	2	35		4
	16/08/2021		27		9
	23/08/2021	1	27		5
	30/08/2021		29		2
2021/22	06/09/2021	1	31		4
	13/09/2021	1	41		4
	20/09/2021		10		21
	27/09/2021		1		35
	04/10/2021		2		39
	11/10/2021				44
	18/10/2021		4		34
	25/10/2021	1	33		13
	01/11/2021	1	38		5
	08/11/2021	1	32		4
	15/11/2021	1	30		3
	22/11/2021		34		14
	29/11/2021		42		8
	06/12/2021		38		9
	13/12/2021		35		9
	20/12/2021	1	52		

Figure 55 FOI data on hospital deaths

Note that ***every death up until 21 June 2021 was recorded as unvaccinated*** simply because hospitals in this Trust were using the NIMS system for classifying deaths which was not up and running until then. But, of course, an unknown number (probably most) of these 742 people were vaccinated.

There are plenty of other anomalies in the data. Note the improbable, sudden and dramatic trend changes:

1. A steady decline in "unvaccinated" deaths from 21 June until 13 Sept. In week ending 13 Sept only 4 out of 46 (less than 9%) were unvaccinated.

2. The next week (20 Sept) the unvaccinated are suddenly the majority again with 21 out of 31 deaths (68%), and this increases so quickly that just 3 weeks later (11 Oct) all 44 deaths (100%) are 'unvaccinated'.

3. But then we get a sudden and rapid decline in the unvaccinated deaths. Just 2 weeks later (25 Oct) the unvaccinated are 13 out of 47 deaths (28%) and by 20 Dec none of 53 deaths (0%) were unvaccinated.

Such changes can only be the result of changes in definition of who should be classified as unvaccinated.

It is easy to see how the Government could cherry pick this kind of data to present the narrative they wanted. When the text messages were being sent out in November 2021 it is reasonable to assume that they were using the cumulative data up to, say, mid-October. Then using the data in the table up to and including 18 Oct 2021 we count:

- 1051 "unvaccinated" (including 17 with just a single jab)
- 370 "vaccinated" (with 2 jabs).

That gives 74% of all hospital deaths classified as "unvaccinated".

But this is all an illusion. In fact, counting just the final three weeks of the data (6-20 Dec), just 18 out of the 144 deaths (12.5%) were unvaccinated.

It is also worth noting that the same NHS Trust provided the following information on "new COVID positives" in its hospitals between 19th Jan 2021 and 19th Jan 2022 (Figure 56).

Age Band	Single vaccinated	Double vaccinated	Triple vaccinated	Not vaccinated	Total
0-10				96	96
11-20	10	9		66	85
21-30	17	43	9	106	175
31-40	14	55	7	130	206
41-50	17	73	10	126	226
51-60	22	104	22	157	305
61-70	31	158	33	135	357
71-80	23	157	42	127	349
81-90	33	115	41	91	280
90 and over	10	35	17	35	97
Total	177	749	181	1,069	2,176

Figure 56 New Covid-19 positives

Given what we know about national vaccination take-up rates, and this Trust's own death data, it is likely that the majority of those classified as 'unvaccinated' here would have been vaccinated (with the exception of those in the 0-20 age categories the vast majority of whom would not have been eligible for vaccination).

So, instead of the '50% of new covid cases' being among the unvaccinated - the 'official' narrative pushed from this data - the true narrative should have been that the vast majority of new covid cases were vaccinated.

13.1.3. FOI email exchange with UK hospital trust

Figure 55 showed the 2021 deaths by vaccination status data provided in response to a Freedom of Information Request to one undisclosed UK Hospital Trust. We present below, without comment, the (email) correspondence in date order related to a request for the updated data.

Subject: New FOI request 7092 (sent to Trust, 22 February 2023)

> "Under a fresh FOI request, please may I have the up to date version of the attached spreadsheet provided under FOI 6400. Namely:
>
> 1. Deaths in XXXXXX Trust (all causes of mortality) between 19th Jan 2021 and most recent date available
>
> 2. New COVID positives in XXXXX Trust between 19th Jan 2021 and most recent date available
>
> If it is more expeditious, the dataset financial week 42 2021/22 to financial week 43 2022/23 will suffice as I already have data for the preceding year (kindly provided)
>
> 3. With regard to 1. above, are these the numbers being reported by the hospital trust to UKHSA and ONS?
>
> Many thanks,"

Trust Response (7 Mar 2023)

> "Vaccination status is no longer recorded so we are unable to provide this information.
>
> Best regards
>
> The Freedom of Information Team"

Follow-up to Trust (7 March 2023)

> "Thanks for the update, XXXXXX
>
> Can I have the data up until the time vaccination status was not recorded ?
>
> Cheers,

Trust Response (9 Mar 2023)

> "Dear XXXXXX
>
> We no longer hold any of this information, current or previous, as we have no legal basis to do so.
>
> Best Regards

13.1.4. Why does it matter?

It matters a lot because, despite being completely bogus, these kinds of ludicrous figures were so consistently repeated that the message "vaccines stop you being hospitalised and dying from covid (even if they don't stop infection and transmission)" was almost universally accepted. Even the strongest critics of the Government's covid response consistently repeated this mantra, as shown in Figure 57.

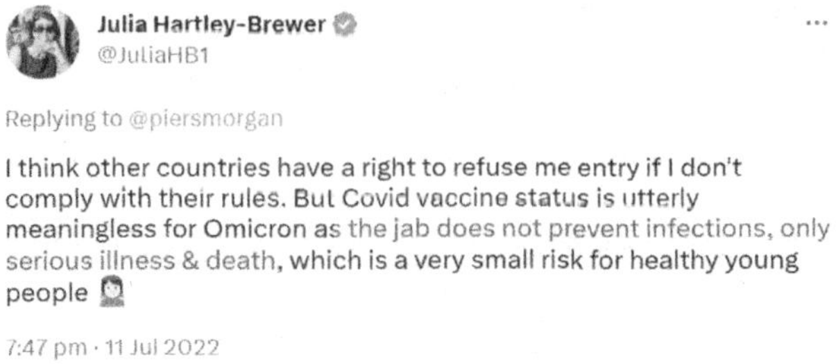

Figure 57 Government critic repeats the mantra

The figures were also used as the basis for the bogus studies claiming millions of lives were saved by the vaccine.

So, yet again, we can see that statistical data was used to create an illusion of vaccine hospitalisation and mortality efficacy by the simplest of means: deliberately murky record keeping ensuring that the vaccinated get recategorised as unvaccinated when they die or are hospitalised.

13.2. The 'fact checkers' can't find the target never mind hit it

3 March 2023

One of the most tiresome features of the covid era has been the growth industry of 'fact-checkers' generously funded by Government, Pharma companies and the likes of Bill Gates to silence anybody challenging the 'official narrative'. The Law, Health and Technology Newsletter has covered this extensively. [447].

There have been a few ludicrous attempts to 'fact-check' our own work but, as an example of how biased and incompetent these people are, we present a request received today from an AFP fact-checker asking Norman to help 'debunk' something .... and Norman's self-explanatory response to it (he has spared the 'fact-checker' personal embarrassment by removing their name).

> **From:** XXXXXX
> **Sent:** Thursday, March 2, 2023 9:17 PM
> **To:** Norman Fenton
> **Subject:** Media Request (AFP) - Addressing Misinterpretations of ONS Covid-19 Data
>
> Hello professor,
>
> I hope you are well. I am a fact-check reporter at AFP based in Washington DC. I am working to debunk online articles that claim English health data indicates that fully vaccinated people are far more likely to die of Covid-19 than those who have not received the shots. Several articles have made this allegation, citing this ONS dataset [448].

For reference, I will archive examples of these articles making the claims *here* [449] and *here* [450].

Based on this *ONS insight* [451] and a previous *bulletin* [452],which says the data is not intended to show vaccine efficacy, it seems like the article is misinterpreting the dataset. Would you be able to offer comment with a brief explanation as to how this sort of data is supposed to be read and used?

Thank you for your consideration,

XXXXXXXX

Agence France-Presse (AFP)

Office #: (202) 414-0527

This was the response:

From: Norman Fenton
Sent: Thursday, March 2, 2023 9:44 PM
To: XXXXXXX
Subject: RE: Media Request (AFP) - Addressing Misinterpretations of ONS Covid-19 Data

Dear XXXXX

Like all mainstream "fact checkers" you clearly have no understanding of what it is you are checking.

The ONS dataset is so flawed and biased that even the Statistics Regulator agreed with us that it could not be used to make any inferences about vaccine efficacy or safety. But you are missing the big problem here.

Instead of focusing on those who are using the data to suggest the vaccine is not as safe and effective as claimed, what you should be focused on are the government and mainstream media who (against the advice of the Statistics Regulator) are using the ONS data to claim the vaccine ***is*** safe and effective. Have a look at this article in the Daily Mail [453] – this is one you should be fact checking (Figure 58). Why aren't you doing that?

Our most recent article covers this whole issue of the ONS data.

In fact, if you make adjustments for the multiple flaws and biases in the ONS data, then it is increasingly clear that the vaccinated have a higher all-cause mortality in many age groups, especially the under 50's. In other words, the evidence increasingly points to the need for the covid vaccine programme to be shut down completely. But that isn't the message you want to portray is it, because your funders are the ones pushing the vaccines?

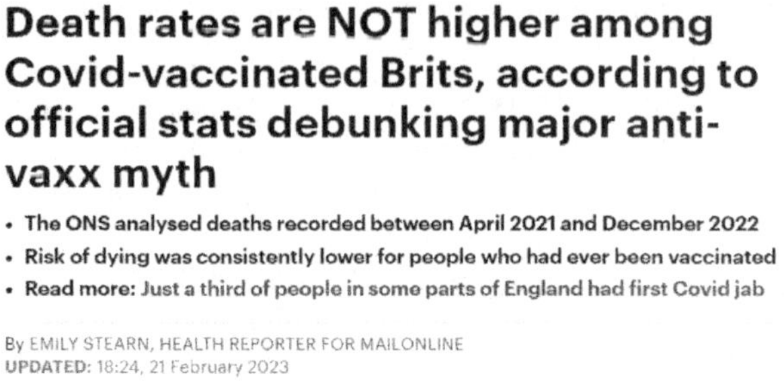

Death rates are NOT higher among Covid-vaccinated Brits, according to official stats debunking major anti-vaxx myth

- The ONS analysed deaths recorded between April 2021 and December 2022
- Risk of dying was consistently lower for people who had ever been vaccinated
- Read more: Just a third of people in some parts of England had first Covid jab

By EMILY STEARN, HEALTH REPORTER FOR MAILONLINE
UPDATED: 18:24, 21 February 2023

Figure 58 Daily Mail defending the narrative

Only one of the links to examples of reports you were seeking to 'debunk' seems to be working, namely the article in The Expose. The claim there is that the ONS report reveals that "the Vaccinated account for 9 in every 10 COVID Deaths over the past TWO Years". Based on the ONS dataset this is correct. Of course, without knowing the true proportion of vaccinated in each age group, we still cannot conclude that the vaccinated are at higher risk of death from covid. But the article is not claiming that, it is simply stating the FACT that a far higher number of vaccinated people have died of covid than unvaccinated since Jan 2022. That the number of vaccinated people who have died of covid is 25,768 is relevant, because we were told by people like you that this could not possibly happen; the vaccines were supposed to have 'stopped hospitalisation and death from covid'.

Yours

Norman Fenton

Chapter 14. Censored by academia and the media

But the vaccine deaths cannot be ignored

14.1. Retrospective censorship

12 April 2023

They're now coming after our pre-covid and non-covid publications (full version of this article with relevant screenshots is here [454]).

Those who wish to silence and cancel people who raise concerns about the 'official covid narrative' (especially those questioning the 'safe and effective' vaccines) are resorting to new, more inventive ways, to attack us. Not content to simply ensure that dissenting research papers on covid data never get published, they are now trying to delegitimise published non-covid papers produced by covid dissenters.

A prominent and disturbing example of this is the retrospective attack [455] on Paul Marik and his 2017 paper on Vitamin C and sepsis - an attack clearly chosen to delegitimise Marik simply because he has been a prominent advocate for early treatment protocols for covid. Fortunately, that attack seems to have finally failed [456]. But this is not going to stop the censors who are determined to silence any dissenters.

In the last few months, Norman has received multiple emails from journals where he had previously published non-covid papers asking him to respond to complaints that he failed to declare conflicts of interest. Invariably these complaints have said that he did not inform readers that he was a member of the HART group [457] or PANDATA [458].

For example, the complaint, sent to the journal that published this article [459] in August 2022 co-authored by Norman (that is totally unrelated to covid or vaccines) stated:

> "Readers of this article are not informed that author Norman Fenton is a member of the HART groups source https://www.hartgroup.org/bios/
>
> "Readers of this article are not informed that author Norman Fenton is a member of ('DATA Scientist') of PANDATA, see https://web.archive.org/web/20221009064651/ttps://counterdisinformationproject.substack.com/p/the-pandata-file"

This is one of many similar reports to journals that he has been asked to respond to. The frustrating thing is that, rather than ignore this nonsense, journals require a formal response, resulting in an exhausting time-suck. And this is the reason why the complainants do it - to grind you down.

In fact, not only is the article that was the subject of the above complaint nothing to do with covid or anything related to the activities of HART or PANDATA, but the complaint is factually wrong. While Norman has spoken twice at PANDA meetings, he was never a 'member'. Indeed, whereas the link [460] provided to HART is to the members list which he is on, the link [463] to PANDATA in the complaint is to a hysterical hit piece about PANDATA in which Norman is not named.

So, what should we declare?

If dissenters are now required to declare affiliations to any group to which we belong or whose objectives we approve of, does this mean that Norman has to declare on each authored paper that he is a Spurs season ticket holder? Or that in his youth he attended meetings of the International Socialists? What about his Amazon prime membership? Or the fact that he owns the entire X-Files series box-set? Or that he has seen Les Misérables 53 times in the theatre?

Do science journals still value quality and accuracy?

The fact is that, while Norman has published over 300 peer-reviewed papers, none of the many dozens [464] he has written about covid data after summer 2020 have even got to the serious review stage when submitted to any journal. For bogus reasons like those described in a previous chapter.

As in the case of our submission [465] to The Lancet nobody ever challenges the accuracy of our work; it is sufficient for them to know 'who' is writing it in order to know it must be banned. And, since people like the Government approved spokesperson for jabbing pregnant women tell everybody that Norman is a 'rabid misinformation merchant', that seems to be sufficient 'evidence' to reject our work (Figure 59).

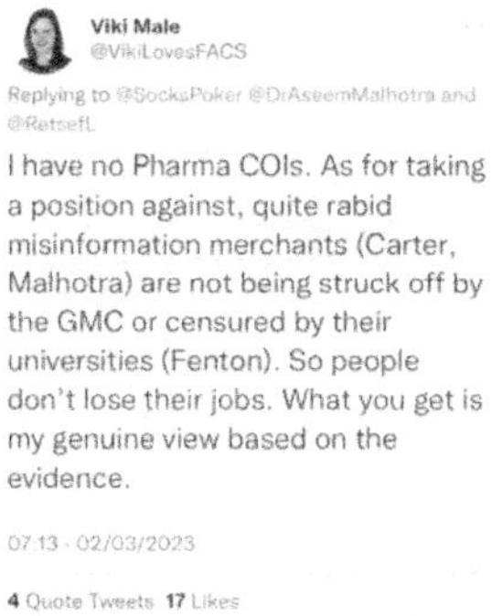

Figure 59 Accusations of being a rabid disinformation merchant

In the very rare cases where papers that seriously challenge the official covid narrative have been accepted or published in a peer reviewed journal, the organised attacks begin instantly. Some of the best-known examples include:

- The first published paper highlighting myocarditis risks post-vaccination by Jessica Rose and Peter McCullough was published online in Oct 2021 but then almost immediately (and permanently) withdrawn [466] by the publishers without any explanation provided to the authors.

- The paper [467] by Hui Jiang and Ya-Fang Mei which proved that the SARS Cov-2 spike protein stops DNA repair (i.e., induces cancer risk) in lymphocytes. It was only after Jiang admitted that, because the vaccine spike was the same as the virus spike, the vaccine had a real risk of causing cancer-inducing changes in DNA that the demands to retract the paper began - as explained here [468] with details of the scandalous retraction politics here [469].

- The paper [470] by Mark Skidmore which estimated over 200,000 people killed by the vaccines has now been retracted by the journal. The 'concerns' [471] leading to the retraction were either easily fixed or bogus, including a claim that there was insufficient ethical approval for the survey on which it was based and failure to declare the views of the person who funded the survey (Catherine Austin-Fitts). Steve Kirsch has announced [472] he is going to mount a legal challenge to this retraction.

For many the covid era has destroyed the trust in many if not all institutions - the government, the pharma industry, the social media giants, and the mainstream media generally. In saner times we would have at least expected academia to rise above the lies and corruption and, especially, the censorship. Yet, academia has spearheaded the censorship of dissenting voices and, by censoring research based on who wrote it or who they are associated with, rather than on its quality and accuracy, any respect for the notion of 'peer review' has been destroyed and may never recover.

14.2. Misinformation from the Times and other media sources

16 May 2023

Within 60 seconds of uploading a two-minute clip from Norman's testimony to the Corona Investigative Committee, Germany, YouTube removed it and gave Norman a strike and one-week suspension.

Full testimony (presented 12 May 2023) is here [473] (testimony starts at 2:29:28).

We look forward to YouTube explaining which claims in the video "contradict expert consensus from local health authorities or the World Health Organisation (WHO)".

- Was it The Times (March 2021) article that described the AstraZeneca vaccine as "100% effective", while also stating that "academics back bizarre claim that vaccines may kill"? (See Chapter for the full details about this and our involvement in it)

- Was it Norman's statement that the online version of the article named him as one of the academics making the "bizarre claims that vaccines may kill" and that he wasn't even an author of the paper that made the claims (see here for the full story about that article), but that we ***had*** indeed found data which suggested there was evidence the vaccines may already have led to deaths?

- Was it Norman's statement that one of Norman's own family members suffered a serious adverse reaction to the AstraZeneca vaccine in April 2021?

- Was it the Daily Express (Dec 2021) article stating that the AstraZeneca vaccine had "disappeared" or Norman's additional statement that, in fact, the vaccine had effectively been withdrawn from GPs in the UK from June 2021?
- Was it national newspaper articles stating that coroners had found that Lisa Shaw and Michelle Barlow died of covid vaccine complications?

In fact, within 3 minutes of Norman appealing the removal of the video (by asking exactly these questions) YouTube responded stating:

> "We have reviewed your content carefully, and have confirmed that it violates our medical misinformation policy"

Perhaps if the voices of us "conspiracy theorists" with our "bizarre claims" (at the start of 2021) that the vaccines could kill had not been censored, while claims that the vaccines were 100% effective were widely promoted, then the thousands of deaths and injuries from the vaccines would have been avoided. And people like Lisa Shaw, Michelle Barlow, Zion, and Stephen Wright - none of whom had any medical need to take this vaccine - would still be alive today.

14.3. The scandal of the AstraZeneca vaccine

From the Emergent Biosolutions plant in Baltimore (24 May 2023)

We have previously reported (here [474] and here) on the problems caused by the AstraZeneca vaccine in the UK and how it was quietly withdrawn even before Dame Sarah Gilbert was given a standing ovation [476] at Wimbledon in June 2021 for leading its development.

What has not been reported in the UK (we could not find a single mainstream media outlet report) was the scandal involving the known faulty AstraZeneca vaccines produced in Baltimore that were exported to Canada and Mexico (and note that AstraZeneca never got approval [477] for their covid vaccine in the US)

The following information was sent to us by a Canadian who was injured by the AstraZeneca vaccine that was 'donated' to Canada from the United States. It highlights the myriad problems experienced at the Baltimore plant that resulted in it being shut down by the FDA and having to dispose of 500 million vaccine doses.

> "This overview is intended to highlight some of the many problems with the AstraZeneca vaccine that was produced at the Emergent Biosolutions plant in Baltimore. AstraZeneca vaccines from this plant were used in the Canadian market until May 11, 2021 when they were pulled.
>
> This article [478] from the National Post that was published on April 4, 2021 had the headline "U.S. removes AstraZeneca from plant that ruined 15 million doses of COVID-19 vaccine". It highlights the cross-contamination with Johnson and Johnson. The cross contamination ruined 15 million doses of J and J. AstraZeneca ended up being removed from production from the U.S plant.

But this article [478] on 23 April 2021 by Tom Blackwell with the headline "More than half of Canada's AstraZeneca vaccine came from U.S. plant accused of quality-control problems" revealed that more than half of Canada's AZ vaccine came from the Baltimore plant. The article contains details of the many concerns the FDA had about the plant.

Law professor and drug policy expert from the University of Ottawa Amir Attaran said [479], "No way should Canadians be offered these doses."

This [480] is the press release from Health Canada from April 25, 2021 where they reassured Canadians about the safety of the product, which Dr. Attaran refutes.

"OTTAWA, ON, April 25, 2021 /CNW/ - Health Canada is aware of the U.S. Food and Drug Administration's (FDA) recent inspection of the Emergent BioSolutions facility in Baltimore, Maryland, which noted multiple areas of concern.
Health Canada would like to reassure Canadians that all AstraZeneca vaccines imported into Canada from this facility are safe and of high quality. Janssen vaccines produced at this site have not entered the country.

Health Canada has verified that the 1.5 million doses of AstraZeneca vaccine imported into Canada from this facility meet quality specifications. The Department reviewed test results of all vaccine lots that came into Canada, as well as the company's quality control steps implemented throughout the manufacturing process to mitigate potential risks of contamination."

Essentially, they were relying on AZ for their quality control information. That same week, Health Canada held off and ultimately rejected doses of Johnson and Johnson made from the same plant.

This article [481] from the New York Times, May 12, 2021 with headline "Vaccine Made at Troubled Baltimore Plant Were Shipped to Canada and Mexico" states that the U.S government was unaware that the factory had previously discarded millions of possibly contaminated doses of AZ. The American government did not vouch for the quality of AZ doses from the Baltimore plant and had left it up to the Canadian/Mexican governments and AstraZeneca quality assurances. Canada had been informed about the manufacturing problems but was allowed to proceed. Prime Minister Trudeau still assured Canadians the vaccine was safe.

This article [482]from the Washington Post/National Post on 20 May 2021 with headline "Johnson & Johnson recorded contamination risks at Baltimore plant seven months before vaccine was ruined". It cites extreme contamination and manufacturing problems at the plant. There was even a house panel investigation chaired by Representative James Clyburn into all of the problems.

On July 29, 2021, the National Post reported [483] with headline "Millions of AstraZeneca doses shipped to Canada from U.S. plant before complete inspection". The acceptance of the AstraZeneca vaccine was based on an inspection from the European Medicines Agency (EMA) but the EMA had not actually inspected the area where the AstraZeneca vaccine was being produced. Again, Professor Attaran cites glaring holes in the process.

A report [484] by the House of Representatives Select subcommittee on the Coronavirus Crisis in May 2022 showed that Emergent had destroyed up to 400 million doses and attempted to cover it up.

By June 8, 2022 J and J had ended [485] their agreement with Emergent Biosolutions.

By August 2022, a congressional committee [486] showed that more than a half billion doses from the Baltimore factory had to be discarded and the company had covered it up. The FDA also had issued a warning letter to the company.

Data [487] from Health Canada and Public Health Ontario indicates AstraZeneca had far greater rates of adverse reactions compared to Pfizer or Moderna. Expanding Figure 2 "Text descriptions" we can see the total adverse event reports per 100,000 does which (as of 23 May 2023) – see Figure 60.

Adverse event reports per 100,000 doses

	Serious	Non-serious
AstraZeneca	34.2	122.9
Pfizer	11.8	40.7
Moderna	8.35	58.8

Figure 60 Adverse event reports Health Canada and Public Health Ontario

Further details can be found here [488] although the results (page 4) are slightly different.

Despite all of these issues, none of this has ever been raised in the House of Commons or brought to the Standing Committee on Health.

I have not included all documentation, but this gives a very good overview of all the problems at the Baltimore plant and the AstraZeneca doses received from that plant. Hundreds of thousands of Canadians received doses from that factory and potentially millions of Mexicans."

Curiously, further information can be found in the New York Times [489].

We don't know how many Canadians were killed by the AstraZeneca vaccine (although as we reported [490] just yesterday the excess deaths in Canada are sky-rocketing).

14.4. How many deaths were caused by the covid vaccines?

4 April 2023

14.4.1. Overview

We thought it would be useful to do an approximate analysis using minimal assumptions, along these lines:

- Contrary to the claims made by covid vaccine proponents there is hard evidence that most reports of vaccine deaths to the USA VAERS and UK Yellow Card systems are genuine. At most 30% of these reports can be ruled as likely not to have been caused by the vaccine.
- There is also evidence that the reporting rates for deaths and adverse events to these systems is very low. It is likely that fewer than 10% of deaths and other adverse events ever get reported.
- With these minimal assumptions we estimate there have been:
    - approximately 120,000 deaths in the USA directly caused by the covid vaccines (between Dec 2020 until 23 March 2023) and 16,000 in the UK (between Dec 2020 until 29 Sept 2022).
    - over 103 deaths per million doses of the covid vaccines in the UK with big differences between the three main vaccines (187 for AstraZeneca , 68 for Pfizer and 35 for Moderna). For AstraZeneca that amounts to 1 death in every 5348 doses.
- Taking account of the small proportion of people reporting serious adverse reactions that may have subsequently led to early deaths, there are likely to have been an additional 70,000 deaths in the USA and 35,000 in the UK indirectly caused by the vaccines. This would mean deaths caused directly or indirectly by the vaccines account for about half the excess deaths in the UK since Jan 2021.

14.4.2. Norman's personal story

At the beginning of January 2021, a friend's father was one of the early recipients of a covid vaccine in the UK. He was 90 years old but, for his age, in reasonable health. He died less than 24 hours later. My suggestion of a possible link to the vaccination was treated with total incredulity by the family. In Jewish tradition he was buried the day after his death and, of course, no postmortem was ever considered. The vaccination was never mentioned again, and it was assumed by all that his death was natural and inevitable.

Since then, I have lost several friends at relatively young ages from cancer and heart attacks. All were fully vaccinated. Two of the cancer victims had been in remission before the vaccinations. Again, not a single family member considered any possibility of a link to the vaccination and none of these cases were reported to the UK Yellow Card system for possible vaccine adverse reactions.

However, I know of one extremely serious and traumatic adverse reaction that followed shortly after the second dose of the AstraZeneca vaccine in April 2021 that *was* reported to the Yellow Card system.

It is one I reported myself as it happened to a very close family member and the effects of this have been life-changing to the victim as well as myself.

I found the Yellow Card system extremely difficult to navigate and it did not allow me to input highly relevant specific information. It seemed designed not to collect such data. I suspect that many people attempting to navigate the system will have given up and not finalised and submitted their report. I have never received any confirmation or follow-up to my report. Furthermore, my GP and specialists involved in the case were dismissive of my claim of a vaccine link.

A family member of Martin's also suffered an adverse reaction which was reported to the Yellow Card system.

6 April 2023 Update: At 45 minutes in on this UK Column programme [491] there is some extremely revealing information on just how bad the Yellow Card scheme is.

14.4.3. How many 'officially reported' deaths occurred?

Except for a tiny percentage of deaths occurring shortly after vaccination, doctors have been extremely reluctant to properly investigate claims of serious adverse reactions from covid vaccines by patients or their relatives. This reluctance to investigate happens even when deaths have been reported to the VAERS or Yellow Card systems. As such, only a tiny minority of cases have ever been subject to formal medical verification, and it is this tiny number that Governments are keen to promote to sustain the false argument that the benefits of vaccination far outweigh the harms. For example, in the UK only coroner confirmed deaths qualify for the Government's £120,000 compensation payment scheme and (as of 3 March 2023) only 52 such deaths [492] were officially classified as having been caused by covid vaccines. This is despite the fact that as, of 29 Sept 2022, there had been 2,272 covid vaccine deaths reported [493] to the Yellow Card scheme.

In the USA things are even worse because, despite 17,315 deaths being reported to VAERS (as of 23 March 2023), it seems that no deaths have been 'officially' recognised as directly caused by covid vaccines. And any attempt to use VAERS as the basis for estimating the true number of such deaths have been simply quashed by the 'fact checkers' as misinformation on the grounds that these are simply 'unconfirmed reports' [494].

Can we estimate the unreported number of deaths from VAERS and the yellow card systems?

We want to make the fewest assumptions possible to estimate the unreported number of deaths from those reported. To do this we need two measures:

1. The *reporting rate* (also often called, somewhat confusingly, the *under-reporting factor)*: What proportion of vaccine deaths are actually reported to VAERS and Yellow Card? If, for example, only 10% of all vaccine deaths are reported then the reporting rate is 10%.
2. The *false positive rate*: What proportion of vaccine deaths actually reported to these systems are not caused by the vaccine. If, for example, 40% of all deaths reported as vaccine deaths were not caused by the vaccine then the false positive rate is 40% while 60% are true positives.

Covid vaccine sceptics claim that the reporting rate is very low due to a combination of:

- People having never heard of the reporting system or assuming someone else would complete it;
- Difficulty in completing the form;
- No surviving relative to complete the form;

- No surviving relative willing to complete the form;
- Failure to contemplate that the cause of illness or death may have been related to the vaccine.
- Compared to previous vaccines, the likely way in which harm is mediated by the mRNA vaccines means adverse events are much more spread out over both time and also the organs affected. This inevitably reduces attribution compared to previous vaccines and suggests under-reporting could be greater.

It has been claimed that (for all types of vaccines) as few as 1% [495] of vaccine injuries are reported to VAERS. A more recent analysis claimed [496] a figure of 1 in 41, i.e., 2.4%. I think that 10% is a conservative estimate, although I will consider a range of values. Whatever the actual under-reporting figure is for VAERS, it is likely to be even lower for the Yellow Card scheme which is especially difficult to submit a report to.

Vaccine 'proponents' often claim that the false positive rate for the VAERS and Yellow Card systems are very high because of either false/malicious reporting or the supposed lack of clinical knowledge of the reporters. However, when the first batch of deaths were reported in VAERS for the covid vaccines McLachlan et al undertook a detailed analysis (with a 2023 update here [497]) of a sample of 250 reports and concluded that less than 15% could be dismissed as invalid.

A reader has now alerted us to a much older paper [498] from 1982 published in the BMJ that provides further valuable insights into the false positive rate for reported serious vaccine adverse reactions. Although the sample size was small (57 reports to the Yellow Card scheme in the UK), it shows that 40 were true positives (77%) while none of the remaining 17 could be proved to be false positives. So, in the absence of evidence to the contrary, it seems reasonable to assume that at least 70% of death reports to the Yellow Card and VAERS systems are genuine, and it is reasonable to assume a false positive rate less than 30%.

14.4.4. Estimate of direct deaths caused by the covid vaccines

Taking account of the 30% false positive rate (70% of the reported vaccine deaths were caused by the vaccine), and different possible under-reporting factors Figure 61 shows the estimates of number of covid vaccine deaths based on Yellow Card and VAERS for the UK and USA.

Hence, with a 10% reporting rate we estimate nearly 16,000 deaths in the UK and over 120,000 deaths in the USA. While these numbers may look high, they are only a tiny proportion of all deaths registered since Jan 2021 (when the vaccine programmes were fully rolled out). For example, in The UK there were over one million deaths in total registered between Jan 2021 and end of Sept 2022, so 16,000 covid vaccine deaths would, as far as excess deaths are concerned, barely be noticed (less than 1.6%).

	UK (up to 29 Sept 2022)	USA (up to 23 March 2022)
Number of deaths reported	2,272	17,315
True positives reported (assuming 70%)	1,590	12,121
Actual number of deaths assuming reporting rates		
1%	159,040	1,212,050
5%	31,808	242,410
10%	15,904	121,205
15%	10,603	80,803
20%	7,952	60,603
25%	6,362	48,482
30%	5,301	40,402

Figure 61 Estimate of direct deaths in UK and USA

14.4.5. Impact of serious adverse events reported on indirect deaths

The number of deaths reported to VAERS is just a small percentage of the total adverse events reported. As of 24 March 2023, the totals in the USA were 947,487 of which 17,315 were deaths, 77,454 were hospitalisations, 114,247 were urgent care and 188,844 involved a doctor's visit.

Many of the more serious adverse reactions will increasingly contribute to early deaths that will never be directly attributed as caused by the vaccines. Of course, whereas as noted above the number of deaths directly caused by the vaccines will barely make a dent on total excess deaths numbers, it has been hypothesised [499] that the large recent increases in excess deaths in highly vaccinated countries is due to the increasing number of deaths indirectly caused by the vaccines. What we really need to know is what proportion of those people reporting serious adverse events (approximately 200,000) have died earlier than they otherwise would have. If the figure is 5% then that would be 10,000 deaths. Based on the 70% true positive rate and 10% reporting rate that would mean an extra 70,000 deaths indirectly caused by the vaccines.

14.4.6. Serious adverse events reported in the UK?

This is where things become curious. In March 2023 the UK Government decided to stop properly updating the Yellow Card figures. In fact, the latest report [500] does not even provide the updated death numbers. Nor does it provide the details of the proportion of reports that are classified as 'serious' in any easily searchable form. The only relevant numbers that are relatively easy to find are shown in Figure 62.

	Number of reports	Number of events	Number of doses	Reports per 1000 doses	Events per 1000 doses
Pfizer	177,925	511,776	84,700,000	2.1	6.0
AZ	246,866	874,912	49,159,700	5.0	17.8
Moderna	47,045	151,628	16,400,000	2.9	9.2
Other	2,182				

Figure 62 SAEs in the UK

The total number of reports (summing the first column) is 474,018 which we can assume correspond to different people reporting. If we assume that 20% of these 474,018 suffered at least one serious adverse event (as per VAERS proportion) then that would amount to 94,804 people. If 5% of these 'died early' then that would be nearly 5,000 deaths. Based on an assumed 70% true positive rate and 10% under-reporting factor that would mean an extra 35,000 deaths indirectly caused by the vaccines. Together with the above estimate of 16,000 deaths directly caused by the covid vaccines, a total of 51,000 would result. This is a significant proportion of the approximately 120,000 excess deaths recorded since Jan 2021.

14.4.7. Death rates per million doses

Applying the same true positive rate and reporting rates to the data from the Yellow Card system (as of 29 Sept 2022) we get the death rate in the UK expressed in per million doses for all vaccinees (see Figure 63).

	Number of deaths reported	Number of deaths based on 70% true positives and 10% under-reporting	Number of doses	Number of deaths per million doses
Pfizer	826	5,782	84,700,000	68.3
AZ	1,314	9,198	49,159,700	187.1
Moderna	82	574	16,400,000	35.0

Figure 63 Deaths per million doses in the UK

In total we see 103 deaths per million doses, i.e., over 1 in 10,000, with big differences between the three main vaccines (187 for AstraZeneca , 68 for Pfizer and 35 for Moderna). For AstraZeneca that amounts to 1 in every 5348 doses. It is little surprise that the AstraZeneca vaccine was quietly and unofficially withdrawn in the UK as early as June 2021 (it had already been suspended [501] from many European countries as early as March 2021).

14.4.8. Conclusion

With a minimal set of conservative and reasonable assumptions we estimate that, since the end of December 2020 approximately 16,000 people in the UK have died directly from covid vaccines, while in the USA the figure is approximately 120,000. An interesting validity check is that the US population is five times that of the UK. Taking account of the later date of the USA figures and the fact that the under-reporting is likely to be lower in the USA, the mortality rate is reasonably consistent between the two countries.

With respect to the additional number of those who may have died indirectly following serious adverse reactions, we have estimated 35,000 in the UK and 70,000 in the USA. This larger number (relative to population size) for the UK may be partly due to the widespread use of the especially problematic AstraZeneca vaccine in the first half of 2021. Luckily for the Americans, this vaccine was not used in the USA. Three times as many adverse reactions per dose were reported for this vaccine than for the Pfizer vaccine and over twice as many per dose than for the Moderna vaccine. However, as reported here, all follow up reports are deleted from public VAERS, which means that many reports in VAERS are actually their least serious version. There are approximately 140,000 missing IDs, and each could be a deleted follow up report.

While AstraZeneca has effectively been discarded worldwide the roll-out of yet more boosters of the other vaccines continues unabated. Yet even before these vaccines were shown to be ineffective in stopping infection and transmission there were already sufficient safety signals that should have led to their suspension. In the USA, the CDC's own analysis [503] of the Pfizer and Moderna vaccines found hundreds of safety signals, while an analysis [504] of the original controlled trials data from these companies also revealed unacceptably high rates of serious adverse reactions. The recent Rasmussen poll [505] as well as the insurance data [506] from the USA provide strong evidence that the estimates we have made of deaths from the vaccines really are very conservative. With evidence of the increasingly low risk that covid poses to any age group, there is no scientific basis for anybody to get another dose of a covid vaccine. This calamity needs to stop now.

Chapter 15. The cheap trick, exaggerated mortality and FDA lies

15.1. The Cheap Trick

The illusion of vaccine efficacy revisited (2 May 2023).

Or:

> "How to make a placebo look 95% effective and guarantee repeat business…"

We have provided numerous explanations (see here [507], and here [508]) and videos (see here [509] and here [510]) explaining why a vaccine that is actually merely a placebo will inevitably appear to have high efficacy if there is a time delay after vaccination during which the participant is classified as 'unvaccinated'. A full example was provided in Chapter 5.

Some people have claimed that the examples - using hypothetical data - are unrealistic and that, with different assumptions about the underlying infection rate, the illusion would not happen. Not true.

This example (full details in the online version [511] of this article) simulates a vaccine roll-out and efficacy evaluation which is essentially how all the 2021 observational studies of the covid vaccines were conducted. We make the following assumptions:

- The entire population starts week 1 as unvaccinated and by week 14 about 90% of has received a single jab (note that we start with a population of one million, but the efficacy results are exactly same irrespective of the starting population).
- Vaccination roll-out starts with 1% of the unvaccinated population vaccinated in week 1 and peaks at 35% in week 8 falling back to 10% in each of the last 3 weeks.
- There is a constant weekly infection rate throughout the period (in the example below it is 2% but, as the video shows, the 'efficacy' numbers are the same no matter what the fixed rate is).
- Any vaccinated person who becomes infected within the first two weeks of their vaccination is classified as unvaccinated (in fact, as can be seen here [512], the Office for National Statistics classifies as person infected within the first three weeks of their vaccination as unvaccinated. And also note this is the case in Sweden [513]).

For simplicity (it makes little difference to the overall results) we also ignore the fact that people are unlikely to get infected twice during a 14-week period.

15.1.1. 86% effective under 14-day rule

To calculate the infection rate for week n for those classified as vaccinated we divide the cumulative number of people classified as infected and vaccinated by week n by the cumulative number of people classified as vaccinated by end of week n.

For example, by end of week 4 at total of 161,147 people have been classified as vaccinated of whom a total 596 have been classified as infected. So, the week 4 infection rate is 596/161,147 which is 0.37%. We do the same for those classified as unvaccinated, so the week 4 infection rate for the unvaccinated is 2.22%. Note that, although the real weekly infection rates of the vaccinated and unvaccinated are always the same 2%, the infection rates after the 'classification' are always lower than 2% for those classified as 'vaccinated' and higher than 2% for those classified as 'unvaccinated'.

To calculate the week *n* efficacy rate, we divide the vaccinated infection rate by the unvaccinated infection rate and subtract this from 1, expressing the result a percentage. Hence, the week 4 efficacy rate is 1 - (0.37/2.22) = 0.834 = 83.4%.

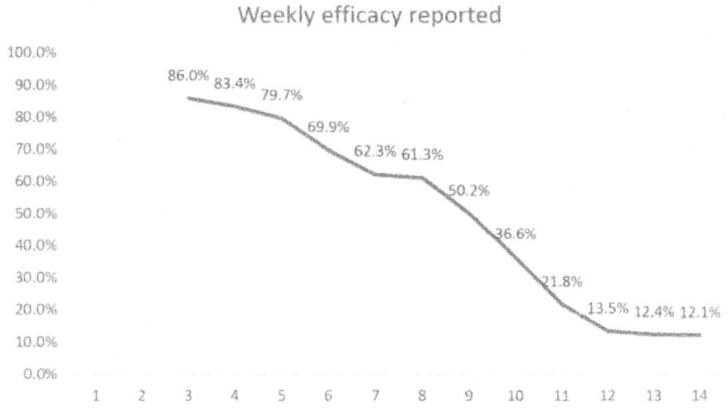

Figure 64 Simulated vaccine efficacy for placebo vaccine under 14-day rule

Now we see in Figure 64 that a completely useless (with true efficacy 0%) vaccine appears to have very high efficacy in the first few weeks. Although it continually wanes it is still above 50% after week 9. By week 14 the efficacy is still positive but only 12.1%, hence the need for a new booster dose! These simulated results are very similar to the real-world efficacy rates that were observed in the first three months of a new vaccine or booster.

15.1.2. 95% effective under 21-day rule

Using the same assumptions but now with those infected within the first 20 days of vaccination classified as unvaccinated, we get a similar graph as Figure 64 but starting at week 4 with efficacy almost 95% before tapering off to 15% by week 14. So now they could claim the vaccine starts with 95% efficacy, but again you need the booster after 3 months for vaccination to be truly effective.

For those who doubt the ONS calculate vaccine efficacy here is what their document [514] that describes the method says:

> "We calculated vaccine effectiveness for different doses (first, second and third dose or booster) and time since dose, to observe how the effectiveness changes over time. The vaccination statuses used were:

- unvaccinated (those with no vaccination or who were vaccinated with a first dose less than 21 days ago)
- first dose (those who were vaccinated with a first dose at least 21 days ago to earliest of less than 91 days after first dose or less than 21 days after second dose)
- ...

15.1.3. Even negative efficacy can be made to look 95% effective!

Note that for a placebo vaccine it is impossible to get negative efficacy. However, if there is a slightly higher infection rate for the vaccine compared to no vaccine then, the same assumptions still yield high efficacy initially before eventually becoming negative. Even if the vaccine actually increases the infection rate by 50% (so a 3% infection rate in the vaccinated rather than the assumed 2% in the above simulations) then under the 21-day rule in week 4 efficacy is over 92%. It dips again but is still positive (over 30%) in week 10. It does not dip below 0% until week 11 despite the fact that, in reality its efficacy its consistently -50%

15.1.4. Caveats and Conclusions

In practice there are a number of factors which, if we included them in the simulation, would produce an even higher efficacy rate than could be claimed for a placebo vaccine. For example:

- The 2021 UK roll out happened during a period when the covid infection rate was declining.

- Asymptomatic unvaccinated people were much more likely to be required to take PCR tests (to go to work or attend events, restaurants etc) than asymptomatic vaccinated people, since the latter only had to show their proof of vaccination. In Israel during this period an unvaccinated person was six times more likely to have to be PCR tested than a vaccinated person. The high false positive rate for asymptomatics would therefore artificially increase the infection rate of the unvaccinated.

- People who were (or had recently been) PCR positive were not allowed to be vaccinated until 14 days after a negative test. This means the vaccinated cohort contained a higher proportion of people who already had natural immunity.

- The so-called 'healthy vaccinee effect' whereby it is claimed that the vaccinated are more likely to be more 'health conscious' and from a higher socio-economic class meaning that they are less likely to get infected.

As we have shown the illusion of high efficacy is also present if the vaccine is worse than a placebo. In particular, we know that, for the covid vaccines, there was a disproportionately high infection rate within the first 14 days after vaccination. Given all of those infected within the first 14 days are classified as unvaccinated, this would lead to even higher efficacy rates than shown in our simulation.

On the issue of immunity, one simplification made in the simulation is that it does not take account of the fact that those who become infected during the period (whether vaccinated or not) would almost certainly not become infected again (and therefore should be removed from the count in subsequent weeks). However, unless the general infection rate is very high this has minimal impact on the efficacy results.

It may be reasonable to allow a certain amount of time for a vaccine to 'work'. However, classifying a person who becomes infected within 14 or 21 days of vaccination as an 'unvaccinated case' in the calculation of vaccine efficacy is nothing short of a scam. It guarantees that any vaccine which is no different (or even worse) than a placebo will be seen to have high initial efficacy.

By using the 21-day period before considering a person vaccinated - as the ONS, and others do, for the covid vaccines - means fraudulently high artificial efficacy rates are guaranteed. The apparent, but completely artificial, 'waning' of efficacy can also be used deviously to support the idea that after 3 or 4 months another dose of the vaccine is required to regain protection. Since the same delay in classification is used for those who receive a further dose it is then guaranteed that high efficacy can again be claimed for the subsequent doses.

All of this creates a repeatable business model for Big Pharma.

Whatever efficacy was claimed for the covid vaccines, we have the evidence of our own eyes and ears. While cases of covid in unvaccinated people who were previously infected are rare, it is the vaccinated who are the ones who are subsequently suffering from repeated bouts of covid.

15.2. When lack of safety means safety

27 May 2023

A new FDA study [515] claims to show covid vaccines are safe for children even though the study shows significant increase in serious heart conditions.

Norman was contacted by both the Epoch Times and the Children's Health Defence (CHD) to comment on the article. Some of his comments and those of other colleagues are included in both the Epoch Times article [516] and the CHD article [517], but not all the problems we raised are included. For the record, here are the full set of comments we made.

Norman said:

> "I've had a quick look through it.
>
> The conclusion that "these results provide additional evidence that COVID-19 vaccines are safe in children" is pretty ludicrous given the fact that a) they show the safety signal for myocarditis and pericarditis is very strong (and is likely underestimated given some obvious weaknesses of the study); and b) the lack of any benefits of the vaccine to children of this age since they are at no risk from covid and (as others studies show) are actually more likely to get covid with the vaccine.
>
> Issues about the study:

There is a clear 'healthy user' bias (or other systemic bias like misclassification or under-reporting of outcomes) in the sample and analysis methods as can be seen for the conditions excluding myocarditis, pericarditis and anaphylaxis. Unless the vaccine has magical health benefits why would incidence of things like bells palsey and appendicitis be so much lower in the vaccinated? In fact, the authors admit that they were unable to follow up extensively on the outcomes.

I don't like the fact that, where number of outcomes is "<11", the exact number is not provided.

Given that the types of outcome are inevitably going to be rare in children I'm a bit concerned that the separation into 3 age groups is diluting the results. For example, I suspect that if the groups were combined there could be a significant safety signal for Anaphylaxis based on the reported risk ratios for the 12-15 and 16-17 groups.

There may be conflicts of interest among the authors."

Dr Scott McLachlan said:

"The "risk window" for some events seems arbitrarily too short.

It feels to me that all they are really giving us is "myocarditis" - likely because we already know (and they already admit to) that one. For everything else it just feels like they tried to hide the noise in the numbers.

Another bias is that they included patients on an insurance plan (who are therefore more likely to have a higher socioeconomic status because their parents are employed and therefore provided with or able to afford expensive health insurance). I think the outcome numbers would be vastly different in a group of children whose parents are not as well off.

It is also retrospective (health records) based. I don't believe they declare what happens when a parent loses their job (and therefore their health plan) and the child ceases to be an active health plan member. I have seen studies out of Optum and Kaiser Permanente in California and Boston in the past where they assume the health plan member had no reaction simply because nothing was written in their health record, but it was assumed they were still a member - sometimes in error. In America this is an incorrect assumption because if you can't afford to attend the Health Plan doctor, you have to go to a community clinic, or the doctor funded by your new health plan provider. That whole "the absence of something is not proof it didn't happen" thing springs to mind."

Dr. Josh Guetzkow said:

"I agree with Norman that the main weakness of this design is the comparison they are doing. They are comparing a highly select group of child and adolescent insured vaccine recipients to a historical baseline population consisting of everyone in the relevant age group who were insured. But the people who get vaccinated tend to be healthy, sometimes much healthier, than others. The Nature paper on increases in

POTS after vaccination [518] showed this very clearly because the baseline risk values for the unvaccinated were many times higher than for the vaccinated group.

Amazingly, this limitation isn't even mentioned in the article!

I also agree with Scott that the risk windows are rather short and arbitrary. Narcolepsy is a perfect example: the narcolepsy cases following the Swine Flu vaccine in 2009 took months to manifest and be diagnosed. If this was the same then you wouldn't expect to see the incidence increase 42 days after jabbing.

Another thing that is arbitrary are the ratios they establish that would trigger a signal. This is in the protocol [519] of the study, Table 5 page 15

Why, for example, is the ratio for appendicitis 1.09, for DVT it's 1.25 and for GBS it's 2.38 (for the .5-4 year olds)? That means that in order for a 'safety signal' to trigger, you'd need a ratio of 2.38 the incidence rate of GBS among vaccinated compared to expected pre-COVID 'background' rate and the ratio would need to be statistically significant. Oh but wait a second! Why don't the authors include sequential test results for GBS in their study? It's in the protocol. They have the background rates. So why no comparison to background rates? The same can be said of some of the other AEs for which there is only descriptive results. You can triangulate between the study protocol (linked above), the published tables (especially in the supplement) and the protocol [520] for establishing background rates to see exactly which ones should have a sequential comparison but instead are only descriptive.(MIS-C is an exception since that is a new diagnosis developed after COVID started.)

Also, according to the protocols, they are supposed to have some 'negative case' controls -- AEs that would be unrelated to vaccination but could detect other differences, like care-seeking. Why aren't those results reported?

Finally, I think the idea that they look at only 20 very specific AEs then declare them safe upon not finding anything is very myopic. There are many different ICD 10 codes for blood clots or strokes, for example, but here they look at very specific ones like DVT. What might they find if they looked at, for example, a broader range of blood clot diagnoses grouped together?

Also (and related), they say in the protocol that they would add AEs to look at based on signals identified from other sources. What about all the concerning safety signals identified by the CDC for these age groups?"

15.3. The UK Government's flawed Covid-19 death numbers

12 June 2023

For well over two years into the covid era the 'headline' number of covid deaths (and the one most prominent on the UK Government covid dashboard) [521]) were those defined as "anybody dying within 28 days of a positive PCR test". While the chart of such "covid deaths" is still prominently displayed on the dashboard to this day, it is no longer the first chart shown. Instead, the first shown is now the (more reasonable) number of deaths "with covid on the death certificate". But looking at the dashboard today filtered for England [522] there is an uncanny likeness between the two different ways of counting covid deaths. As can be seen in the full version of this article [523], while the graphs are very slightly different, the cumulative totals of deaths are almost identical:

- England: Total deaths with covid on death certificate: 192,231
- England: Total deaths within 28 days of positive test: 192,320

This is a freakish likeness of numbers which should surely be very different. In an earlier version of this article we assumed these figures must be wrong because when we looked at the dashboard [524] filtered for the whole of the UK it appeared that the whole UK total for deaths within 28 days of a positive test (178,407) was lower than for England (192,320). But what we failed to notice is that, unlike the England data, the UK total for deaths within 28 days curiously only goes up to May 2022.

But, even if we assume that the UK figures are correct, there remains a fundamental problem. We would expect the total deaths within 28 days of a positive test to be much greater than the total dying with covid on the death certificate. This is because surely almost all of the latter would have tested positive within 28 days of death; and we would expect many of those dying within 28 days of a positive test to have died from causes other than covid and hence that covid should not be on the death certificate.

So why are these numbers essentially identical? In fact, it gets even stranger because if we look at the cumulative totals up the end of 31 Dec 2021 (i.e., a period that covers the main two years of the pandemic 2020-2021) we find (for England) that the total with covid on the death certificate is over 20,000 ***higher*** than the total within 28 days of a positive test:

- Total deaths with covid on death certificate: 151,088
- Total deaths within 28 days of positive test: 130,756

This is partly explained by the fact that in the first few months (before mass PCR testing) some people dying with covid were diagnosed based on symptoms alone. But since August 2020, with everybody entering hospital for any reason being tested almost daily, it is inconceivable that a person could die with covid listed as a cause unless they had tested positive within 28 days.

While the number of deaths within 28 days of a positive test has been gradually 'catching up' (to be exactly equal as of today) the only way to explain why the numbers are still so similar is that:

- almost every person dying within 28 days of a positive test must, for a very long period, automatically have had covid listed as a cause written on the death certificate. This is something we were assured was not happening; and
- even after the introduction of mass PCR testing many people were somehow determined to have died because of covid without any test.

And, of course, there is other data which confirm that the figures for total deaths with covid on their death certificate must be a massive exaggeration of the true number of covid deaths.

Consider, for example, the total (mentioned above) of 151,088 deaths in England up to 31 Dec 2021 with covid on the death certificate. This figure is nonsensical given this response [525] to an FOI asking for number of deaths where covid was the only cause mentioned on the death certificate. The response confirmed that less than 5% of all officially classified covid deaths in England and Wales up to 31 Dec 2021 listed covid as the only cause of death on the death certificate.

What can we conclude from all of this?

- It is a statistical freak only that, as of today, the total number of England deaths with covid on the death certificate is equal to the total number of deaths within 28 days of a positive test.
- The covid death numbers for the UK as stated on the UK Government dashboard have been - and continue to be - massively exaggerated.

15.4. The Very Best of Cheap Trick

29 July 2023

Our team first exposed the practice of deliberate miscategorisation of vaccine status on December 3rd, 2021, in a tweet [526] that got 3 million impressions. The tweet was based on our paper lodged on the ResearchGate archive, here [527] (this and an earlier version got approximately half a million reads).

The 'cheap trick' is simple: categorise those who are vaccinated as unvaccinated up until some arbitrarily defined time period after vaccination takes place. The time period might be 7, 14 or 21 days. The supposed justification for this practice being that the benefits of the vaccine do not accrue until it has had time to 'kick in'. And before it becomes effective on day seven, fourteen, or whatever, the recipient is considered to be unvaccinated.

At the time of our original work, we were not at all sure how globally widespread this selection bias was. Recently the Dark Horse podcast [528] covered the issue and shortly after Bret Weinstein asked me if there was a comprehensive list of studies that had deliberately committed this cheap trick.

This article is our first attempt to provide such a list. It contains a mix of observational and other studies that have employed the cheap trick when assessing vaccine effectiveness for either infection, hospitalisation or death.

Note that as well as numerous and varying time periods that the trick might be employed, there are four ways in which this kind of selection bias might take place:

1. **Miscategorised**: Vaccinated are categorised as unvaccinated (or twice vaccinated categorised as single vaccinated Etc.)

2. **Unverified**: Those who are vaccinated but cannot be verified as such are categorised as unvaccinated.

3. **Excluded**: Those who are vaccinated but are infected before 14 days (or whatever) are allocated to neither the unvaccinated nor vaccinated categories but are instead simply removed from the analysis.

4. **Undefined**: The definitions of vaccinated and unvaccinated are left intentionally undefined.

This third version of the trick - exclusion - has tended to have been overlooked.

Note that Hulscher et al [529] systematic review of autopsy studies found that the average time from injection to death was 14.3 (mean), 3 (median) irrespective of dose.

Also, it is worth pointing out that miscategorisation of vaccine status is not a phenomenon unique and new to covid but has a long history going back to at least the 19th century, when in 1889 Alfred Wallace [530] documented cases where deaths were registered as unvaccinated when they had been vaccinated.

To compile this list, we looked through our own records and also consulted this Lancet meta-analysis [531]on vaccine effectiveness.

The list is organised by authors and publication venue (Lancet, New England Journal of Medicine (NEJM), Journal of Vaccines Etc).

Andrews et al UK study – NEJM [532]

> "Duration of Protection against Mild and Severe Disease by Covid-19 Vaccines"
>
> Only "those at least 28 days after first dose were considered vaccinated:
>
> Vaccine effectiveness was assessed for each vaccine separately and according to intervals after vaccination of at least 28 days after the first dose and at least 14 days after the second dose.

Baum et al Finland study - BMC Infection Diseases [533]

> "High vaccine effectiveness against severe COVID-19 in the elderly in Finland before and after the emergence of Omicron"
>
> Definitions are vague but it appears anybody with first dose within 21 days was classified as unvaccinated.

Buchan et al Ontario study – JAMA [534]

> "Estimated Effectiveness of COVID-19 Vaccines Against Omicron or Delta Symptomatic Infection and Severe Outcomes"
>
> We excluded .... individuals who had received only 1 dose or 4 doses of COVID-19 vaccine or who had received a second dose less than 7 days before being tested.

Corazo et al Quebec study – Lancet [535]

> "Protection against omicron (B.1.1.529) BA.2 reinfection conferred by primary omicron BA.1 or pre-omicron SARS-CoV-2 infection among health-care workers with and without mRNA vaccination: a test-negative case-control study".

We defined mRNA vaccination as receipt of one dose at least 14 days before specimen collection or two or three doses at least 7 days before specimen collection, with the first and second doses administered at least 21 days apart. People who had a SARS-CoV-2 test within these intervals, who had an invalid vaccination date, or who received a non-mRNA vaccine were excluded.

Chung et al Ontario study - Open Forum Infections diseases [536]

"Effectiveness of COVID-19 Vaccines Over Time Prior to Omicron Emergence in Ontario, Canada: Test-Negative Design Study"

We excluded tests from individuals who, on the testing date, had previously tested positive for SARS-CoV-2 or had received only a single vaccine dose, had received 2 doses but were <7 days from the second dose, had received any non–Health Canada–approved vaccines (including the Johnson & Johnson/Janssen Ad26.COV2.S vaccine, which was approved but rarely used in Ontario), or had received 3 doses.

Pálinkás and Sándor Hungary study – Vaccines [537]

This was a study into Covid-19 vaccine effectiveness in Hungary.

They admitted they simply excluded those people who were 'partially' vaccinated:

Partially vaccinated people who received the vaccine during the follow-up period but did not become protected during the study period (did not receive the booster or died before the 7th day after complete vaccination) were excluded from the investigation.

Dagan et al Israel study – Lancet [538]

This study by Dagan et al from April 2021 in the NEJM looked at Covid-19 vaccine effectiveness in Israel.

In the paper the authors said:

"We considered three periods: days 14 through 20 after the first dose of vaccine, days 21 through 27 after the first dose (administration of the second dose was scheduled to occur on day 21 after the first dose), and day 7 after the second dose until the end of the follow-up....The period immediately after the first dose, when immunity is gradually building, was excluded in the main analyses".

Mark Reeder in his paper [539] on the Dagan study carefully documented this and other sources of selection bias.

Haas et al Israel study – Lancet [540]

The Hass et al study, published in the Lancet has been the subject of a long-running saga here [541] on our substack. It looked at effectiveness in those who were twice vaccinated (after 7 days had passed) versus the unvaccinated:

"....Covid-19-related hospitalisation, severe or critical hospitalisation, and death was calculated on the basis of incidence rates in fully vaccinated individuals (defined as those for whom 7 days had passed since receiving the second dose of vaccine) compared with rates in unvaccinated individuals (who had not received any doses of the vaccine)."

Ferdinands et al USA study – BMJ [542]

"Waning of vaccine effectiveness against moderate and severe Covid-19 among adults in the US from the VISION network: test negative, case-control study".

"We excluded individuals who... received only one dose of an mRNA vaccine less than 14 days before."

Lyngse et al Denmark Delta study - Nature Communications [543]

This study from Denmark only considered 'fully vaccinated' against 'unvaccinated' with neither term defined anywhere in the paper. The authors also admit that that the 'unvaccinated' were likely to have been subject to more frequent PCR tests than the 'fully vaccinated'.

Nordström et al Swedish study – Lancet [544]

"Risk of infection, hospitalisation, and death up to 9 months after a second dose of COVID-19 vaccine: a retrospective, total population cohort study in Sweden"

Compares only those "Vaccinated" which is defined simply as 'two doses' against 'unvaccinated'. No definition of either is given anywhere in the paper.

Rosenberg et al USA study – NEJM [545]

Very high efficacy rates were reported in this paper but "vaccinated" here refers to: fully vaccinated (≥14 days after receipt of the final dose)

while "unvaccinated" refers to anybody who did not have a matching Covid-19 vaccine record according to the NYSIIS and CIR databases.

Petráš et al Czech study – Vaccines [546]

"The Effectiveness of Post-Vaccination and Post-Infection Protection in the Hospital Staff of Three Prague Hospitals: A Cohort Study of 8-Month Follow-Up from the Start of the COVID-19 Vaccination Campaign (COVANESS)"

This paper is remarkable in that it considers three categories of vaccination status (unvaccinated, partially vaccinated, full vaccinated) without providing any definition of what any of these categories mean.

Thomas et al International RCT – NEJM [547]

This was a placebo-controlled trial, but efficacy was only assessed based on cases at least 7 days after the second dose:

BNT162b2 efficacy against laboratory-confirmed Covid-19 with an onset of 7 days or more after the second dose was assessed.

Australia New South Wales - official study [548]

"Vaccination among COVID-19 cases in the NSW Delta outbreak Reporting period: 16 June to 7 October 2021"

Unvaccinated cases were defined as either those with a) no vaccine record in NCIMS and unable to link to a record of any COVID-19 vaccination in AIR, or b) within 21 days of first dose.

Double vaccinated cases were defined as those as least 14 days after second dose and a minimum of 14 days between doses.

Robles et al Puerto Rico study – Lancet [549]

This appallingly biased study was actually used to impose vaccine mandates in Puerto Rico. The authors' state:

The decision to impose mandates, as well as current Department of Health recommendations related to boosters, were guided by the data and the effectiveness estimates presented here.

But the very high efficacy rates published were based on comparing 'fully vaccinated' with everybody else:

We denoted an individual as fully vaccinated two weeks after the date they received the final dose in the COVID-19 vaccine series.

So, anybody not 'fully vaccinated' was essentially classified as unvaccinated.

Swedish Ministry of Health [550]

The Swedish doctors appeal uncovered the scandal that the Swedish ministry of health had miscategorised over 900 deaths:

The Swedish Public Health Agency has misled the public about the benefits of vaccination against Covid-19 by recording Covid-19 deaths amongst the vaccinated as unvaccinated. Over 900 deaths with Covid-19 have been misrepresented as occurring in the unvaccinated, thereby greatly distorting the effectiveness of the vaccination programme, for which the Swedish Public Health Agency is responsible.

USA CDC definition [551]

The US CDC defines Covid-19 cases by vaccine status using a two-week rule:

Vaccinated case with a primary series: SARS-CoV-2 RNA or antigen detected in a respiratory specimen collected ≥14 days after verifiably completing the primary series of an FDA-authorized or approved COVID-19 vaccine.

Vaccinated case with a monovalent booster: SARS-CoV-2 RNA or antigen detected in a respiratory specimen collected in a person verified to have received a primary series of an FDA-authorized/approved vaccine and ≥14 days after receipt of at least one additional dose of any monovalent FDA-authorized/approved COVID-19 vaccine ....

Vaccinated case with a bivalent booster: SARS-CoV-2 RNA or antigen detected in a respiratory specimen collected in a person verified to have received a primary series and ≥14 days after receipt of one additional dose of any bivalent FDA-authorized/approved COVID-19 vaccine .....

Partially vaccinated case: SARS-CoV-2 RNA or antigen detected in a respiratory specimen collected from a person who received at least one FDA-authorized or approved vaccine dose but did not complete a primary series ≥14 days before collection of a respiratory specimen with SARS-CoV-2 RNA or antigen detected.

The CDC classify the unvaccinated as:

Unvaccinated case: SARS-CoV-2 RNA or antigen detected in a respiratory specimen from a person who has not been verified to have received any COVID-19 vaccine doses before the specimen collection date.

The crucial thing about the unvaccinated category is that it hinges on verification. So, if someone cannot have their vaccination status verified, they will likely be listed as a an unvaccinated Covid-19 case/death despite being vaccinated.

Also note that those who are categorised as ≥14 days might not be classed as unvaccinated (or as partially vaccinated if they have taken a second dose) but might instead simply be excluded from any statistics or efficiency calculations altogether.

Bermingham et al UK ONS study - official report [552]

Estimates of the risk of hospital admission for coronavirus (COVID-19) and death involving COVID-19 by vaccination status, overall and by age group, using anonymised linked data from Census 2021:

We calculated vaccine effectiveness for different doses (first, second and third dose or booster) and time since dose, to observe how the effectiveness changes over time. The vaccination statuses used were: unvaccinated (those with no vaccination or who were vaccinated with a first dose less than 21 days ago)

UKHSA - official response [553]

In response to a FOI request made by Joel Smalley the UK Health Security Agency (UKHSA) admitted to a similar practice when recording those who had received two vaccine doses as having received a single dose.

Individuals who have received 2 doses but less than 14 days before the specimen date of their positive Covid-

19 test are included in the 'Received 1 dose ≥ 21 days before specimen date' category.

Pilishvili et al USA study – NEJM [554]

This paper in the NEJM on the vaccination of US Healthcare personnel and employed the trick there:

"The effectiveness of a single vaccine dose was measured from 14 days after receipt of the first dose through 6 days after receipt of the second dose (partially vaccinated)."

Bermingham et al UK ONS study – preprint [555]

The observational study by Bermingham et al looked at vaccine effectiveness against hospitalisation and death using the ONS data set. The pre-print is available on medrixv.

Whilst the paper defines exposure as first dose, second dose and third dose Covid-19 vaccination the unvaccinated category is conspicuous by its absence of *any* definition.

However, perhaps partly in reaction to our past criticisms the authors did perform a sensitivity analysis by omitting those vaccinated 'within 21 days' from the unvaccinated category:

The impact of including the first 21 days after a first dose of a vaccine in the 'unvaccinated' category was investigated by omitting these days from the 'unvaccinated category' (treating the 21 days after first dose as a separate vaccination status).

Clearly the default categorisation is that 21 days after first dose is counted as being unvaccinated and removing this group from the unvaccinated category is treated as a deviation from normal practice This is confirmed elsewhere by the ONS's own admitted practice [556].

In the paper's discussion section, they then make a Freudian slip by referring to the 'unvaccinated vaccination' category!

In addition, we also show in a sensitivity test that including the first 21 days after the first dose, when protection is rising, in the unvaccinated vaccination produces results consistent with the main analysis.

Angel et al Israel study – JAMA [557]

The main results stated (which equated to a VE ratio of 83%) were based only on "fully vaccinated" against never vaccinated where:

Full vaccination was defined as more than 7 days after receipt of the second vaccine dose.

Arbel et al Israel study – NEJM [558]

In September 2022 the NEJM published a study by Arbel et al, who investigated nirmatrelvir as a treatment for Covid-19. Subsequently Hoeg et al [559] submitted a letter to the NEJM editor complaining about confounding and healthy vaccine bias in the data.

However, unfortunately Hoeg et al failed to pick up on the obvious miscategorisation bias in the Arbel et al study. This was instead reported by Retsef Levi on twitter [560].

Subsequently the authors of the study responded to the letter from Hoeg et al, casually admitting the miscategorisation:

The authors and colleagues reply: With regard to a potential healthy vaccinee bias, all participants in our study started at an "unboosted" status, which was changed to a "boosted" status 7 days after vaccination....

Lyngse et al Denmark Omicron study - Nature Communications [561]

This is similar to the other Lyngse et al paper except it focuses on the omicron variant.

We classified individuals into three groups: (i) unvaccinated; (ii) fully vaccinated; or (iii) booster vaccinated. The definition of fully vaccinated included individuals that had been infected more than 14 days previously, but was otherwise defined according to the vaccine used as follows: 7 days after second dose of Comirnaty (Pfizer/BioNTech); 15 days after second dose of Vaxzevria (AstraZeneca); 14 days after second dose of Spikevax (Moderna); 14 days after vaccination with Janssen (Johnson & Johnson); 14 days after the second dose for cross vaccinated. Booster-vaccinated was defined as 7 days following the booster vaccination.

Paternina-Caicedo et al Colombian study – Lancet [562]

Paternina-Caicedo et al published this study about vaccine effectiveness in Colombia. M. Nathaniel Mead sent us this communication about the study:

As an aside, I recently confirmed this misclassification practice with Dr. Angel Paternina-Caicedo, lead author of a cohort study in Colombia (n=720K). He openly admitted to me that this is what they were doing. In their study, the magnitude of the claimed Pfizer vaxx "death vaccine effectiveness" is so high 93% (men) and 94% (women), that if these values were true, the Pfizer jabbed countries (e.g., Israel) would have Covid deaths rates that should have stopped in their tracks - 93% reduction. So, it simply cannot be true! It's like running a clinical trial where everyone is in the control group, then changing groups conditional on surviving 2 weeks after people taking a drug. I have many thoughts about this study but won't go into them.

Stock et al. Vaccination in pregnant women in Scotland - Nature Medicine [563]

In this study which claimed lower covid infections rates and better outcomes for women vaccinated in pregnancy compared to those unvaccinated, the unvaccinated were defined as:

no previous COVID-19 vaccination before the date of onset of COVID-19 or with one dose of vaccination ≤21 d before the date of onset.

Mitchell et al Canadian Nosocomial Infection Surveillance Program – JAMA [564]

This study concluded:

"Admission to the ICU and in-hospital all-cause death rates were significantly higher among those who were unvaccinated against COVID-19 when compared with those who were fully vaccinated"

But in a response to Alberto Donzelli, the lead author Robyn Mitchell replied:

"My sincere apologies for my delayed response, I found your email in my junk folder unfortunately.

Yes, you are correct – in the methods under definitions:

Fully vaccinated was defined as a patient with symptom onset or specimen collection date that was 14 or more days following receipt of a second dose of a 2-dose COVID-19 vaccine or a single dose of a 1-dose COVID-19 vaccine.

Fully vaccinated with an additional dose was defined as a fully vaccinated patient with symptom onset or specimen collection date that was 14 or more days following receipt of at least 1 additional dose of a COVID-19 vaccine.

Additionally, as noted for Figure 4 - Partially vaccinated patients (defined as patients with a symptom onset or specimen collection date that was 14 days following receipt of a first dose of a 2-dose COVID-19 vaccine or <14 days after receiving a second dose) were excluded from these analyses.

To answer your question, yes we considered any patient who did not meet the above criteria as unvaccinated. In our surveillance protocol the definition we applied for unvaccinated:

Unvaccinated = Patients with a symptom onset date or test date that was 0 to <14 days following the first dose of a two-dose COVID-19 vaccine or patient had received zero doses of a COVID-19 vaccine.

Thank you for raising this question as we should have considered including this definition in our manuscript.

Kind regards,

Robyn"

Kashif Ali et al Evaluation of covid vaccines in adolescents - New England J Medicine [565]

The figures for vaccine efficacy in prevention of SARS Cov-2 infection were based on considering as vaccinated only those 14 days after vaccination.

The WHO Public health surveillance for COVID-19, 22 July 2022 [566]

States: "a person is defined vaccinated when they have completed the primary vaccination series."

Yau et al Singapore study – Lancet [567]

Patients who were partially vaccinated or did not receive any vaccination were deemed 'not fully vaccinated.'

M. Nathaniel Mead (Nutritional Epidemiologist, Consultant & Science Editor Editorial Board Member, *Integrative Cancer Therapies*) asked corresponding author Joachim Yau how "vaccination status" was defined in their study. Specifically, asking whether a person was considered "vaccinated" only 14 days after the injection. He confirmed that this was indeed the case, that his study uses the same 14-day rule used by Singapore as per CDC guidelines.

Tan et al Study of effectiveness of covid vaccines in cancer patients JAMA, 2023 [568]

This study claims to provide "evidence of the clinical effectiveness of mRNA-based vaccines against COVID-19 in patients with cancer". But, after Alberto Donzelli wrote asking for clarification about definitions not provided in the paper, author Raghav Sundar replied:

For persons who are vaccinated with only 1 dose (0-7 days), they are classified as unvaccinated and for those who are vaccinated with 2 dose (0-7 days), they are classified as zero/single dose, whereas those who are boosted (0-7days) are classified as vaccinated with 2 does (>150 days).

Chapter 16. Blasphemer's begone! Censorship, secrets and it gets personal

16.1. Blasphemers begone: cancelled by the NHS!

22 June 2023

16.1.1. The invitation and cancellation

A few weeks ago Norman was invited to present our work on Bayesian networks for the NHS Health and Care Analytics Conference 2023 [569]. This is a large and important conference chaired by Ben Goldacre (the author of the best seller 'Bad Science' [570])- sold out with over 400 delegates and a similar number online.

The conference organisers tweeted [571] about Norman's presentation:

> "The brilliant @ProfNFenton will be sharing his expert knowledge on Bayesian networks and how they can improve your decision quality"

Norman was neither offered, nor asked for, any fee for doing this. In the last week he spent many hours preparing a presentation to ensure it properly addressed the conference theme and contained our latest research with examples of Bayesian network risk models for a range of chronic diseases (diabetes, rheumatoid arthritis, multiple sclerosis and Alzheimer's). The title, abstract and bio that were agreed and approved (see full article [572]) confirm that the talk was nothing to do with any work he had undertaken on covid or the vaccines.

On Tuesday (20 June 2023) - ironically just seconds after recording a video for Michael Shellenberg's [573] Censorship Files documentary - he received this email from the person who had originally invited him to make the presentation (we have redacted the name of that person and the other recipients):

> From: XXXX
> Sent: Tuesday, June 20, 2023 4:32 PM
> To: Norman Fenton
> Cc: XXXX, XXXX, XXXXX
> Subject: Session on BN for NHS conference
>
> Dear Norman
>
> I hope you are well.
> I am sorry to say that the conference organising committee have just been alerted to the controversy around vaccinations on your twitter account and fear that this may distract from the conference. They have asked that we not proceed with the planned session on Bayesian Networks. This is very unfortante <sic> given your expertise in BN.

> With sincere apologies
> XXXXX

So, Norman was cancelled not for the content of his talk but because he had done other work raising concerns about covid vaccine safety.

After an immediate response that he sent on 20 June stating that he intended to make this public (for which there was no response), he sent the following more formal follow-up at 09.00 on 21 June:

> "Following on from my response yesterday, I would like to know more about how the decision was made to cancel my presentation and who initiated it and approved it (including if any of the recipients of the email approved the decision). Was there any attempt by any NHS staff to reverse the decision given that it is clear that my voice has been suppressed simply for raising safety concerns in the public interest? I am asking this because it has become a matter of public interest to publish this story of censorship. I would be grateful if you could reply within 24 hours as I intend to publish this tomorrow.
>
> I also require a copy of all the communications referred to ("the conference committee have just been alerted to") by return under GDPR."

More than 24 hours have passed, and Norman has still received no acknowledgement or reply.

Of course, this is just the latest - albeit a particularly nasty - example of the censorship and cancellation I've suffered for the last three years.

As Martin noted [574] on twitter:

> "Note that in censoring Norman they are also censoring research undertaken by young researchers who have not uttered a public word on the subject of vaccines. Also bear in mind the results of this research were largely funded by the public purse, hence the event committee are denying the NHS access to research results funded by another arm of government. The decision is not only unethical and irrational, it is deliberately vindictive."

Some relevant information on Ben Goldacre here [575] and here [576].

Norman sent the following (more or less the same) subject access request letter to the various organisations involved in the conference, namely Birmingham University who hosted the conference, The NHS Strategy Unit, who organised the conference, and the various NHS Trusts supporting the conference.

> "Dear Sir or Madam
>
> **Subject access request (relating to cancellation of my presentation to Health and Care Analytics Conference 2023.**
>
> Following the cancellation of my presentation on Bayesian networks to the Health and Care Analytics Conference 2023 as described in this

> article: https://wherearethenumbers.substack.com/p/blasphemers-begone please supply copies of all emails and other available electronic communications between conference committee members (including the co-chair Ben Goldacre) and others in which my name or conference contribution is mentioned.
>
> Yours faithfully
>
> Professor Norman Fenton"

16.1.2. The Birmingham University subject access request response

On 31 July 2023 Norman got a formal response from Birmingham University (which, in its previous replies to many of his supporters who wrote to them to complain, responded with a form message simply saying that the decision to cancel Norman had nothing to do with them).

Here is the Birmingham University cover letter [577] which sets out what they claim are the limits to the information they can provide. And here is the 12-page (heavily redacted) report [578] containing the relevant emails and correspondence about him. Some 'highlights' include:

> A heavily redacted email sent by a person in the NHS Midlands and Lancashire Commissioning Support Unit on 23 June at 15:22 that included the statement: "*We were alerted to his twitter profile and its anti-COVID vaccine response and an internal decision was made to uninvite him. He has called us out on twitter and on his blog about it, and there is a medium sized backlash which we're ignoring (if he contacts us directly we will respond).*"
>
> Another heavily redacted email from somebody at Birmingham University made it clear that Birmingham University received a lot of emails complaining about the decision to cancel Norman: "*Would you let me know what has happened with Norman Fenton please? Was there any specific reason he was dropped from the conference, we have received some (not) nice emails about this XXXXX*"

There follows several examples of the emails they received, but the most revealing information is this 'Teams data' transcript at the end; dates are not provided (we assume the 'Monday' messages were 19 June) except for the last one dated 20 June at 15:43. This is where Norman is referred to as a "hardcore anti-vaxxer". The email informing him of his cancellation was sent just minutes later at 16:08 on 20 June.

> Teams data
> Monday 08:56: Seen the emails about Norman Fenton for NHS.
> Monday 12:35: Causing us all the issues with Norman
> Monday 08:35: Looking through the emails, there is one from redacted who is blaming the university for the Norman Fenton thing.
> Monday 08:54: We've had a really tricky one from Norman himself
> Monday 08:58: We can reply to say that we weren't involved in the decision and our only involvement was to remove him from the programme.
> Monday 11:53: This Norman thing is causing a lot of backlash.

> Monday 12:19: Asked Norman for a few details – we have a draft we can go with but thought invite him to share the info.
> Norman does some things around Covid counting. How stats have been used and whilst its all accurate and from a mathematician's perspective, there is an angle.
> 20 June 15:43: Someone has just flagged on Twitter that Professor Norman Fenton is a hardcore anti-vaxxer

We look forward to the eventual responses from the NHS organisers and especially any correspondence involving the event co-chair Ben Goldacre who has so far refused to respond to the many people who have written to him about this.

16.1.3. NHS response

18 August 2023

The NHS Midlands and Lancashire Commissioning Support Unit say they need more time to provide the information (they are now long past the 20 days within which they should have provided it). When Norman reminded them of the delay they said:

> We have received some records that we are reviewing but we have just enquired with the relevant people to make sure we have received all records applicable for the processing of this SAR.

Yet, interestingly, D Jackson submitted a Freedom of Information Request asking about the reasons for the cancellation and they have published their response to it here [579].

According to this, the cancellation was triggered by a single twitter message (with all names redacted) alerting the 'conference team' to Norman's twitter account. The message was dated 3:33pm, 20 June 2023. The email [580] sent to Norman telling him he was cancelled was sent at 16:08 on the same day, just 35 minutes later.

Well, first of all, it is very simple to check who sent this redacted tweet since it is still public [581] on twitter. Just in case it is deleted by the time I publish this, Figure 65 is a screenshot of the tweet [*within a couple of hours of this article being published the tweet was indeed deleted and now the whole account is 'protected'!*]

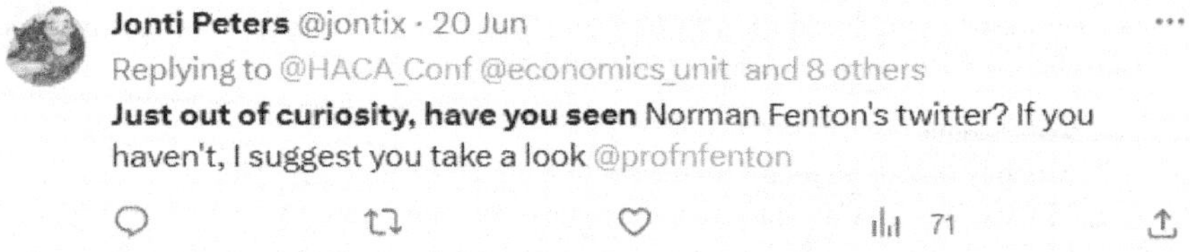

Figure 65 Non-redacted version of tweet

Among those tagged in the tweet were 8 NHS organisations, namely: Health and Care Analytics Conference 2023 (@HACA_Conf); Health Economics Unit (@economics_unit); NHS Midlands & Lancashire CSU (@MLCSU); NECS (@NHSnecs); SCW (@NHSscw);

NHS Arden and GEM CSU (@ardengem); Strategy Unit (@StretegyUnit; Midlands Decision Support Network (@MidlandsDSN).

The FOI states (obviously [name] is Norman):

> The conference team were in a meeting at the time of receiving the above and scrolled through [name]'s Twitter feed. It was felt comments made by [name] on Twitter, conflicted with NHS values regarding vaccination, and thus would not be in keeping with our values as an NHS organisation.
>
> There was no further analysis, and the decision was made in the meeting to cancel the session.

So, according to this narrative, in just 35 minutes between 15:33 on 20 June (when Jonti Peters posted the tweet) and 16:08 on 20 June when Norman received the cancellation email:

- the conference team just happened to be all meeting;
- someone in the team saw the tweet;
- they all looked through Norman's twitter feed
- they made their decision to cancel Norman;
- they agreed on the wording of the cancellation email;
- someone wrote the email and sent it to Norman.

That means that within a period of at most a few minutes unspecified comments made by Norman on twitter regarding vaccination were deemed by the conference committee to be 'not in keeping with our values as an NHS organisation'. This is a slightly different reason for cancellation than that previously provided which was that Norman's 'presence would be a distraction' at the conference. But it shows how little effort is required to cancel someone.

Disagree with NHS policy on one medication and you are unpersoned. That is totalitarianism.

Before Jonti Peters deleted his tweet and set his whole account to 'protected' we managed to get a screenshot (see full article [582]) of the very curious ("Digital Intelligence Unit") tweet [583] that a reader here alerted us to. The tweet from Jonti Peters said:

> Two great opportunities to work within the Digital Intelligence Unit <links to position for "Full Stack Developer" and "Senior Full Stack Developer" were provided>
>
> Feel free to DM me if there's anything you want to know, or to have a chat about them <gif of Bart Simpson cartoon with caption "JOIN US">

16.1.4. NHS finally responds

28 August 2023, plus updates

On 28 August 2023 Norman finally got a response from the NHS to his own subject access request about the cancellation. For legal reasons he never reported on that or what happened thereafter because The Free Speech Union lawyers submitted a formal request for an apology on his behalf and a small payment to a charity. Because there has as yet been no resolution there are still limits to what we can say publicly. But we can reveal some snippets of what the NHS and their lawyers said.

The NHS response to the subject access request contained a covering letter and 17 different heavily redacted documents, each of which contained a thread of one or more emails about Norman. Four of the documents were simply email threads in which Norman had participated before and after the cancellation - so nothing new there. Nine of the documents were correspondence from, presumably, members of the public who had made formal complaints to the NHS about his cancellation.

It was nice to know that people had complained on Norman's behalf, but the most interesting aspect of the exchange was that the documents contained no responses from the NHS and no information as to whether the NHS ever did reply to these complaints.

The remaining four documents were internal communications announcing, and later confirming, that Norman's talk was cancelled, instructing people to remove his name, close down the associated Eventbrite announcement, etc. Hence, there was little new in the subject access request response to shed light on the real reasons and process that led up to their decision to cancel his appearance. And, to this day, the Conference Chair Ben Goldacre has refused to respond to any of the multiple requests for information about this.

However, following the Free Speech Union letter the NHS lawyers sent a lengthy response that contained many remarkable and offensive statements about Noman. First, they inexplicably referred to tweets he had made AFTER the cancellation announcement on 20 June 2023 (so, comically, they are using tweets posted months after the lecture as their first reason for cancelling his lecture!). They stated (in point 6 of their letter):

> Since 20 June 2023, the Defendant has been aware that the Claimant also maintains an active profile on Twitter as a controversialist. For example, in recent weeks, he has repeatedly tweeted arguments against the conviction of NHS nurse Lucy Letby for the murder of seven babies. He is a climate crisis denier, tweeting and retweeting about climate change as "climate catastrophe propaganda" and criticising "the tyrannical Net Zero policies being foisted upon us all under the guise of solving the non-existent 'global boiling crisis'".

While Norman certainly stands by the claims about "climate catastrophe propaganda", the statement that he "repeatedly tweeted arguments against the conviction of NHS nurse Lucy Letby for the murder of seven babies." is false. It seems to be based on the fact that he had simply posted a video interview he made with a colleague who raised concerns about the conviction and followed that up with links to his articles about it.

In point 7, apart from the fact that they object to tweets which simply state the truth about covid, they bizarrely imply that Norman is some kind of Hitler fan for using the 'clown world' icons in tweets. This is despite the fact that he had very publicly stated in a viral video [584] in March 2023 that he was a Jew whose father was the sole survivor in his large family of the Nazi Holocaust:

> The Claimant's tweets about Covid 19 are less moderate than his "position" as expressed in your letter. He tweets allegations that the "mainstream media" or

> "MSM" has lied about Covid, that death tolls have been inflated and even that there has not been a pandemic. For example, he tweeted that the "MSM" have "frame[d] Trump as a liar when he was the one telling the truth about it". He regularly ends his tweets about Covid with the clown emoji followed by the world emoji, meaning "clown world" ("🤡🌎"). This is an alt-right internet meme, which originated in 4chan and is also known as the "Honkler" or "Heil Honkler" sign1 within the American white supremacist movement. Honkler joins "Honk" with "Hitler". It is a dog whistle conveying that "the left" are creating a "clown world".

The reference to Trump above concerned the media's response to his statement in 2020 that he believed the claimed 3.4% covid fatality rate was too high. Trump was of course right, and the mainstream media were wrong.

In point 8 they attempt to paint Norman as an ignorant anti-vaxxer, and totally misrepresent some tweets he posted:

> In particular, the Claimant often tweets inflammatory messages condemning the basic interventions supported by the NHS and health services all over the world. This includes explicitly anti-Vaxx tweets, not only challenging vaccination for younger age groups (as mentioned in your letter) but for all age groups. For example, he recently tweeted about the NHS winter Covid booster campaign, which only targets older age groups and those at risk: "They'll repeat the mantra 'they stop hospitalisation & death'. So, here's a reminder of why that's garbage too." In the same tweet thread, he stated "every Covid test is an unnecessary medical intervention", accompanied by a child's face, crying and covered in blood.

The explanation for his cancellation is contained in point 11 of their letter, which amusingly refers to The Great Reset as a 'well-known covid conspiracy theory'

> On 20 June 2023, the HACA Conference organisers were in an internal meeting when a Twitter user tweeted at them asking if they had seen the Claimant's Twitter feed and suggesting that they should take a look. Some present at the meeting immediately did so and were very concerned by what they saw, which included sensationalist material, dog whistles and conspiracy theories. For example, they saw a tweet praising a project to "disrupt global tyranny", advertised by the slogan "resist the great reset", which refers to a well-known covid conspiracy theory. They saw another tweet alleging that "data scams have sustained 'official' narratives" in respect of Covid. Those present at the meeting felt the implication of many of the tweets was the NHS and Government is actively lying about harming patients with COVID vaccines as part of a globalist takeover of democratic governments. It was decided that inviting the Claimant to speak at this NHS conference would be inappropriate and would conflict in a damaging way with the NHS position on vaccination. They were also concerned that inviting the Claimant would implicitly endorse his public persona, which might deter NHS staff from attending the conference.

In Points 18 and 20 they provide the following further rationale for the cancellation:

> First, and most importantly, the decision furthers the objective of protection of health. All NHS bodies (and UK public authorities more widely) maintain clear and consistent messaging on the importance of vaccination against Covid 19 and other diseases. Since the pandemic, there has been a significant rise in the anti-Vaxx movement, which in turn risks jeopardising the vital public health benefits of high vaccine uptake. There are grave public health risks arising from any declining trust in vaccines and in NHS advice more generally. Put bluntly, a refusal to accept vaccination risks lives. The anti-Vaxx and Covid-sceptic movement has been fuelled by the kind of inflammatory tweets found on the Claimant's Twitter feed. As is well known, media platforms (particularly social media platforms such as Twitter) have been enormously influential in the spread of vaccine hesitancy. Such platforms have been used to spread widespread disinformation about the effectiveness or safety of vaccination both by individuals and by hostile state actors such as Russia. The influence of commentary upon social media platforms is magnified, where those who post on such platforms speak from a position of apparent authority.
>
> Second, the decision furthers the objective of the protection of the MLSCU's reputation. MLSCU's functions include advancing innovation and research within the NHS. In order to carry out this function effectively, it needs to maintain the trust of NHS professionals. It does this by inviting credible individuals to share their research. While the Claimant has conducted well-respected research as an academic, his public profile contains extremist, controversialist positions, including alt-right memes and conspiracy theories. MLSCU was entitled to take the view that its own reputation and ability to carry out its functions could be undermined by hosting the Claimant. Further, any erosion in the credibility of the MLSCU could have an indirect adverse impact on the protection of health, if NHS professionals were to forego the opportunity to access important research shared by the MLSCU.

Further reasons are provided in points 27, 28:

> The decision is justified by reference to his inflammatory and controversialist profile on Twitter, covering a wide range of subjects on which the Claimant has no particular academic expertise and expressed in a style that extends to far right dog whistles. Both the content and style of large numbers of tweets by the Claimant mean that they clearly are not "academic expression".
>
> This decision addresses the risk that placing the Claimant on an NHS platform would be reported or perceived by anti-Vaxxers and the public as an endorsement of his extreme statements on Twitter, as well as leading to potential loss of trust in MLCSU. This risk would subsist regardless of whether he spoke on these issues at the conference. There would be no way of ensuring that the Claimant's presence at the conference was always reported on social media with a relevant disclaimer.

For the record here [585] is the actual talk Norman had planned to give.

16.2. Censored by the academic preprint servers

5 July 2023

MedRxiv and arXiv are systematically rejecting academic papers that do not fit the narrative.

We were asked today if it was true that the preprint server medRxiv (which is supposed to accept unreviewed papers relating to health and medicine) was automatically rejecting all our covid papers. In fact, we have reported on such rejections several times before (see, for example here and here). As we have made clear, initially when we were not challenging the 'official' covid narrative in the spring of 2020 we had no problems getting our research papers accepted in peer reviewed journals as well as preprint servers like medRxiv and arXiv. Indeed, we have just checked and all of the papers (which were mainly focusing on covid risk factors) in 2020 were published on medRxiv:

- Butcher, R., & Fenton, N. E. (2020). Extending the range of symptoms in a Bayesian Network for the Predictive Diagnosis of COVID-19, medRxiv [586].
- Prodhan, G., & Fenton, N. E. (2020). Extending the range of COVID-19 risk factors in a Bayesian network model for personalised risk assessment. medRxiv [587].
- Fenton, N. E., McLachlan, S., Lucas, P., Dube, K., Hitman, G., Osman, M., Kyrimi, E., Neil, M. (2020). "A privacy-preserving Bayesian network model for personalised COVID-19 risk assessment and contact tracing". MedRxiv [588].
- Neil, M., Fenton, N.E, Osman, M., & McLachlan, S. (2020). "Bayesian Network Analysis of Covid-19 data reveals higher Infection Prevalence Rates and lower Fatality Rates than widely reported". Journal of Risk Research [589], 23 (7-8), 866-879. Preprint: MedRxiv [590].

But every paper submitted after that has been rejected and, on reflection, it is surprising just how many there were and at the 'reasons' given. For the record, the full list from medRxiv with the associated rejection letters is provided in the full version [591] of this article (in each case we also link to the article as published on ResearchGate). Here is a selection of the responses we got:

> "We regret to inform you that your manuscript is inappropriate for medRxiv. It is primarily a review/viewpoint not a research article with new data and therefore out of scope."
>
> "Thank you for your submission to medRxiv. Unfortunately, during the screening process, we determined that this manuscript is not suitable for medRxiv. It is not a clinical research paper so out of scope."
>
> "Thank you for your submission. As part of our process, all submissions are screened to ensure they match medRxiv posting criteria and scope (see https://www.medrxiv.org/content/about-medrxiv). During our screening process, your manuscript was judged to be primarily a viewpoint rather than a clinical

research article with new data and is thus not within medRxiv scope (see https://www.medrxiv.org/about/FAQ), so will not be posted."

> "Thank you for submitting your manuscript to medRxiv. We regret to inform you that your manuscript is inappropriate for posting. medRxiv is intended for research papers, and our screening process determined that this manuscript fell short of that description."

> "Thank you for submitting your manuscript to medRxiv. We regret to inform you that your manuscript will not be posted. A small number of papers are deemed during screening to be more appropriate for dissemination after peer review at a journal rather than as preprints." (This exact response was received twice)

> "Thank you for submitting your manuscript to medRxiv. We regret to inform you that your manuscript will not be posted. A small number of papers are deemed during screening to be more appropriate for dissemination after peer review at a journal rather than as preprints."

> "Thank you for submitting your manuscript to medRxiv. As part of our process, all submissions are screened to ensure they match medRxiv posting criteria and scope. During this process, we determined that your manuscript is not suitable for medRxiv. It is not a clinical research article with new data and therefore it is out of scope and will not be posted."

> "Thank you for submitting your manuscript to medRxiv. We regret to inform you that your manuscript will not be posted. A small number of papers are deemed during screening to be more appropriate for dissemination after peer review at a journal rather than as preprints. Please be assured that this conclusion is not a judgment on the merits of the work described."

What is also interesting is that every single ***non-covid*** paper we have submitted to medRxiv during this time period (all using similar techniques such as Bayesian network modelling, albeit none with Norman as lead author) has been accepted.

It is more difficult to get the arXiv rejection information because they remove all information about rejected submissions from a user's account and the email rejections do not even state the name of the paper rejected. But, as a flavour, here are some of the email rejections we had saved:

For the paper [591]: What proportion of people with COVID-19 do not get symptoms? Norman Elliott Fenton, Martin Neil, and Scott McLachlan

> "Our moderators have determined that your submission is not of sufficient interest for inclusion within arXiv. The moderators have rejected your submission after examination, having determined that your article does not contain sufficient original or substantive scholarly research. As a result, we have removed your submission.
>
> Please note that our moderators are not referees and provide no reviews with such decisions. For in-depth reviews of your work, please seek feedback from another forum.

> Please do not resubmit this paper without contacting arXiv moderation and obtaining a positive response. Resubmission of removed papers may result in the loss of your submission privileges."

For the paper [592]: Discrepancies and inconsistencies in UK Government datasets compromise accuracy of mortality rate comparisons between vaccinated and unvaccinated, Martin Neil, Norman Fenton, and Scott McLachlan:

> "We regret to inform you that arXiv's moderators have determined that your submission will not be accepted and made public on arXiv.org
>
> Our moderators determined that your submission does not contain sufficient original or substantive scholarly scientific research and is not of interest to arXiv.
>
> arXiv moderators strive to balance fair assessment with decision speed. We understand that this decision may be disappointing, and we apologize that, due to the high volume of submissions arXiv receives, we cannot offer more detailed feedback. Some authors have found that asking their personal network of colleagues or submitting to a conventional journal for peer review are alternative avenues to obtain feedback."

There were various repetitions of the above rejections but recently we have been getting the following reason (despite the fact that we only submit papers to arXiv that are fully within their stated scope (which is different to medRxiv with more focus of the computing/statistical analysis):

> "Our moderators have determined that your submission is on a topic not covered by arXiv or that the intended audience for your work is not a community we currently serve."

Matthew Brett, who is the person who asked about our experience with medrXiv, has investigated [593] the acceptance criteria that these organisations seem to have introduced since covid.

Finally, at least we are it seems in good company. John Ioannidis of Stanford - one of the most highly cited scientists in the world - has had a very similar experience [594].

16.3. Why is the MHRA hiding critical vaccine safety data?

2 August 2023

16.3.1. Background and summary

We have reported before [595] on the basic failings of the MHRA in their duty with respect to safety monitoring of the covid vaccines. Now, we can reveal a new scandal as a result of a Freedom of Information Request by the tenacious Cheryl Grainger about the 2000 pregnant women who were vaccinated in the first half of 2021 who the MHRA were supposed to have been monitoring.

Following Cheryl's FOI of 13 April 2023 asking for the outcome data on the monitored pregnant women, on 19th July 2023 the MHRA stated that they had all of the information

Cheryl requested but refused to release it, citing exemption under Section 22 of the FOI Act; this exemption applies when a 'future' report is to be issued containing the relevant information.

Even though all the relevant pregnancy outcomes data would have been known by mid-2022, the MHRA provided no information as to when this 'future' report would be issued.

The MHRA did, however, send Cheryl a copy of a redacted report dated July 2021 marked "Not for Publication" sent to the Pharmacovigilance Expert Advisory Group (PEAG) for advice.

This report to the PEAG provided information about the adverse drug reactions (ADRs) reported up until 30 June 2021 by the Yellow Card Vaccine Monitor (YCVM) Group (a self-selected group of 30,000 people who registered to provide regular updates of any adverse reactions to their vaccinations).

An astonishing 53% of all those in the YCVM reported at least one ADR (adverse drug reaction). Of those receiving the AZ vaccine 59.2% reported at least one ADR, compared to 38.8% for Pfizer and 59.3% for Moderna.

There were 1366 pregnant women in the YCVM. Of those who received the AZ vaccine a whopping 66% (124 out of 203) reported at least one ADR; 38% of the Pfizer recipients and 61% of the Moderna recipients reported at least one ADR.

Because of the timing of the report to the PEAG there is only minimal information on the pregnancy outcomes (only 6 births in total had been recorded by 30 June 2021).

Despite the report making clear the high importance of continuing the YCVM the scheme appears to have been halted shortly after the July 2021 report. This suggests that the promised report being withheld now under Section 22 of the FOI Act must have been completed well over a year ago.

Despite the obvious safety signals in the 'not for publication' report sent to the PEAG in July 2021 we do not know what the PEAG response was. It is possible that the quiet (still not officially announced) withdrawal of the AZ vaccine around this time was one result of the report, but it begs the question why the entire vaccine programme was not halted at this point.

16.3.2. Cheryl Grainger's FOI to June Raine of the MHRA

13 April 2023

"Dear Dame June Raine

FREEDOM OF INFORMATION REQUEST

"On 17th November 2022 you gave a recorded lecture at the All-Wales Therapeutics and Toxicology Centre at the AWMSG 20th Anniversary Conference - The Nicola Wheatley Memorial Lecture. During that lecture you spoke of the Yellow Card Monitor as an active surveillance of specifically identified cohorts and specifically mentioned a group of **2000**

pregnant women who shared their data via the monitor. You were very pleased that this specific group gives you a denominator to presumably work out more accurate data analysis.
FOI Questions on active surveillance of 2000 pregnant women:

1. How were the pregnant women monitored, how often did they report and how long were they followed for?
2. When were they vaccinated, in which trimester, and how often were they vaccinated and with which vaccine?
3. What was the % of the 2000 pregnancies experiencing:
    a. miscarriage?
    b. still births?
    c. spontaneous abortions?
4. What was the % of the 2000 pregnancies that delivered:
    a. to full-term?
    b. pre-term?
5. Was there any congenital malformation?
6. What were the serious adverse side effects for:
    a. Mother?
    b. Baby?
7. What were the less serious adverse side effects for:
    a. Mother?
    b. Baby?
8. Were there any women followed up whilst breast feeding?
    a. Were any AEs recorded?
    b. Any breast milk discolouration, paresis, suppressed lactation, pain?
9. Did this cohort of 2000 pregnant women influence the MHRA risk/benefit analysis in pregnancy?

I believe that I should receive a response within the 20-day period from receipt.
Yours sincerely
Cheryl Grainger BSc"

The MHRA responded on 19 July 2023:

> "We confirm that we hold the information you have requested. However, we consider the information to be exempt under Section 22 (Information held with a view to its future publication) as we are working on a scientific publication in relation to the information you have requested.
>
> Section 22 is a qualified exemption and as a result we have considered the public interest in applying this exemption. We acknowledge that there is significant interest in the safety of medicines in those who are pregnant, including vaccines for COVID-19. However, we do have publicly available information on our position on the use of COVID-19 vaccines in those who are pregnant. This position is based on analysis of all Yellow Card data and relevant data from other sources rather than the subset of data which relates to Yellow Card Vaccine Monitor, to which your request relates. Given this we do not consider that the public interest is best served by releasing the information to you ahead of its formal publication.

Our position on the safety of COVID-19 vaccines in pregnancy can be found on our website via the link below (please follow the link and scroll down to the section entitled 'Comments on safety in specific populations'):

https://www.gov.uk/government/publications/coronavirus-covid-19-vaccine-adverse-reactions/coronavirus-vaccine-summary-of-yellow-card-reporting [596]

It may be helpful to explain the process for assessment of data arising from the Yellow Card Vaccine Monitor programme. Data arising from this element of the Covid-19 vaccine surveillance strategy [597] is continuously assessed alongside other data we collect or have access to, to support our signal detection activities, as such there are not regular reviews of this data source in isolation. The MHRA is developing a scientific publication of Yellow Card Vaccine Monitor, which will discuss the totality of the data collected including the specific points you have requested above. However, in order to provide some information in the interim we have attached an interim review of the Yellow Card Vaccine Monitor data that was presented to our Pharmacovigilance Expert Advisory Group in July 2021. You will note that at this stage 1197 individuals had reported that they were pregnant. Final numbers of registrations as well as analysis of outcomes will be included in our scientific publication in due course. Please note that there is some information redacted in this document. We have applied these redactions under Section 40 (2) of the Freedom of Information Act. The redacted information is personal data (names of members of staff), and its disclosure would lead to the identification of individuals. The staff names withheld are those of members of staff below a certain level of seniority; this is consistent with our approach to the disclosure of staff names.

If you are dissatisfied with the handling of your request, you have the right to ask for an internal review. Internal review requests should be submitted within two months of the date you receive this response and addressed to: info@mhra.gov.uk

Please remember to quote the reference number above in any future communications.

If you were to remain dissatisfied with the outcome of the internal review, you would have the right to apply directly to the Information Commissioner for a decision. Please bear in mind that the Information Commissioner will not normally review our handling of your request unless you have first contacted us to conduct an internal review.

ours sincerely

MHRA Customer Experience Centre

The 'not for publication' redacted report for the PEAG is here [598].

16.3.3. Key points and conclusions to note in the report for the PEAG

Here are some key points about this report:

- This particular report is the same one that Nick Hunt was sent earlier this year - see his article [599].

- 600,000 people were 'invited' to register for the YCVM scheme with the aim of contacting registered vaccinees at set intervals ("for example 7 days, 14 days, 3-6 months"). Of these 29,832 vaccinated subsequently registered but only 24,611 responded. Of those for who the vaccine make taken was known 67% were AZ, 32% Pfizer and 1% Moderna. The YCVM Group was disproportionately elderly, with 61% being over 60 years old.

- This report also provides some basic information about ADRs reported up until 30 June 2021 the Yellow Card Scheme (i.e. all other reports of ADRS submitted to the notoriously complex to complete MHRA Yellow card scheme.

- In the YCVM Group 53% reported at least one ADR by 30 June 2021. Of those receiving the AZ vaccine 59.2% reported at least one ADR, compared to 38.8% for Pfizer and 59.3% for Moderna. A major safety signal all round but especially for AZ.

- In the Yellow Card scheme there were 303,203 individuals reporting ADRs by 30 June 2021. Despite the fact that it was the over 60s who had been primary vaccinated by then an astonishing 78% of those reporting ADRs were under 60. This contrasts with 47% in the Monitor group (which was disproportionately elderly). Another major safety signal. Curiously, unlike for the YCVM, there is no breakdown on ADRs reported for the different vaccine makes.

- In both the YCVM group (65%) and the Yellow Card Scheme (75%) far more women than men reported ADRs.

- While the report notes 82 million doses of the vaccine had been delivered by end of June 2021 (perhaps implying that the 303,203 individuals reporting ADRs was therefore not excessive) it fails to draw the obvious conclusions about under-reporting of the notoriously difficult to use Yellow Card scheme. Since 53% of those in the YCVM group reported ADRs there is no reason to believe that a significantly different proportion of individuals would have reported ADRs if they had been actively monitored. Assuming about 30 million people had been vaccinated by 30 June 2023 this means we might have expected 15 million to have had an ADR rather than the 303,203 who did report. The 303,203 who did report represent only about 1% of that 30 million vaccinated people, rather than the 53% rate (~15 million) implied by the YVCM data.

- The main report and appendix provide inconsistent numbers about vaccinated pregnant women in the YCVM Group, but as the appendix provides greater details, we use the data there. We note there that there were 1366 reports of maternal exposures during pregnancy up to 30th June 2021, including data from 187 recipients of the Oxford-AZ vaccine, 1003 recipients of the Pfizer-BioNTech and 95 recipients of the Moderna vaccine. Of these, 565 participants reported

ADRs following vaccination up to 9th July 2021. Thus, 66% (n = 124) of recipients of the Oxford-AZ vaccine, 38% (n = 383) of recipients of the Pfizer-BioNTech and 61% (n = 58) of recipients of the Moderna vaccine reported ADRs and were included in the analysis. The fact that, when this report was completed most of the women were still pregnant (a total of only 8 live births among the 565 reporting ADRs had been recorded by 9 July 2021) makes the need to answer the questions asked by Cheryl Grainger so imperative.

- Point 26 in the report states "Given the volume of pregnant women enrolled in the YCVM, we have an important future data source to support continuous and long-term monitoring of pregnancy outcomes and will provide an update to the VBR in due course." Yet the MHRA is still refusing to publish the results of these outcomes two years later.
- While the report stresses the high importance of continuing and improving the Monitoring Scheme, Nick Hunt believes [600] the Target Active Monitoring (YCVM) was quietly dropped in Mid-2021. He comes to two conclusions: either the MHRA is not doing the Covid vaccine surveillance as promised; or it is doing it and not making the results publicly available. Certainly, the promised update report with the pregnancy outcome data being withheld now under Section 22 of the FOI Act must have been completed well over a year ago. Buttressing this conclusion is the fact that, in her lecture on 17 Nov 2022, MHRA CEO June Raine made a statement about the YCVM in pregnancy.

16.4. AstraZeneca's second most lethal batch

8 August 2023

A personal story from Norman.

In a recent report [601] I revealed publicly for the first time that my wife was diagnosed with frontotemporal dementia (pre-covid, 2019) but there was a rapid deterioration in her condition following two doses of the AstraZeneca vaccination in March and April 2021 (taken against my advice, but it was the only way she could travel to see her family who all live in Israel) – see Figure 66. Her GPs and dementia specialists of course would not countenance the notion that the vaccine played any role in her deterioration, so I knew there was little point in applying to the (dysfunctional) vaccine injuries compensation scheme. I did, however, with enormous difficulty submit a Yellow Card report (which was never acknowledged, and which does not seem to appear in any search result).

It turns out that, thanks to a tweet [602] by Jules Serkin showing the results of an FOI, we now know that the PV46664 batch used in my wife was the second most lethal of the AstraZeneca batches, as shown in Figure 67.

We have previously reported (here [603] and here [604]) on the problems caused by the AstraZeneca vaccine in the UK (and elsewhere [605]). Just last week we reported [606] on how the MHRA knew full well the scale of the problem with the vaccine in June 2021 but kept this information hidden. That is almost certainly why it was quietly withdrawn even before Dame Sarah Gilbert was given a standing ovation [607] at Wimbledon on 28 June 2021 for leading its development (from the photo of this event, it looks like Sarah Gilbert really knew how undeserved her many accolades were and how her useless, dangerous 'vaccine' was destroying the lives of real people for no good reason

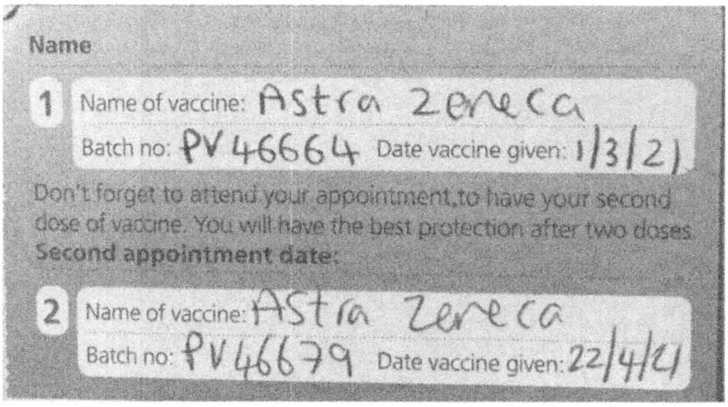

Figure 66 AstraZeneca vaccine card

Table 2: Total number of UK spontaneous Adverse Drug Reaction (ADR) reports for the 10 most reported batch numbers for the COVID-19 AstraZeneca vaccine up to and including 30/04/2023.

Batch number	Number of ADR reports	Number of fatal ADR reports
4120Z003*	7394	18
PV46664	6648	17
PV46671	5341	15
AB0012	4966	13
PV46672	4753	6
PW40009	4445	13
PV46669	4002	10
AB0011	3913	19
PV46673	3901	5
PV46663	3802	15

*Please note that the increase in the number of reports for batch 4120Z003 when compared to the figure given in FOI 22/611 is due to a change in the search criteria for this batch, which now includes variations between the number 2 and the letter Z.

Figure 67 AstraZeneca batches with ADRs and fatal ADRs

Chapter 17. Were Covid-19 respiratory symptoms caused by bacterial pneumonia?

17.1. Why this hypothesis?

30 August 2023

We have investigated the pneumonia hypothesis: that the proportion of Covid-19 deaths associated with respiratory symptoms (rather than deaths coded as Covid-19 because of a positive PCR test, that are absent symptoms), were caused by bacterial pneumonia, and that bacterial pneumonia was the primary, not the secondary, infection. This hypothesis is important because it challenges what the true causative agent behind the 'pandemic' was – a bacterium, a virus, both or neither? It also brings into question how the agent was spread, and challenges how and if it was appropriately treated. Ultimately, we ask: do we really know what happened and is there a risk we have everything wrong or back to front?

The reason we are focusing only on cases and deaths where people presented with respiratory symptoms associated with bacterial pneumonia is because it is these cases that were used as the spark to create fear of the 'pandemic', via news videos and reports. As such, they deserve special attention. Of course, many other causes of death other than bacterial pneumonia were misattributed as Covid-19. This is simply one distinct category.

The seminal work of Rancourt et al from October 2021 [608] is perhaps the first to identify a strong link between Covid-19 and bacterial pneumonia, making the case that many Covid-19-assigned deaths may be misdiagnosed bacterial pneumonia deaths and attributing observed excess deaths as partially explainable by a reduction in antibiotic prescriptions.

False attribution/conflation of pneumonia deaths to a virus is not a new phenomenon. James Lyons Weiler reports [609] on a long history of manipulation of definitions and statistics to inflate the perceived danger from the flu, when the actual danger is bacterial pneumonia. Pneumonia deaths were henceforth coded as influenza/pneumonia.

When medics say 'pneumonia' they can mean cause, effect and/or mechanism (all at once or single or in arbitrary pairings). This confusion and conflation of causality is typical in medicine and leads to both muddled definitions and a vulnerability that is exploitable by people with a sharper appreciation of the power of language and definitions. Names have power, after all.

Allegorically speaking, events are akin to a scene from an Agatha Christie 'Whodunnit'.

This chapter is based on a fuller article with relevant screenshots here [610].

17.2. Mens rea: "the act is not culpable unless the mind is guilty".

Before SARS-CoV-2 came on the scene, there was a belief in pharmaceutical circles that the flu wasn't perceived to be dangerous enough and a concern that flu vaccination rates were dropping. To some it may have looked like the vaccine enterprise and pharmaceutical industry itself might be in danger of terminal decline. In October 2019, there were calls for a universal high-tech flu vaccine [611] to face upcoming viral threats and 'blow up' the existing system, with the necessity of having many people dying for the sense of urgency to occur.

The reduction in the public's perceived threat of flu may have prompted the pharmaceutical industry to attempt a rebranding of the threat along with a new suite of marketable products to respond to that threat. Rick Bright suggested the problem of long-term development might be sidestepped if:

> "....there were an urgent call for an entity of excitement that is completely disruptive and is not beholden to bureaucratic strings and processes."

Anthony Fauci said in response:

> "So, we really do have a problem of how the world perceives influenza and it's going to be very difficult to change that unless you do it from within and say, I don't care what your perception is, we're going to address the problem in a disruptive and in an iterative way because she does need both......
>
> ...But it is not too crazy to think that an outbreak of a novel avian virus could occur in China somewhere. We could get the RNA sequence from that to a number of regional centers if not local, if not even in your home at some point, and print those vaccines on a patch of self-administer."

17.3. Whodunnit opening scene – the first victim

Let's look at the opening scene of our whodunnit. The first victim is: "Patient Zero" in China. On 26th December in Wuhan, China, patient zero was admitted to hospital experiencing a 'severe' respiratory syndrome that included fever, dizziness, and a cough.

Patient zero's symptoms are typical of any respiratory infection. Patient zero is relatively young, with no significant health problems. Yet patient zero was subjected to a battery of tests, including very expensive genetic sequencing of fluid removed from his airways, that (we are told) ultimately led to the discovery of a new coronavirus subsequently dubbed SARS-CoV-2. This is not a routine medical response to a typical respiratory infection.

As described in the seminal paper in Nature published 3 February 2020 [612], the clinical features of the illness of the alleged patient zero, from whom the genome of the "novel virus" was said to have been sequenced, are perhaps more suggestive of a regular, bacterial pneumonia:

- The patient's X-ray / CT findings also seem to suggest an unremarkable pneumonia: "bilateral focal consolidation, lobar consolidation and patchy consolidation, especially in the lower lung."
- Chest radiographs were abnormal with air-space shadowing such as ground-glass opacities. However, this is not unique to Covid-19. Ground glass opacities are also commonly associated [613] with influenza infections [614] and with a wide range of other [615] lung conditions, including pneumonia.

Given this evidence, it is reasonable to ask whether patient zero may have been a case of bacterial pneumonia? A substack reader pointed out that the metagenomic sequencing of Wuhan-Hu-1 lung samples of COVID patients run discovered a large number of Prevotella reads (Prevotella is a gram-negative bacteria).

This Nature paper was circulated widely to medical practitioners worldwide and has subsequently earned a place in the top 100 most widely cited scientific papers to date. Despite the importance of the findings, it remains largely unchallenged in academic literature and has simply been accepted at face value.

17.4. Scene two: Panic!

Weeks later, Sky News' Chief Correspondent Stuart Ramsay reporting from the main hospital in Bergamo, Italy, provided a series of apocalyptic warnings of what was to come, but this puzzling statement also slipped out:

> "It is ***not*** like flu, **it is chronic pneumonia**, and it is killing hundreds each day."

You can find this statement at 1:16 in his video report on YouTube [616].

And at 1.40 he interviews the head of emergency care, Dr Roberto Cosentini:

> Ramsay:
>
> > "People keep describing this as like the flu. It's worse than that, no?"
>
> Cosentini:
>
> > "No, it's totally another thing. I think it is (mumbles) pneumonia because most people get pneumonia, and as I have said before it is a very severe pneumonia..."

Makes you think, doesn't it? Here we have one of the most widely promoted videos from Spring 2020, one that helped trigger pandemic response globally, and the first word which springs to mind describing what is going on is *pneumonia*, not Covid-19. Further, they are at pains to confirm that it isn't flu.

Given they are proposing it is pneumonia, we can see why they would treat it with oxygen (the right thing). But why move to intubation (the wrong thing)? And why are they at pains to say it isn't caused by flu? Are such pains a red herring – or are they genuine clues as to what was really going on?

In another interview [617], Dr Cosentini says his hospital has admitted "900 patients with a pneumonia needing oxygen" and that "the virus circulated among us before we recognized it." He advises that UK hospitals "prepare for the struggle" by reorganizing emergency departments "to become great respiratory units with different level of intensity" and mentions needing to "pre-empty the hospital" in this effort. He also mentions "a young patient with severe pneumonia," but makes no connection to Covid-19 or to whether the young patient has tested positive for the virus.

Of course, as we've observed with the Wuhan patient zero, a possible explanation is that bacterial pneumonia was a secondary consequence of the initial viral infection. If this is the case, why didn't Dr Cosentini make this clear? Moreover, if bacterial pneumonia was the proximate cause of illness and deaths witnessed in the hospital, then surely this would relegate Covid-19 to the class of 'just another respiratory virus', like flu, that can weaken the immune system to the extent that it may help pneumonia flourish, but is eminently treatable in most cases with antibiotics?

The patient zero evidence along with what happened, and what was said in Bergamo, is an indication that bacterial pneumonia may have been the primary infectious pathogen, and that SARS-Cov-2 was a coincidental infection simply present at the time.

17.5. Which was first on the crime scene: SARS-CoV-2 or pneumonia?

What else is odd about the narrative? Have you ever read much discussion of pneumonia vaccines? No?

A purported preventative of one of the major causes of bacterial pneumonia is said to be the pneumococcal vaccine [618]. This is sometimes given to the elderly and vulnerable, although these vaccines get much less public attention than influenza vaccines.

Lewnard et al [619] looked at the interaction between bacterial pneumonia and SARS-CoV-2 and found some interesting results, especially when investigating whether vaccination for pneumonia reduced the risk of Covid-19 disease.

They observed:

> "Evidence that upper respiratory commensal bacteria promote viral infection dates at least to 1987 …, with studies demonstrating that enzymes expressed by bacteria (including pneumococci …) enhance influenza virus replication and pathogenicity. More recently, blunting of innate immune responses to influenza virus during pneumococcal colonization has been demonstrated in human challenge studies …. Such mechanisms of interaction may account for epidemiologic observations of enhanced virus acquisition and symptom risk among carriers of pneumococci and other respiratory commensal pathogenic bacteria.."

This raises an interesting question: Does pre-existing exposure to bacterial pneumonia lead to a higher propensity to acquire, and/or fail to mount a strong immune response to, a viral infection, such as influenza or SARS-CoV-2? If this were the case, then bacterial pneumonia might be better considered to be the primary infection and the virus the secondary, rather than the other way around. If we put the chicken before the egg, the root cause of illness, hospitalisation or death might be pneumonia (inadequately treated), and not whatever virus occupies the nasopharynx or lungs at the time.

Note that the main aim of their study was to examine the effects of two types of pneumonia vaccinations, PCV13 and PPSV23, on Covid-19 diagnosis, hospitalisation and mortality. The authors found that bacterial pneumonia vaccination reduced the risk of Covid-19, and by a statistically significant margin (but note that we are not making any claims here about the efficacy or safety of pneumonia vaccination but are instead simply pointing out evidence that contradicts the central covid narrative). Given the desperation for a covid vaccine, why didn't the authorities consider rolling out a bacterial pneumonia vaccine globally?

This might show that the actual burden of risk to patients is not SARS-CoV-2 at all but bacterial pneumonia. And that SARS-Cov-2 is secondary to bacterial pneumonia, or it masks bacterial pneumonia, not the other way around. Given this, it might be the case that bacterial pneumonia is acquired in the community rather than in hospital, and that viral infection follows bacterial pneumonia infection.

Vardhaam et al [620] say this about the etiology of community acquired pneumonia (CAP):

> "It is often observed that viral species colonize nasopharynx of patients with CAP. Whether they are the primary cause or contribute to the pathogenesis by secondary bacterial causes is still being investigated."

Howard et al [621] say:

> "...interactions between viruses and pneumococci in the nasopharynx during asymptomatic periods might have a role in onset of subsequent acute respiratory illness. The mechanisms for these interactions, along with other potentially associated host and environmental factors, and their role in ARI pathogenesis and pneumococcal transmission require further elucidation."

Also, this paper by Lu et al [622] found that the presence of Prevotella bacterium, and other bacteria, in SARS-CoV-2 patients:

> "The oropharyngeal microbiome characterization was different between SARS-CoV-2 infection and infections caused by other viruses. *Prevotella* could act as a biomarker for COVID-19 diagnosis and of host immune response evaluation in SARS-CoV-2 infection. In addition, the cross-talk among *Prevotella*, SARS-CoV-2, and sphingolipid metabolism pathways could provide a basis for the precise diagnosis, prevention, control, and treatment of COVID-19."

Finally, Upadhyay et al [623] report on the use of an expanded PCR panel testing for the identification of respiratory pathogens and coinfections in influenza-like illness:

> "A detailed analysis of the detected pathogens showed that *S. aureus* was the most prevalent on both platforms (~30%) followed by SARS-CoV-2 (~25%), HRV (~15%) and HHV-6 (~10%).....Coinfections between viruses and bacteria were the most common (~69%), followed by viral–viral (~23%) and bacterial–bacterial (~7%) coinfections......
>
> ...*S. aureus* was the most prevalent bacterial coinfecting pathogen, where SARS-CoV-2/*S. aureus* coinfections were the most common (~30%).
>
> S. aureus (Staphylococcus aureus) is a Gram-positive spherically shaped bacterium, is frequently found in the upper respiratory tract and on the skin. It is a recognised cause of bacterial pneumonia."

Finally, this paper from 2016 by Han and Mallampalli [624] report the biggest common risk factor of acute respiratory distress syndrome is acute sepsis which explains 79% of cases:

The incidence of this clinical syndrome has been on the rise, now reported up to 86.2 per 100,000 person-years [625], which totals about 200,000 cases yearly in the United States. The hospital mortality is high at 38.5% and has not significantly improved for the past several decades. The most common risk factor is severe sepsis with either a pulmonary or non-pulmonary source, explaining 79% of the cases.

These are recent papers so are representative of the state of medical knowledge around bacterial and viral interaction. And what is the state of knowledge? It is obvious that, despite billions in research funding, the medical community really knows very little with any certitude. However, research does suggest that:

- sequential infection: pneumonia infection followed by viral infection, or
- parallel infection, both at once,

are both possible. Yet, the default operating assumption in the medical literature and in practice is the opposite: viral then bacterial infection.

17.6. But the pneumonia coinfection rates were low!

Zahin et al (UK) [626] and Langford et al (USA) [627] report that the risk of death increases many-fold for those patients co-infected by SARS-CoV-2 and bacterial pneumonia but note that despite the rate of coinfection being low (3.5% of patients with confirmed covid), co-infections were mainly in intensive care patients (8.1%). Hedberg et al [628] found the coinfection rate for bacteria with SARS-CoV-2 was 4% in 2020, compared to 27% for influenza. So, one might conclude that there is no reason to blame deaths on pneumonia because it was largely absent.

One might think this proves that SARS-CoV-2 is the deadly causative agent and not pneumonia. But if SARS-CoV-2 was (relative to bacterial pneumonia) a benign but very widely prevalent coronavirus, or if most cases in intensive care are simply PCR false positives or are from a 'bystander' virus, then the opposite conclusion can conceivably be true. After all, as Monotti [629], notes:

> "if we were to have routinely tested everyone for spike proteins or other coronavirus target genes before 2020, we would have found them in approximately one third of what we call winter colds or flus if not higher.
>
> This is just to say that there is no public health emergency any different than any other year. There are approximately 200 respiratory viruses that can lead to respiratory disease. Many are coronaviruses."

Let us explain. Many people will be in hospital for a non-respiratory comorbidity but labelled as suffering from Covid-19 because of a PCR positive test and may go on to die of that comorbidity. These deaths will be categorised as SARS-CoV-2 virus deaths without pneumonia coinfection. However, those people carrying pneumonia as a primary pre-condition, but as yet undetected, may also receive the Covid-19 label by the same mechanism and die of what looks like secondary pneumonia. In aggregate the percentage of coinfections will appear small because the proportion of detected pneumonia cases was small to begin with. The same would occur if we labelled everyone in the hospital as "human genome" positive: then all deaths would be caused by the "humanity virus".

In case this isn't clear, imagine out of 100 "Covid-19" deaths 10 were actually found to have bacterial pneumonia, and 90 didn't. But of that 90, 85 die of a comorbidity, having been classified as Covid-19 merely by virtue of a positive test (tests in hospital were frequently repeated until a positive one was "found"). Simplistically, one might conclude that 10%, i.e., 10 out of 100 covid deaths, were bacterial. But the correct way of looking at this is to exclude the deaths which really had no respiratory component at all, which leaves 15. So, in fact, 10 out of 15 (i.e., 2/3) of true covid deaths had a bacterial component.

Here is another mechanism. In published observational studies those suffering pneumonia will have an intrinsically higher mortality risk because they are already in intensive care. This introduces the obvious potential for selection bias. If the background mortality rate in intensive care is higher for pneumonia patients than for patients suffering other non-respiratory or other conditions, then it is inevitable that mortality for 'pneumonia plus Covid-19' will be higher than for 'another non-respiratory or other condition plus Covid-19'. Especially if other selection factors are at play.

Let's look at other studies. From Korea Hyobin et al [630] found results that stand in stark contrast to those presented by Langford and Zahin:

> ".....(COVID-19 associated co/secondary infection prevalence is up to 45.0%). In the COVID-19 pandemic, *Streptococcus pneumoniae* is the most common coinfecting pathogen. Half of the COVID-19 mortality cases showed co-infection, and pneumonia-related COVID-19 mortality in patients >65 years was 23%."

So, the Korea researchers found 45% of the patients showed coinfection but, in the USA, it was reported as less than 3.5%. How can the same pathogen have such a different coinfection profile? And from the Korean study the fatality rate for elderly was 23% if they had pneumonia coinfection, but it was much less in the USA.

Again, things don't add up. Pneumonia coinfection rates might be reported as low, but this could be artefactual. Is there any evidence of selection and observational biases that might explain misleadingly low coinfection rates?

We have teams of researchers claiming wildly different coinfection and mortality rates for pneumonia and Covid-19 and these differences get little attention in medical academic literature. This has not gone unnoticed with Weidmann et al [631] who published a highly detailed paper looking at the rates of microbial testing, for Covid-19 and non-Covid-19 cases. They say this about other studies:

> ".....none of these studies have assessed the concurrent rate of bacterial CAP, HAP, and VAP rates compared to non-COVID patients for whom respiratory cultures were ordered during the same period. In addition, no previous studies have assessed whether respiratory culture ordering was appropriate based on rates of positivity in the setting of COVID-19 for these groups. This lack of a direct comparison between COVID-19 and non-COVID-19-infected patients makes it difficult to determine

> whether the highly disparate reported rates of bacterial coinfection represent the heterogeneity of the patient populations studied or a truly elevated risk of bacterial pneumonia associated with SARS-CoV-2 infection."

When reporting for their own hospital, Columbia University Irving Medical Center (CUIMC) located in New York City, they report that respiratory cultures were ordered for test in 16% of SARS-CoV-2 positive patients compared to 6.2% in negative patients. So, as the overwhelming majority of Covid-19 patients were not tested for competing pathogens, it cannot be ruled out that those showing respiratory symptoms attributed to SARS-CoV-2 might have been suffering from another viral or bacterial coinfection.

Likewise, it looks like the majority of respiratory culture tests were performed post intubation. Unfortunately, any positive culture tests found for intubated patients collected at least 2 days prior to intubation were excluded from the study (because they would not qualify under the class "ventilator acquired pneumonia" versus hospital or community acquired). It is thus possible that cases which would have tested positive for competing pathogens contracted before ventilation but were only discovered during ventilation and classified as a secondary pneumonia, were actually a primary pneumonia contracted in the hospital or in the community. They also say:

> "....between March 10th and 23rd, testing was performed by clinical suspicion due to limited testing capacity...."

So, there was an absence of rigorous data collection at the height of the 'pandemic' in NYC and at other times the rates at which culture testing is done appears selective, and cases appear to have been removed from the analysis due to classification requirements. This suggests that the rates at which bacterial and viral coinfection, and the stage at which infections are detected (community, hospital ICU) are highly sensitive and dependent on local testing and record keeping practices, and also differences between practices extant prior to the 'pandemic' and during it.

Weidmann et al [631] found that hospitalised patients with Covid-19 were 1.5-fold more likely than non-Covid-19 patients to have positive respiratory cultures, which was higher for patients requiring intubation. They also noted that a significantly higher proportion of patients had ventilator acquired pneumonia relative to non-Covid-19 patients.

Typical bacterial pneumonia is notoriously difficult to detect, as reported by Wagner et al [632] ,who say:

> "In addition to common viruses and bacterial pathogens (e.g. *Streptococcus pneumoniae*), fastidious respiratory pathogens like *Chlamydia pneumoniae*, *Mycoplasma pneumoniae* and *Legionella* spp. can cause severe atypical pneumonia. They do not respond to penicillin derivatives, which may cause failure of antibiotic empirical therapy. The same applies for infections with *B. pertussis* and *B. parapertussis*, the cause of pertussis disease, that may present atypically and need to be treated with macrolides. Moreover, these fastidious bacteria are difficult to identify by culture or serology, and therefore often remain undetected."

Finally, Platt et al [633] compared the premortem with the postmortem detection of pulmonary co-infections in 55 fatal Covid-19 cases from March 2020 to March 2021 and found:

> "The concordance in the premortem versus the postmortem diagnoses and the pathogen identification were evaluated. Premortem pulmonary co-infections were extracted from medical charts while applying standard diagnostic definitions. Postmortem co-infection was defined by compatible lung histopathology with or without the detection of an organism in tissue by bacterial or fungal staining, or polymerase chain reaction (PCR) with broad-range bacterial and fungal primers. Pulmonary co-infection was detected premortem in significantly fewer cases (15/55, 27%) than were detected postmortem (36/55, 65%). Among cases in which co-infection was detected postmortem by histopathology, an organism was identified in 27/36 (75%) of cases. *Pseudomonas*, *Enterobacterales*, and *Staphylococcus aureus* were the most frequently identified bacteria both premortem and postmortem. Invasive pulmonary fungal infection was detected in five cases postmortem, but in no cases premortem....
>
> Bacterial and fungal pulmonary co-infection are under-recognized complications in critically ill patients with Covid-19."

A sad example of the consequences of a failure to test for bacterial pneumonia was reported by, Rebecca Charles, whose daughter very sadly died whilst under the care of Northwell Health. They did not perform tests for bacterial pneumonia and an autopsy determined that this was a factor in Danielle's death. The full story can be read here [635].

17.7. Pneumonia has 'previous'

Bacterial pneumonia has a track record of previous/prior convictions yet appears to get off the hook in 2020 as well as during previous influenza seasons. We have argued that the steepness of the mortality spikes in Lombardy, Italy and New York City do not reflect those we might expect from a virus. Hence, we must look elsewhere for an alternative explanation. Might they be better explained as localised pneumonia outbreaks?

Fauci et al [636] believe that the 1918 pandemic was largely caused by pneumonia; indeed, an NIH News Release dated 19 August 2008 had the headline:

> "Bacterial Pneumonia Caused Most Deaths in 1918 Influenza Pandemic".

The similarity of the mechanism between 1918 and 2020 is uncanny. The flu pandemic might be more accurately called a pneumonia pandemic. In 1918, influenza was blamed, but pneumonia did the deed. Yet with 1918 and 2020-2023, the historical lesson from public health is that people need to fear viruses, yet pneumonia does not get public attention.

As Lewnard et al [637] said, upper respiratory commensal bacteria promote viral infection. Infection with a virus might therefore be a necessary but not sufficient condition for illness and death, and in the absence of serious bacterial infection a viral infection, in itself, may not present a serious hazard to health. Given there are millions of (known and unknown) circulating viruses and virus variants it might not even matter what the virus is. It is the severity of the bacterial infection and vulnerability of the host to this infection that matters.

It is also to be noted that in this [638] study carried out in Japan and published in Nature, nearly all face coverings retrieved from a series of users in Japan had evidence of potentially pathogenic - and mainly commensal - bacterial and fungal colonies, which might have been particularly dangerous for the immunocompromised, such as the elderly.

17.8. Evidence from the crime scene

The data shown in the chart [639] for respiratory disease as an underlying cause of death for New York City hospitals for 2020 (J00-J98) does not include Covid-19 (code U07.1 in the ICD Chapter "Codes for Special Purposes"). Digging further into specific codes, we find much of the increase in deaths was accounted for by deaths attributed to other non-influenza viral and bacterial pneumonias. Could a high proportion of these deaths be ventilator associated pneumonia deaths?

The chart [639] for weekly number of hospital deaths with respiratory disease as a cause, compared against Covid-19 death, shows a startlingly high number in the spring of 2020 for which most are Covid-19. However, given that New York City's largest healthcare systems reported administering thousands of SARS-CoV-2 PCR tests a day early on, both in hospitals and in other settings, it should not be a surprise. Furthermore, given that these tests generated exceptionally high positivity rates, that climbed to 70% and higher, it should be clear that the observed Covid-19 case count was dominated by testing rather than a genuine respiratory illness. However, we can see that genuine bacterial pneumonia cases remain prominent in NYC despite the explosion of Covid-19 cases generated by PCR testing. To date the global mortality burden shows that Covid-19 is a respiratory illness comparable to and less risky than flu for all but the sickest/oldest people. However, from this chart we can see the respiratory disease mortality burden exponentially increased— and did so toward the end of flu season, when the people most susceptible to a respiratory illness would have already succumbed to flu or similar. This NYC data is entirely inconsistent with previous viral or pneumonia outbreaks, including that seen in 1918, suggesting some other mechanism is needed to explain the entirety of the mortality pattern.

In the UK the ICNARC report [640] for Covid-19 in critical care charts the "all pneumonias" and Covid-19 admissions for 2020 to January 2023. This show that pneumonia was effectively replaced with Covid-19 diagnosis (the majority of the Covid-19 admissions may have been simply positive PCR tests rather than symptomatic respiratory conditions).

The global downward trend in bacterial infections, as well as in virtually all other infections during spring 2020 is amply illustrated by the BioFire syndromic trends [639] reporting system and shows the USA percentage detection rate of pathogens by BioFire clinical diagnostic systems (PCR), from 2019 through to 2021. The reported rate of bacterial pathogens detected at least halved after SARS-CoV-2 appears on the scene in the USA, UK and Europe in February 2020.

Given that the claim of interference frequently made refers to interference between viral (and not bacterial) infections, then any claim that SARS-CoV-2 out-competed pneumonia does not hold water. The reduction in bacterial infections can only be attributed to changes in diagnostic testing, treatment and case definitions.

17.9. A pinpoint pandemic?

Bacterial pneumonia is said to be the most common kind of pneumonia and is claimed to spread by droplets and fomites [641]. It is also generally viewed as the most serious kind of pneumonia. It doesn't spread like a respiratory virus, through the air, but spreads by touch or via surfaces. Therefore, outbreaks are highly localised.

The pattern of spread, and the geographical concentration of the Covid-19 mortality toll is not what one would expect from a respiratory virus. Deaths were highly localised in care homes and hospitals, within elderly age groups and those suffering multiple comorbidities and in specific cities and regions such as New York, Lombardy and Madrid. For instance, by May 2020 the 'pandemic' in the USA had only occurred around a few points that could have been pinned on a map, and everywhere else failed to experience it. If the pneumonia was caused by the newly-named pathogen, then how was it introduced to "localised populations"? If we cannot count on a natural explanation, then perhaps a man-made one is worth considering.

Given pneumonia spreads by droplets we searched for experiments that attempted to determine how bacterial pathogens spread through a population over a geographical area. Luckily for us (but not for the unwitting and unknowing participants in the experiments) the US Navy conducted such experiments (in secret). One, Operation Sea Spray, was a 1950 U.S. Navy secret biological warfare experiment in which *Serratia marcescens* and *Bacillus globigii* bacteria were sprayed over the San Francisco Bay Area in California, to determine how vulnerable a city like San Francisco may be to a bioweapon attack.

None of these experimental results have been released so we have no evidence to determine whether and how a bacterial pneumonia outbreak might occur and spread. It certainly doesn't look like the experiments caused any global bacterial outbreaks or pandemics. We suggest that, under modern sanitary conditions, very large-scale pneumonia outbreaks in highly concentrated areas look to be unlikely to occur naturally. After all, we haven't seen one since 1918, which was also a time of malnutrition and insanitary post war conditions, combined with huge movements of people and experimental vaccination in at least a few U.S. locations. We must therefore look elsewhere for explanations, including the possibility of human agency.

Given that rates of pneumonia deaths in 2020 [642] were similar to those seen in previous years then, changes in ventilation policy and practices coupled with new PCR testing, would be enough to cause the pin-point pandemic effect.

17.10. The EPIC and other studies

Chapter 19 covers the interview with ex-CDC scientist Dr. Norman Pieniazek where he cited two studies by the CDC in 2015 (one for adults [643] and one for children [644]). In these studies, the CDC acknowledges the inability of swabs to collect causative agents. Hence, a positive result gained from a sample taken from the upper throat or nose does not mean an infection is caused by the detected pathogen. These quotes from each paper are especially informative and relevant:

> "molecular detection of viruses and atypical bacteria in the nasopharynx and oropharynx does not necessarily indicate causation and could represent infection that is limited to the upper respiratory tract or convalescent-phase shedding."

> "The detection of pathogens in nasopharyngeal or oropharyngeal swabs with the use of a PCR assay could represent infection limited to the upper respiratory tract or convalescent-phase shedding, and thus detection may not denote causation."

In August 2020 Rasoul et al [645] published on bacterial coinfections with SARS-CoV-2, reporting the very high incidence of coinfection, not only for SARS-CoV-2 but for other coronaviruses. They also say that differential diagnosis, between bacterial and viral infection, based on clinical manifestations is not possible.

Finally, Kabrah et al [646] found that 43% of samples from Covid-19 patients contained Klebsiella pneumonia and that all bacteria detected were multidrug resistant.

17.11. Discussion

We asked: does pre-existing exposure to bacterial pneumonia lead to a higher propensity to acquire a viral infection, such as influenza or SARS-CoV-2? We suggest that SARS-Cov-2 infection (or a positive test for it) may be secondary to pneumonia or may mask pneumonia, and not necessarily the other way around. Therefore, was SARS-CoV-2 a coincidental, bystander, infection simply present at the time of presentation or testing and the actual burden of risk to patients is not SARS-CoV-2 (or other viruses) at all but bacterial pneumonia?

We have also found that high rates of ventilator induced pneumonia, attributed to SARS-CoV-2, are confounded by changes in protocols, delays in admission, overuse of ventilation and classification biases and therefore any claim that SARS-CoV-2 was uniquely dangerous cannot be relied upon. Bacterial infection is ever present at the scene.

The pattern of spread of SARS-CoV-2 in spring 2020, and the geographical concentration of the SARS-CoV-2 mortality toll is not what one would expect from a respiratory virus. It is highly localised in specific geographically distant regions and cities. It is a pin-point pandemic. Under modern sanitary conditions large scale pneumonia outbreaks in highly concentrated areas are unlikely to occur naturally. Changes in ventilation policy and practices coupled with new PCR testing, would be enough to cause the pin-point pandemic effect.

The central question remains: Was SARS-CoV-2 used as a decoy and were bacterial pneumonia deaths used as proof that SARS-CoV-2 was a deadly respiratory pathogen?

Allegorically speaking, events are akin to a scene from an Agatha Christie novel where SARS-CoV-2, a bystander used as a decoy, is guilty of the crime, with ventilation as the accomplice, but the actual criminal, who has got off scot-free, is in fact bacterial pneumonia. In other words, SARS-CoV-2 has been framed.

Chapter 18. Why more ventilation and opioids but fewer antibiotics?

18.1. How did antibiotics use change?

3 October 2023

After reading our 'whodunnit' [647] (Chapter 17) article on pneumonia Dr David Wiseman recently sent us an email asking about antibiotics:

> "Senator Johnson asked [648] me the other day about reports of lowered antibiotic use during the pandemic. I have probably missed those reports, but I mentioned your work on the co-prevalence of various respiratory infections. He was certainly interested."

So, if it is true that antibiotic use went down this could have contributed to mortality/morbidity by failing to deal with the otherwise antibiotic sensitive components of the mixed infection.

We realised that we didn't have a list of articles to hand covering the relevant topics:

- National policy changes affecting antibiotic prescriptions and administration.
- Time series statistics on changing prescription patterns in different countries.
- Success stories where antibiotics were given to Covid-19 patients, resulting in positive outcomes.

Hence, this chapter is a (definitely incomplete) list of the above materials and covers, examples of successful application, academic papers and statistical charts. It is also based on material from a number of articles with relevant charts and tables here [649] and here [650].

Antibiotics are essential in a pandemic. This view is motivated by the fact that in his 2008 article [651] in the Journal of Infectious Diseases (which reported on autopsies of well-preserved victims of the Spanish Flu pandemic), Anthony Fauci concluded that:

> "Prevention, diagnosis, prophylaxis, and treatment of secondary bacterial pneumonia, as well as **stockpiling of antibiotics** and bacterial vaccines, should also be high priorities for pandemic planning."

What happened to those stockpiles during the covid 'pandemic' – or were these never actually created?

18.2. Policy for the treatment Covid-19

The most damning evidence can be found in this NICE Rapid Guideline (NG163) [652] (published 3 April 2020) that has since been deleted. However, it can be found via the wayback machine here [653]. NG163 is effectively a palliative care pathway that did not recommend the use of antibiotics. It did, however, recommend the use of midazolam for treating patients aged 18 or over with 'anxiety' even though midazolam did not have a UK marketing authorisation for this purpose. Specifically, Table 6 of the report states:

> Anxiety or agitation and unable to swallow: ***midazolam injection***. Midazolam 2.5 mg to 5 mg subcutaneously every 2 to 4 hours as required. If needed frequently (more than twice daily), a subcutaneous infusion via a syringe driver may be considered (if available) starting with midazolam 10 mg over 24 hours.

Moreover, the 'Notes' with this table states:

> "At the time of publication (April 2020), midazolam and levomepromazine did not have a UK marketing authorisation for this indication or route of administration (see General Medical Council's guidance [654] on prescribing unlicensed medicines for further information)."

The BMJ published the NICE NG163 guidance [655], in 20 April 2020. In reaction, a rapid response letter [656] was sent by eminent experts in palliative care warning of the dangers of administering treatment more appropriate for end-of-life care to Covid-19 patients.

As well as NG163 there is also the NICE guidance NG165 [657] issued at the same time on managing suspected or confirmed pneumonia, which explicitly forbade the use of antibiotics in Covid-19 cases. It states:

> "Antibiotic treatment
>
> 4.5 As COVID-19 pneumonia is caused by a virus, antibiotics are ineffective.
>
> 4.6 Do not offer an antibiotic for treatment or prevention of pneumonia if:
>
> - COVID-19 is likely to be the cause and
> - symptoms are mild.
>
> Inappropriate antibiotic use may reduce availability if used indiscriminately, and broad-spectrum antibiotics in particular may lead to Clostridioides difficile infection and antimicrobial resistance."

The current US policy on treating adults for Covid-19 is provided here [658] by the NIH, with full 466 pages available here [659]. The policy on "Pharmacologic Interventions for Critically Ill Patients" states:

- In the absence of a proven or suspected secondary infection, the COVID-19 Treatment Guidelines Panel (the Panel) recommends against the use of empiric broad-spectrum antimicrobials in patients with severe or critical COVID-19 (BIII).
- As with any hospitalised patient, patients with COVID-19 who receive antimicrobials should be reassessed daily to minimize the adverse consequences of unnecessary antimicrobial therapy (AIII).

Where antibiotics are considered, they are recommended too late, when the patient has acquired pneumonia in hospital or when on a ventilator:

> "The use of antibiotics in patients with severe or critical COVID-19 should follow guidelines established for other hospitalised patients (i.e., for hospital-acquired pneumonia, ventilator-associated pneumonia, or central line-associated bloodstream infection)"

18.3. Changes in antibiotic prescribing patterns

In this twitter post [660] Jikkyleaks looked at UK antibiotic prescribing practice from 2017 to 2022 using the UK online open prescribing system and compared it against projected usage based on historical patterns. This made clear that antibiotic prescriptions reduced dramatically in the UK from Spring 2020 to Summer 2021 and then again over the winter of 2021/22. The twitter post exposed an academic paper by Zhong et al [661] that claimed there was no evidence of changes in antibiotic prescribing from the start of the 'pandemic'.

Jikkyleaks' claims are verified by the time series chart of antibiotic prescriptions direct from the UK open prescribing system [662].

A paper [663] published in the BMJ in August 2021 provided an analysis of primary care prescription trends in England during Spring 2020 and concluded that there was a dramatic increase in end-of-life care drugs such as Midazolam. It claims that there was no dramatic change in antibiotic prescribing in 2020 but contained a chart showing the reduction in doxycycline hyclate prescribing compared to expected.

King et al [664] reported that US outpatient antibiotics prescriptions changed dramatically during the period January to May 2020, exceeding expected seasonal reductions.

Aerzteblatt [665], the German online journal of medicine and public health reported that:

> The outbreak of the COVID-19 pandemic in March 2020 has also led to significant changes in the burden of disease and thus in the prescriptions of medicines in Germany. This can be seen particularly succinctly in the number of prescriptions for antibiotics. These fell to an all-time low in Q2 2020.

From 29.5 million prescriptions in 2019 the figure in 2020 was only 21.8 million, and this reduction occurred during a 'pandemic'. The effect is highest among 18- to 65-year-olds, where around 4.5 million fewer prescriptions (-26%) were issued in 2020 than in 2019.

Note that we are not claiming that this mechanism would have caused a massive increase in national mortality figures attributed to pneumonia, but it is enough to cause a temporary spike in pneumonia cases/deaths, which would look to hospital staff like it was caused by a novel and deadly new virus for which they were testing, and finding, with a newly launched PCR test.

18.4. Physicians defying public health authorities

When physicians chose to use antibiotics to treat patients in defiance of public health authorities, they reported some startling results.

In contrast to the evidence presented above, physicians in Toledo [666], Spain, empirically administered antibiotics to Covid-19 patients during spring 2020, contrary to official guidance. This resulted in zero hospitalisations or deaths in their care homes after they started routine administration. Their resulting mortality over spring 2020 was approx. 7% versus 28% in other comparable care homes (and the 7% died before they started routine antibiotic use).

Likewise in Romania a physician, Flavia Groşan, was reported in the media [667] as approaching Covid-19 as "atypical pneumonia", saying there were huge mistakes with excessive oxygen therapy and intubation:

> "Too much oxygen for too lengthy periods at a time, says Groşan, can lead to cerebral edema which in turn can cause death."

She gave her patients 'enough' oxygen for their needs, antibiotics and other cheap medicines. On the choice of antibiotics, she said:

> "There are only three antibiotics in the macrolide class, erythromycin, which everyone knows, azithromycin and clarithromycin. I don't like azithromycin because it's a weaker copy of clarithromycin. I worked in some very interesting clinical studies on pneumonia and there I learned about the viral tropism of clarithromycin, as well as the anti-inflammatory role of clarithromycin, which no antibiotic has. I have been working with this antibiotic in viral and atypical pneumonias for 10 years. When the pandemic hit I went for an etiological treatment, clarithromycin. Of course, in addition to this antibiotic, there are several adjuvant treatments, because it can't cope alone. It is a treatment scheme that is my own."

She reported healing 100% of some 1,000 patients using this approach.

At St Paul's hospital in Vancouver, Canada, Russell and Walley learned that Covid-19 is not deadly in itself, but it is sepsis that causes the organ failure leading to death. In this article [668] they say:

> "The pandemic we've all been living through is actually a pandemic of sepsis due to COVID-related pneumonia. Everybody who dies of COVID actually dies of sepsis and pneumonia. Everybody."

Sepsis is the number one cause of death worldwide. They go on to emphasise the importance of antibiotics and other measures in treating Covid-19:

> "It's a complex syndrome that can require antibiotics, oxygen, drugs to stabilize blood pressure, and dialysis to support failing kidneys. In addition to this, there's also no diagnostic test available to detect sepsis, making the diagnosis a challenge."

Also, this study [669] from 2023 found that recovery times were significantly improved by the early administration of antibiotics:

> "..the ethical perspective of using antibiotics to save lives and reduce viral replication on bacterial platforms arises especially in the early spread of the virus.

> The immediate administration of antibiotics at the onset of symptoms may be justified."

The various protocols for use of ivermectin as an early treatment and prophylactic for Covid-19 also include the administration of antibiotics, such as doxycycline and azithromycin, as documented in the Zelenko protocol [670], which for "Moderate / High risk patients" specifies:

- Elemental Zinc 50-100mg once a day for 7 days
- Vitamin C 1000mg 1 time a day for 7 days
- Vitamin D3 10000iu once a day for 7 days or 50000iu once a day for 1-2 days
- Azithromycin 500mg 1 time a day for 5 days or
- Doxycycline 100mg 2 times a day for 7 days
- Hydroxychloroquine (HCQ) 200mg 2 times a day for 5-7 days and/or
- Ivermectin 0.4-0.5mg/kg/day for 5-7 days Either or both HCQ and IVM can be used, and if one only, the second agent may be added after about 2 days of treatment if obvious recovery has not yet been observed etc.

The McCullough protocol [671] also recommends doxycycline and azithromycin.

And, of course, ivermectin is reported to have antimicrobial policies, in itself, as documented here [672].

Finally, there is this [673] evidence that chloroquine is a potent treatment for SARS.

Note that these protocols recommend antibiotics for high-risk patients. Those are the same patients who may be likely suffering from bacterial pneumonia.

It is worth pointing out that ivermectin and many antibiotics often have antioxidant or anti-inflammatory properties that will also help when treating viral and bacterial infections. This is the case with azithromycin [674] and a cursory search of pubMed results in 58 papers [675] on the topic.

A fascinating letter [676] appeared in the Proceedings of the Royal Society of Medicine in 1958 written by a Dr J. Morrison Ritchie in response to an article on the common cold by Hope Simpson. In it he describes a study carried out at the Birkenhead Public Health Laboratory on 1,000 volunteers in the winter of 1955/56 where they applied antibiotics for patients suffering cold symptoms. They reported that:

> "There were 22/581 colds among those receiving antibiotic tablets on the first day, as against 87/338 among those receiving inert control tablets: 3.8 % as against 25.7%, a drop to one-seventh. In the adult industrial population, the proportion was one to nine, and this drop was evident in all the units of the investigation."

Clearly many colds were not viral infections at all but bacterial infections, but such is the overlap in observed respiratory symptoms for these broad classes of pathogen, that absent the administration of antibiotics, this would have escaped attention.

If physicians can easily confuse common cold infections with bacterial infections what is to say they will be able to differentiate between SARS-CoV-2 and bacterial pneumonia?

18.5. Was ventilation an accomplice?

The claim of higher Covid-19 mortality (in comparison to previously experienced respiratory viral infections), despite the best and most expensive treatment regimens (intensive care units – ICUs) that modern healthcare systems have to offer, was based on direct firsthand reports in the media. Fortunately, retrospective studies have now been performed to codify the experience. But unfortunately, they paint a grim picture, not of a pandemic but of potential data bias. Much of this bias involves a medical intervention called ventilation, which we might view as playing the role of the accomplice.

Many of the frightening images being circulated in the media in spring 2020 were from ICUs showing patients being treated on ventilators. It was claimed that people were dying of acute respiratory distress caused by SARS-CoV-2 whilst being ventilated, including non-elderly adults age groups for which the infection fatality rate of the virus is known to be relatively low [677].

Prior to covid, ventilator associated pneumonia (VAP) was a well-known condition, the study of which goes back to 1978 with this paper [678]. According to Wikipedia ventilator associated pneumonia is:

> "a type of lung infection that occurs in people who are on mechanical ventilation breathing machines in hospitals. As such, VAP typically affects critically ill persons that are in an intensive care unit (ICU) and have been on a mechanical ventilator for at least 48 hours. VAP is a major source of increased illness and death. Persons with VAP have increased lengths of ICU hospitalisation and have up to a 20–30% death rate. Critical care physician Paul Mayo [679] summarized the risk well saying, "**Putting a person on a ventilator creates a disease known as being on a ventilator**".

18.5.1. Covid-19 and ventilator acquired pneumonia

Typical of these is that by Rouyer et al [680] who examined patients in the ICU of a 350 acute-care bed hospital in the Ile de France region in France from 1 March 2020 to 1 May 2020, and compared them with non-Covid-19 patients who developed VAP in the ICU from 2011 to 2019 and with patients who did not develop VAP from 1 March 2020 and May 2020. Their hypothesis is that Covid-19 is novel and more deadly:

> "The main hypothesis to verify is that VAP in COVID-19 is a new 'pathology' with some peculiarity that needs different healthcare than VAP in non-COVID-19 patients."

They found that:

> ".....morbidity was principally due to SARS-CoV-2 infection and some other microbiologic characteristics, such as an association with positive blood cultures and polymicrobial cultures rather than patients' related risk factors, such as immune-depression and co-morbidities."

So here the authors acknowledge that other microbiologic and polymicrobial cultures are to be found at the 'crime scene' yet are not directly implicated in the deaths. SARS-CoV-2 is named as the guilty culprit.

However, there are the following problems with this paper, although some of these were inevitable and a consequence of it being a retrospective and not a controlled study:

- The VAP non-Covid-19 group, comprising 37 patients, from spring 2020 disappears from the paper as soon as they are introduced. This means there is no basis for directly comparing treatment regimens in spring 2020 (i.e., during the same period) for non-Covid-19 patients against Covid-19 patients. The justification for this is nonsensical:

  "The choice of comparing two different timeframes was motivated by the following: (i) during the COVID-19 pandemic, the ICU of our hospital was exclusively reserved for COVID-19 patients; (ii) VAP in non-COVID-19 patients is less frequent than COVID-19 patients, and our ICU's capacity is limited. For these reasons, we were forced to select non-COVID-19 patients during a longer timeframe."

- They describe the populations they set out to compare in their study as:

  "From 1 March 2020 to 1 May 2020, 346 patients were hospitalised in the ICU. Among them, 100/346 (29%) were SARS-CoV-2 PCR-positive, 79/100 (79%) received mechanical ventilation, 42/79 (53%) experienced VAP, and 12/42 (28%) had a VAP relapse. From 1 January 2011 to 31 December 2019, 188 patients experienced VAP in the ICU, and 8/188 (4%) had VAP relapse."

  So, over a two-month period in 2020 42 from 79 experienced VAP, yet over a 9-year period 188 patients experienced VAP in the same ICU (the authors fail to provide the denominator). This suggests the chance of a patient being ventilated in spring 2020 was significantly higher than at any time in the preceding decade.

- Everyone in the ICU in March to May 2020 was a Covid-19 patient and all had acute respiratory distress syndrome (ARDS). This was because ARDS and a Covid-19 diagnosis was a mandatory criterion for hospitalisation in the ICU for all Covid-19 patients. Other patients with other conditions were not put in the ICU, whilst historically in the period 2011-2019 only 33% of patients in the ICU were suffering ARDS.

  So, in the spring 2020 cohort all subjects had ARDS and all of them had SARS-Cov-2, yet it is SARS-CoV-2 that was found to be statistically significant. The mere act of universal labelling would achieve the same ends: mark everyone in the ICU with a red sticker and this would be found statistically significant.

- When we look at the microbiological isolates taken from patients suffering from VAP we find that gram-positive bacteria are present in Covid-19 patients at a statistically significantly higher rate compared to non-Covid-19 patients. *Staphylococcus pneumoniae* (pneumococci) are gram-positive. Hence, there is significantly higher presence of pneumonia (caused by this pathogen) in this cohort, which the authors fail to discuss.

It looks like this study suffers heavily from selection bias; it ignores the potential role of bacterial pneumonia strongly suggested by the data, and it has intentionally discarded data that might contradict its conclusions. Given these facts any claim of a higher mortality rate for Covid-19 patients must be in question.

Rouze et al [681] performed a multi-centre study of 1576 patients that had suffered VAP and who had been admitted with SARS-CoV-2, influenza or no-virus. They found that SARS-CoV-2 patients had significantly higher rates of VAP than those with flu or no-virus: SARS-CoV-2 (36%), influenza (22%) or no-virus (16%). Careful reading of the paper shows that the flu and no-virus cohorts were selected prior to spring 2020, before the pandemic. Therefore, again, the study suffers from retrospective selection bias, which at least the authors recognize:

> "Fourth, ICU triage criteria, ICU efficiency, and isolation measures differed between the pandemic and the non-pandemic periods."

It is therefore entirely conceivable that the differences in lethality may be entirely explainable by changes in practice.

Rouze et al [682] also looked at the incidence of VAP and SARS-CoV-2 and found that SARS-CoV-2 patients were around twice as likely to develop lower respiratory tract infections (including VAP). However, again we find selection bias and treatment differences. The authors say:

> "During the pandemic it was impossible to have patients with diseases other than COVID-19, because ICUs were full of COVID-19 patients. Inclusions of patients with influenza or no viral infection, admitted to the ICU before the pandemic, allow a fair comparison of VA-LRTI incidence between COVID-19 patients and other at-risk patients.
>
> .....the higher incidence of VA-LRTI in patients with SARS-CoV-2 pneumonia is probably related, at least in part, to the longer duration of mechanical ventilation."

The act of keeping people on ventilators for longer, perhaps to protect staff as an early FDA statement [683] indicated, confounds any claim that SARS-CoV-2 was more deadly. Lastly, hidden within this paper we also find that the rate of gram-positive microbial infection, including bacterial pneumonia, was twice as high in the SARS-CoV-2 patients (19.5%) than found in historical influenza patients (11%).

Henri-Wicky et al [684] reviewed similarities and differences between ventilator associated pneumonia in SARS-CoV-2 infection and with acute respiratory distress syndrome (ARDS):

> "The increased risk of VAP in SARS-CoV-2 infections, as compared to other ARDS, may have been due to multiple factors including less rigorous use of standard prevention strategies during COVID-19, disease and therapy-associated immune impairment, more prolonged duration of mechanical ventilation, prolonged

use of sedation, more frequent need for prone ventilation, and higher risk for pulmonary infarction with associated superinfection. Although ICU overcrowding could also have been a factor, the study of Blonz et al. was done in an "inundated" region where ICUs had adequate facilities for providing usual level of patient care, and thus there were less potential breaches in contact isolation. Similarly, in another single center study, a VAP rate reaching 74% was observed during both the first overcrowded wave and during the second wave where the ICU beds were sufficient."

Clearly ICU patient care is very complex and challenging. There are myriad factors that affect rates of VAP, including patient positioning, sedation, oxygenation, medication, etc. Outcomes will inevitably be sensitive to any deviation from well-established practices as they relate to any of these parameters. Gao et al [685] looked at the relationship between length of ICU stay and unresolved VAP in a Chicago hospital, using 2018-2020 as a comparison, and concluded that:

> "Unsuccessful treatment of VAP is associated with higher mortality. The relatively long length of stay for patients with COVID-19 was primarily due to prolonged respiratory failure, placing them at higher risk of VAP."

The investigators found nearly half of patients with COVID-19 develop a secondary ventilator-associated bacterial pneumonia:

> "Those who were cured of their secondary pneumonia were likely to live, while those whose pneumonia did not resolve were more likely to die," Singer said. "Our data suggested that the mortality related to the virus itself is relatively low, but other things that happen during the ICU stay, like secondary bacterial pneumonia, offset that."

And:

> "The importance of bacterial superinfection of the lung as a contributor to death in patients with COVID-19 has been underappreciated, because most centers have not looked for it or only look at outcomes in terms of presence or absence of bacterial superinfection, not whether treatment is successful or not".

Both studies suggest that any conclusion that SARS-CoV-2 was the primary causal factor in mortality is heavily confounded, inter alia, by bacterial infection and changes in treatment protocols. Patients were in the ICU for longer and the increase in bacterial pneumonia, from prolonged exposure to ventilation, may well have led to an increased mortality rate and the misattribution of this to SARS-CoV-2.

Furthermore, it appears that established protocols for bacterial sampling were changed to reduce exposure of hospital staff to the virus:

> "Additionally, VAP incidence may vary according to the bacteriological test used. Indeed, to avoid healthcare workers (HCW) contamination when the diagnosis of VAP is suspected, the use of bacteriological samples and bronchoscopy have been reduced, and gram stain examination not performed."

This suggests that bacterial causes for acute respiratory distress might not have been detected at all in many cases, but not because it wasn't present, but because it was never tested for.

Weidmann et al [686] say:

> "Bacterial pneumonia in COVID-19 patients was much more likely to be ventilator associated and less likely to be community acquired when compared to non-COVID patients"

From comments made by the authors about testing and record keeping, it should be clear that it would take only some small shifts in the number of cases from community or hospital acquired pneumonia to make it appear that VAP rates are significantly worse for SARS-CoV-2 positive patients. Delaying or accelerating the culture testing until after a patient has been admitted or intubated might make a big difference to how a patient is eventually categorised, especially during turbulent times or where staff are new or inexperienced.

To further illustrate how sensitive the classification is to secondary (VAP) pneumonia rather than primary (community), according to a report [687] in the BMJ very often patients were rushed onto ventilation:

> "Two thirds (132) of Covid-19 patients who required critical care in the UK had mechanical ventilation within 24 hours of admission, an audit of patients from England, Wales, and Northern Ireland has found."

Any community acquired bacteria pneumonia infection will therefore most likely not be detected for patients rushed into ICU and ventilated. Any hospital infection registered in the system for a patient now ventilated, but ventilated within 48 hours, would then be recorded as a VAP infection. In this way primary bacterial pneumonia infections might be recorded as secondary.

Note that overall similar numbers of pneumonia patients that have tested positive (249) for SARS-CoV-2 as have tested negative (219), in Weidmann et al, suggesting there is a 53% chance their symptoms would be attributed to a positive SARS-CoV-2 test result when in fact pneumonia was always the underlying risk.

In contrast with Italy in spring 2020 there was no evidence of excess mortality in Germany in those months. Was this due to a different policy on ventilation? This report [688] in the Frankfurter Allgemeine suggests this might just be the case. Lung specialist Thomas Voshaar, said:

> "Of the ventilated Covid-19 patients, unfortunately, only between 20 and 50 percent have survived so far. If this is the case, we have to ask: Is this due to the severity and course of the disease itself or perhaps the preferred treatment method? When we read the first studies and reports from China and Italy, we immediately wondered why intubated so often was done there. This contradicted our clinical experience with viral pneumonia."

On the use of ventilators to protect doctors and nurses from the virus he said "We cannot subordinate the well-being of the patient to the well-being of the staff. In terms of content, it is also nonsensical. Experienced pulmonologists and intensive care nurses can keep the aerosol load low."

18.6. Increased Fentanyl and Midazolam use in NYC hospitals

The opioid sedatives, painkillers and muscle relaxant drugs needed to keep patients on ventilators were running low [689] in spring 2020 showing that there was a huge spike [690] in demand for use with the high number of patients put on ventilation in places like New York City. Dabestani et al [691] report on the use of fentanyl in New York hospitals during Spring 2020 Their charts show the almost constant number of patients between March and mid-May 2020 but the disproportionate huge increase in fentanyl and midazolam doses administered from March 27th to 24th April 2020. Figure 1 shows the charts for fentanyl and midazolam.

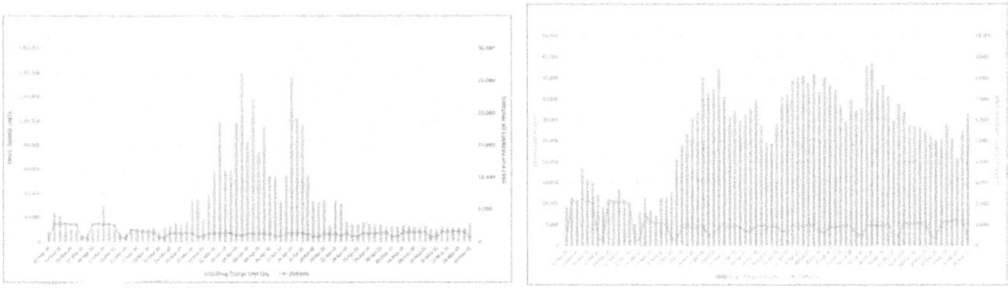

Figure 68 Fentanyl (left) and midazolam (right) doses administered to patients in NYC March to May 2020

Atei et al [692] reported that opioid use acts as a double edge sword. Opioid use at high doses and over several months duration can mitigate the immune system's function, which may complicate the course of COVID-19 disease. Potential suppression of parts of the immune response may be important in prevention, clinical support, and therapeutic use of medications in various phases of the COVID-19. Specifically, opioid use disorders via an inhalation route may enhance the "late hyper-inflammatory phase" or result in end-organ damage. It is well established that opioids decrease ventilation as their effect on the medullary respiratory centers increases the risk of (*bacterial*) pneumonia.

Lastly, even Anthony Fauci [693] admitted that ventilation was over-used:

> "We very, very readily would put people on mechanical ventilation. When we found out through clinical experience it might have been better just to make sure we position them properly in the prone or supine position, and not necessarily intubate somebody so readily, which might have actually caused more harm than good."

After experiencing this spike, hospital ICUs abandoned overuse of ventilation and resorted to other methods to handle Covid-19 patients, as reported here [694] and here [695].

In the BMJ Frazer and Frazer [696] reported on the massive increase in prescription drugs and noted that medications for end-of-life symptom control increased in April 2020, including levomepromazine hydrochloride which increased by 94.7%.

In January 2024 Sy [697] performed a statistical analysis of the role of midazolam and vaccinations on cause of death and concluded:

> "excess deaths remained elevated following mass vaccination in 2021, but were statistically uncorrelated to COVID injections, while remaining significantly correlated to Midazolam injections. The widespread and persistent use of Midazolam in UK suggests a possible policy of systemic euthanasia."

Note that midazolam was stockpiled [698] by the US Army as a mass casualty medical countermeasure; 675,000 multi-dose vials were approved for the strategic national stockpile to be used as an anti-seizure medication for people exposed to chemicals that cause prolonged seizures, in combat, domestically or from an intentional attack. Apparently, this was in response to exposure to chemicals and not biological threats.

18.7. But they were given antibiotics in ICU!

In the VAP studies cited earlier, rates of first line antibiotic treatment were similar across groups, as was targeted treatment with antibiotics. At first glance this appears to falsify the claim (discussed here [699]) that denial of antibiotics caused SARS-CoV-2 respiratory deaths. However, as with all medical treatments the important question is whether, if people had pneumonia, they were given antibiotics on time, in the community or in hospital, before they were presented to the ICU and experienced VAP. Langford et al [700] report that "the majority of patients with Covid-19 received antibiotics" - estimated at 72%. But what if the wrong people got the antibiotics, and those with pneumonia did not? The study authors don't say but the effect of any misallocation would naturally be to increase the mortality rate of those with pneumonia.

Pneumonia symptoms overlap heavily with SARS-CoV-2 symptoms and given the edict that antibiotics do not help in the treatment of SARS-CoV-2, it is inevitable that many patients suffering from pneumonia would have been denied antibiotics until it was too late for them to have a material effect.

In his 2008 article [701] in the Journal of Infectious Diseases (which reported on autopsies of well-preserved victims of the Spanish Flu pandemic), Anthony Fauci concluded that:

> "Prevention, diagnosis, prophylaxis, and treatment of secondary bacterial pneumonia, as well as stockpiling of antibiotics and bacterial vaccines, should also be high priorities for pandemic planning."

What happened to those stockpiles during the covid 'pandemic'–or were these never actually created?

Furthermore, in spring 2020 people were told to self-isolate if they suffered covid symptoms. This would buy time for pathogens to multiply and for a more severe condition to develop, which might be subsequently harder to manage. Many people would have then presented late to ICU, with incipient or lingering pneumonia (perhaps from the previous normal flu season), disguised as Covid-19, and were left untreated with antibiotics until their condition deteriorated further. The reluctance to perform bacteriological investigations may have been a further contributory factor. They would therefore have suffered higher levels of

ARDS than would have been seen historically. Given the lateness of presentation to hospital, and despite the administration of antibiotics, this may have come too late to save them from what was a (detected or undetected) bacterial pneumonia infection. A proportion of these would have been attributed to SARS-CoV-2.

King et al [702] reported that outpatient antibiotics prescriptions changed dramatically during the period January to May 2020, exceeding expected seasonal reductions, as shown in Figure 69.

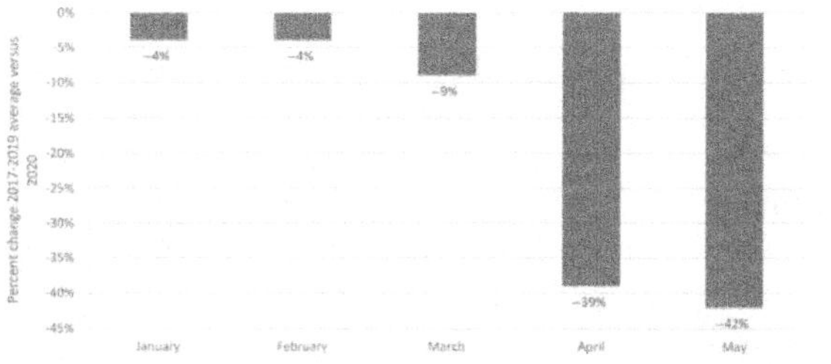

Figure 1. Estimated percent change in the number of patients with antibiotic prescriptions dispensed from retail pharmacies by month, 2017–2019 versus 2020, United States. Only systemic antibiotics were included. Data are from IQVIA Total Patient Tracker (January 2017–May 2020) and were accessed July 15, 2020.

Figure 69 Outpatient antibiotic prescriptions from January to May 2020

We are not claiming that this mechanism would have caused a massive increase in national mortality figures attributed to pneumonia, but it is enough to cause a temporary spike in pneumonia cases/deaths, which would look to hospital staff like it was caused by a novel and deadly new virus for which they were testing, and finding, with a newly launched PCR test.

18.8. DNRs and official recognition of higher mortality

This X/twitter thread [703] by JavRoJav outlines many of the issues and cites numerous papers citing the dangers. This policy change was coupled with DNR (Do Not Resuscitate) orders, which Amnesty [704] revealed as one of the scandals of the pandemic. The 'possible' use of DNRs in the USA was discussed in the Washington Post here [705].

In an article by Griffen [706] in the BMJ it was reported only a third of the excess deaths seen in England and Wales could be explained by Covid-19. Of those 30 000, only 10 000 have had Covid-19 specified on the death certificate. This article also reported a quote from Professor Sir David Spiegelhalter made on May 12th, 2020, who said:

> "over the past five weeks, care homes and other community settings had had to deal with a "staggering burden" of 30 000 more deaths than would normally be expected, as patients were moved out of hospitals that were anticipating high demand for beds.
>
> ......the huge number of unexplained extra deaths in homes and care homes is extraordinary. When we look back . . . this rise in non-covid extra deaths outside the hospital is something I hope will be given really severe attention."

To date the Scottish Covid-19 enquiry is the only public enquiry to allow reports of widespread medical harm. Video of harrowing testimony from the hearings have been reported by biologyphenom here [707].

18.9. Covid-19 ventilation: A policy made in America

The lethal role[1] of ventilation in treating Covid-19 is a hot topic again after Elon Musk raised it in conversation with Joe Rogan on this Spotify podcast [708].

Here is the discussion:

> 0:00 Well, 80% of the people they put on ventilators died.
>
> 0:03 Yeah.
>
> 0:03 So in fact, I actually posted about that because, I, I called doctors in Wuhan and said, what are the biggest mistakes that you made on the first wave?
>
> 0:12 This was early on?
>
> 0:13 And they said we put far too many people on intubated ventilators.
>
> 0:17 So then I, I actually posted on Twitter at the time and said, hey, and what I'm hearing from Wuhan is that they made a big mistake in putting people on intubated ventilators for an extended period.
>
> 0:29 and that this, this is actually what is damaging the lungs, not covid.
>
> 0:32 It's, the treatment is the cure is worse than the disease.
>
> 0:35 And they just, people yelled at me and said, I'm not a doctor.
>
> 0:38 I'm like, yeah, but I do make spaceships with life support systems.
>
> 0:40 What do you do?
>
> 0:42 I twiddle knobs.
>
> 0:44 I'm like, ok, great rock on.

Astute observers will be aware that Elon Musk posted [709] that he was happy to supply ventilators to NYC, sourced from China in March 2020. CNBC reported [710] that he also supplied 1,000 ventilators to California. None of this was mentioned on the Joe Rogan podcast.

There is a deeper, more disturbing, story about the origins of ventilation as a policy response to the 'pandemic' that we are not being told. Likewise, the known risks involved with ventilation, as well as the legal and ethical violations associated with such a response, are largely unknown and undebated.

In this article [711] Michael Senger says that tens of thousands of Americans died after being placed on mechanical ventilators in 2020. He points out that early data from China had suggested that ventilators would need to be used widely in the treatment of Covid-19 patients and this led to a major rush to procure ventilators worldwide. Further he laid the blame for ventilation policy at China's door:

> "This practice of extended intubation was apparently consistent with early guidance coming from China."

But is this true? Can we really blame China for this policy? If not, then where did it originate?

It might come as a surprise that despite China being the first to make widespread use of ventilators evidence suggests that the Chinese may have been following US policy in these matters.

Mass ventilation for respiratory distress is actually a key component in the US, and international, repertoire of what is known as Disaster Medicine, which covers pandemics as well as bioterrorism events.

Disaster medicine has a long history going back to at least 1991 when Heller et al [712] use the example of the first gulf war chemical attacks on Israel to argue that; in the event of a chemical attack, hospitals will need to quickly deploy mechanical ventilation systems to deal with mass casualty events.

By 2005 the infrastructure was in place with Rubinson et al [713] reporting on the 'Working Group on Emergency Mass Critical Care'. On ventilators they say:

> "The Working Group believes that provision of a basic mode of mechanical ventilation (e.g., assist-controlled or pressure-controlled ventilation) for large numbers of patients should be a priority in these conditions. Mechanical ventilators in this setting need not be state of the art but should be rapidly available and portable, should provide adequate gas exchange for a range of clinical conditions that warrant mechanical ventilation, should be safe for patients (disconnect alarm capabilities), should be safe for staff (reduce staff time in patients' rooms if disease is contagious) and should allow for efficient use of staff."

Notice that one of the supposed benefits of ventilation is that it reduces the time staff spend in patient's rooms if the disease is contagious (as we know during Covid-19 staff were made highly anxious and fearful of catching the supposedly novel and deadly virus).

Modelling and planning for pandemics was in full swing by 2006, and that included tracking and managing ventilator stockpiles. The New York City Pandemic Critical Care Capacity Planning Survey [714], from 2006, used the US CDC Disease Control FluSurge [715] model for pandemic influenza planning to determine whether there was sufficient capacity in NYC hospitals to deal with an 'event'. Almost all of the analysis is focused on availability and expected usage of ventilators in the event of a moderate or severe (1918 like) pandemic.

Jumping forward to 2007 Daugherty et al [716] from the Johns Hopkins University School of Medicine, quote SARS and MERS to warn of the looming threat of an influenza pandemic, and the need to focus on large-scale survivable respiratory failure events. Their paper describes recommendations covering strategic stockpiles of ventilators (and how limited they are), sharing ventilators between multiple patients, oxygen stocks and delivery, pulse oximetry and for patient care to be overseen by specialists trained by the Society of Critical Care Medicine Hospital Mass-Casualty Disaster Management.

They also cite Project Xtreme, a program that aims to provide just-in-time cross training of non-respiratory care professionals to assist therapists in caring for surges of ventilated patients (a common practice adopted during the 'pandemic').

Clearly this evidence suggests that much money, energy and thought has been given to disaster planning: ensuring there are enough ventilators in stockpiles, that people are trained, and that supporting equipment is both available and functioning.

Disaster medicine is primarily focused on treating patients in pandemics and bio-terror events, but it also covers ethical standards of care and legal liability of those operating ICUs.

In 2008 Branson et al [717] at the University of Cincinnati did a literature review covering respiratory failure, disaster preparedness, pandemic influenza and mass casualty care. They cite a number of events where manual ventilation was necessary, but they reported that during hurricane Katrina, the Copenhagen polio epidemic of 1952 and the sarin gas attacks in Japan, there was a lack of available equipment. However, in a crucial warning they note that:

> "There is little historical or empirical evidence upon which to base decisions regarding mass casualty respiratory failure and augmenting positive-pressure ventilation capacity."

Ventilation was therefore being recommended with NO consideration of the risks, and with little to no real evidence to support it.

In an editorial for the journal of Disaster Medicine and Public Health Preparedness by Rubinson and Christian [718], published in 2013, they report on the allocation of mechanical ventilators during medical catastrophes:

> "To best use scarce resources, managing medical catastrophes requires deliberate transition from individual-centered to population-focused critical care. In the United States, **the federal government provides neither permission nor definitive guidance for such modifications in care delivery**. Although the federal government has oversight for practices related to health care–relevant federal statutes (eg, the Health Insurance Portability and Accountability Act, the Emergency Medical Treatment and Active Labor Act, and Centers for Medicare and Medicaid Services obligations by health care institutions) and civil rights protections, most health professionals' clinical activities are overseen by states. In recognition of the states' role, the New York State Workgroup developed a process to fairly and justly transition to population-focused care."

Several hugely contentious legal & ethical red flags are being raised here, including the suspension of individual rights with priority being placed on collective protection via population-focused care. Furthermore, they add that their efforts have been influenced by the legal aftermath from hurricane Katrina:

> "In the wake of the response to Hurricane Katrina, the post-event lawsuits and prosecutions have become a significant concern for health care professionals for future disasters. A major advantage of a statewide effort rather than isolated local planning is the **greater possibility for protection from criminal and civil liability for health professionals and institutions** that implement the guidance."

For context the events they are referring to, during and in the aftermath of hurricane Katrina, are covered in this report [719], which describes the incident at Memorial Hospital Center in New Orleans. Mortuary workers recovered 45 bodies from the hospital and toxicology tests were performed on 41 bodies, and 23 tested positive for one or both of morphine and the fast-acting benzodiazepine sedative midazolam. Following an investigation into these deaths, the local district attorney decided there was sufficient evidence to charge three medical staff with four counts of second-degree murder. Charges against two were later dropped in exchange for testimony.

In 2015 New York State issued its policy [720] on ventilator allocation, strongly suggesting they expected a shortage of ventilators. The accompanying detailed guidelines [721] run to 266 pages showing there was a well thought out and extremely detailed plan for the use of ventilators including a 'solid' ethical and legal basis for their use.

However, Michael Senger [722] believes that, even though the public health authorities were obviously well aware of the legal and ethical risks, the information coming from China might excuse them from responsibility or blame:

> "Regardless of how much harm was done, it's simply too difficult to prove that the procedure violated the emergency standard of care given the information coming from China at the time."

There can be no doubt that the well-established US disaster medicine plans were implemented in the 'pandemic' despite the known very high risks presented by ventilation and the acknowledged profound legal and ethical issues in enforcing a 'collectivist' approach in the form of 'population-focused' care.

There is no evidence to support the assertion that ventilation use was reactive and adopted in a panic, or mis-applied *en masse*. On the contrary the expectation was that ventilation was the default, and sole, reaction to a respiratory medical emergency, be it from a natural virus or a bioweapon.

Mass ventilation formed a central plank of the USA's planned response to the Covid-19 'pandemic'. It was 'built-in' to the protocols, procedures and plans, from national to state level. Likewise, given the technological leadership exerted by the USA it would not be surprising that other countries, such as the NATO, EU and Five-eyes nations, would simply follow their lead.

It is therefore not too much of a stretch to assume that, to demonstrate the technological power of the party, that the CCP and China would adopt the same approach. In fact, evidence strongly suggests that the Chinese may have been following – rather than leading - US policy in this critical matter.

There is explicit guidance from China on ventilation policy in the form of the issuance of the 'Handbook of Covid-19 Prevention and Treatment' in March 2020 on ResearchGate [723]. This was widely circulated beforehand via the WHO, as a pdf file [724]. The handbook was edited by Prof. Tingo Liang and initiated by the Jack Ma Foundation and Alibaba. Quite why one of the richest people in China initiated the adoption of Covid-19 treatment protocols, including ventilation, is a bit of a mystery, and why this same initiative was pursued, almost in parallel, by one of the richest people in the USA compounds the mystery. Nevertheless, it doesn't change the fact that ventilation and other pandemic treatment protocols were already 'baked into' the USA's pandemic response pre-2020.

Chapter 19. Celebrating the NHS, informed consent, and eye-opening discussions

19.1. I helped protect the NHS

17 August 2023

A story of self-sacrifice by Martin Neil.

Boris Johnson, the UK prime minister, called on the whole of the UK to protect the NHS from the dangers of the pandemic. As a result, health services were almost completely withdrawn for the vast majority of the over sixty million people living in the UK in 2020.

A 'spontaneous' campaign started where the public were encouraged go out on the doorsteps of their house to clap the NHS to show their appreciation for the heroes protecting us all from covid. This was timed to occur on Thursdays at 8pm, and people were encouraged to 'witness' (surveille?) their neighbours engaged in the 5 minute 'love' session.

However, in the midst of the hysteria those who experienced serious health issues were forgotten about and effectively abandoned. Many had serious illnesses that were not covid. And they had to find ways to get health advice and treatment in a system that was no longer interested in them. I was one of those people. I was expected to sacrifice myself to protect the NHS.

This is the story of my experience trying to find help when I developed skin cancer over the summer of 2020.

In May 2020 I noticed an odd growth on my left cheek which I thought was maybe a bite of some kind. The swelling didn't go down, so I visited my GP who was happy to accept a face-to-face appointment given I mentioned the C-word as a possibility. He agreed I needed a biopsy, just to be safe.

When I visited the local hospital dermatology unit for the biopsy, I was treated by four staff. The hospital was empty, and I was the only case they had that day. We chatted about covid, of which they were all sceptical, but frightened by the overreaction and worried what was happening to the NHS. The 2-weeks guaranteed turnaround time for the biopsy was now 6-weeks because admin staff were working from home (or the lab techs were twiddling knobs on PCR machines).

Five weeks later I got a call to visit the 'big' hospital, which was like a ghost town, and upon my arrival I was met by a MacMillan nurse. MacMillan nurses are special cancer care nurses, funded by charitable donations, trained to impart bad news in smart uniforms. She asked if I had anyone with me and whether I would like to sit down. I said, "no, I'm fine on my own, because I know what's going on". She asked, how and what I knew. I said, "well you are a specialist cancer nurse wearing a smart uniform, that shouts 'you have cancer' so it doesn't take a genius to know its melanoma".

I asked "So, what's next?" she responded - triage. I asked where am I in the triage list, first, second or dead? She couldn't help and didn't really know what the triage process involved because it was all very new, having been put in place to respond to covid. And all the admin staff were working from home so there was no one to ask. She had no ideas about timescales or whether I would be referred to a consultant either.

Realising I was being effectively abandoned I had the presence of mind to ask: "Assuming it involves going under the knife, what kind of consulting surgeon would do the work?" She responded telling me it would be a maxillo-facial consultant. Which hospital I asked? She had no idea. Do you have a list of consultants. Again, no idea. Why, I asked? Covid.

So at least I had something to go on. I was now doing the job of NHS admin, and just needed to find the names of the top maxillo-facial consultants in the southeast of England registered with one of the big private health insurers. So, I looked on the internet. After ringing around, leaving messages and sending emails a consultant's secretary got back to me. She was working at home and was bored as their private patient lists were drying up - everyone was saving the health service by staying at home. But I could have a private appointment in three weeks' time. I said I'd pay cash. No problem. £250.

I barely made the appointment at the bigger hospital with moments to spare, after a 10-hour drive from Glasgow (I was visiting family). The maxillo-facial consultant, who was great, inspected the melanoma, read the notes and recommended surgery as it looked 'nasty'. "Fine" I said. I will pay cash. How much? He said probably about £6,000. Great, let's do it. He said it isn't that easy, because non-NHS private surgery was suspended. I groaned with disappointment thinking I had hit a brick wall. But luckily, he explained that a recent change in government policy meant that the NHS would remain protected, and largely free of patients, but urgent NHS cases could be treated privately in private hospitals. This raised a potential issue: "could I be treated as a private patient, which I was now, in a private hospital that had now been taken over by the NHS?" He said, no - it wouldn't be possible. "So, what should I do?" I asked. He said the simplest way out of this catch-22 is for you to become an NHS patient, for me to bump you up the waiting list and for me to forego private payment. I immediately agreed to this brilliant, much cheaper but also very much more effective, plan.

Around a month later I was given a date for surgery at the bigger Hospital but in the private wing, as an NHS patient. I was advised I would need a PCR covid test, blood tests etc and a CT scan the week before, but that I would need to phone up to arrange this myself. NHS admins were working from home. After a few calls I got some appointments sorted out.

So off I went for a CT scan at the bigger hospital. Again, it was empty. The radiography suite was also empty (I know from my wife's breast cancer treatment 6 months before how busy it should be. It should be rammed). There were only three patients there including me.

Unfortunately, there was a problem: they could not do the scan because they didn't have a photograph from the consultant that shows the melanoma, nor did they have all the notes. He asked, was I a private patient? "No, I am NHS". Maybe the notes have gone missing. NHS admins are working from home don't you know.

In lieu of a photograph of my left cheek I actually pointed at my left cheek and said - "look it's there you can see the thing, why do you need a photograph?" Protocol apparently. I asked, "so if you don't have a photo what happens now?" We'd need to cancel. Really? Yes, really. I quickly responded with "Well how about if I help by getting my wife to photograph it, and I send it by email to the consultant (who I knew was on holiday) and ask him to email you the photograph with any notes you might need? And I can give you his mobile phone number so you can discuss it?" That was acceptable. And that's what happened. I got the scan.

Next hurdle was the PCR test. By that time, I knew quite a bit about PCR. It was very lucky I did. Very lucky indeed. Doing the PCR in some god forsaken car park was routine. What happened next was Kafkaesque.

A week later my surgery was booked for 6am admission, but at 10.40pm the night before I received a phone call from the hospital. There was a serious problem: they had lost my PCR test. Could I come in at midnight to get another one done? I asked why and was told this was because the hospital had a duty to maintain its covid-free status and I couldn't be admitted without a negative test. After a heated one-hour long argument they refused to back down and I finished the conversation by saying: "I will be there with my bag at 6am as planned and you will need to get security to throw me out".

After four hours sleep, I arrived for surgery at 6am. First hurdle was reception. They didn't ask about the PCR test. Excellent, I'm in! I was then shown to my nice private room (a perk the NHS were paying for). I had a chat to the anaesthetist and the surgeon who agreed the covid stuff was bollocks and both were happy to proceed without a negative PCR test. At last, some sanity, but that was short-lived.

Matron arrived. She was very concerned. I was putting the hospital at risk! Why, I asked? She said I might have covid because I didn't have a negative PCR test registered on the system. I explained they had lost it. She was horrified and bluntly stated the surgery would have to be cancelled and I would have to go home. I kept my head and carefully explained the balance of risks from covid versus cancer. It didn't make any difference, she was immovable. I explained that she was being unethical and in breach of her oaths, was opening up the hospital to a legal suit and was endangering my life. I said I'd go to the newspapers. She wasn't impressed by any of this. I said "well, I'm not moving because the surgical team are happy to proceed, and you will have to physically throw me out".

Given I had dug my heels in she was stuck. With great reluctance she said she would deviate from procedure and seek out a new PCR test but warned it had an eight-hour minimum turnaround time. It would have to be analysed in a lab in a hospital 40 miles away. It was 9am. If they got the negative back by 5pm they could do the surgery. My operation was then rescheduled to be the last one of the day.

I sat back thinking these people really want to kill me.

Trying to remain positive I cheered myself up by chatting with one of the nurses. She agreed the covid nonsense was all bollocks and she was working in crazy land but was willing to agree with me that my experience thus far was even more nuts than usual. She also imparted to me that the place was full of NHS patients and those who had private cover were being de-prioritised. I consoled myself by reflecting on lucky I was that my maxillo-facial consultant understood what was happening in a fast-moving administrative admissions policy landscape.

But this got me thinking about the PCR. Was there a way to speed this up? I realised there was. I knew there was a new nudge-DNA test kit that had been introduced to the NHS the week before. This had a turnaround of a few hours.

I buzzed for matron. And asked, "Do you have any DNA nudge PCR kits onsite?" She looked at me in wild surprise and responded by asking how I knew about that. I said PCR was a recent hobby of mine but don't worry about the details, all you need to do is get the head of hospital PCR to obtain one: it's got a fast turnaround time. She said they were still in their boxes, unopened. I suggest using me as a guinea pig. She said she'd talk to the head of PCR.

The head of PCR turned up with a brown box like an excited child with a new toy. He was happy to do the PCR and would swab me on the spot. They would have a result by 3pm.

At 3pm the moment of truth arrived. The matron came and said we had a negative result on our hands and the surgery could go ahead. I was elated but also feeling a little devilish, so I asked, "what PCR test was the negative result from?". She didn't know and didn't think it mattered. I said: "of course it matters, because if it was the first lab PCR test that was a negative and if the DNA nudge PCR test comes back positive then I have clearly caught covid in your fucking hospital! And I will sue your arse and get it closed down!"

After she had slammed the door on the way out, I settled in and enjoyed my well-earned rest before the surgery. It went ahead. It was a great success, other than the fact I had to discharge myself the next day and make my own arrangements for pain killers and to have my stitches taken out.

Did I clap for the NHS? I think you know the answer to that question!

19.2. The scandal of the EU/Pfizer contract is even worse than reported

October 2022 and August 2023

Interesting article in the Daily Sceptic today [725] reveals that in April 2021 the Pfizer EU contract contained the statement:

> "The Participating Member State further acknowledges that the long-term effect and efficacy of the Vaccine are not currently known and that there may be adverse effects of the Vaccine that are not currently known".

The article shows that this paragraph (along with other incriminating material) has now been redacted in the version posted by the European Commission. The fact that such clauses were ever in the contract and that the EU is now trying to cover them up is, of course, a very important story.

But, for the record, in October 2022 (after a tip-off from colleagues in Slovenia) we already published [726] this information about the Pfizer contract (our article included a scanned pdf of all versions of the contract). Our colleagues had received the document following an FOI request to the Slovenian Government. Note also that, whereas the Daily Sceptic article refers to the version of the document dated April 2021, the Slovenian document dated 28 Sept 2021 (when so much more was known about the vaccine adverse effects) contains exactly the same wording.

Here [727] is a (scanned) pdf of the Slovenian Government contracts with Pfizer for their Covid vaccines.

Note that there are 4 different contracts here dated 10 Dec 2020, 4 March 2021, 7 April 2021 and 28 Sept 2021. The documents show the number of doses ordered per month (but the price is redacted). But, note that even the latest of these contracts (dated 28 Sept 2021) contains the following statement in Article 1 (it's on page 17/25 of the scanned document).

> "The ...State further acknowledges that the long-term effects and efficacy of the Vaccine are not currently known".

While that may have been a reasonable statement to include in the December 2020 contract, it is curious that no update at all had been added by the end of September 2021 given all the data on hundreds of millions of doses that had been administered by then.

Regarding the Pfizer contract with the UK (which presumably has the same wording) it is very interesting to note that this UK Government report [728] ("Conditions of Authorisation for COVID-19 Vaccine Pfizer/BioNTech (Regulation 174", updated 16 Aug 2022) says:

> "Pfizer/BioNTech must provide a regular analysis of safety data based on the MHRA's specifications relating to booster or supplementary doses"

19.3. Informed consent statement on covid policies

Affecting children and young adults (9 September 2023)

We provided the following statement to support a case concerned with informed consent relevant to the vaccination and masking of children and young adults. All of the numbered references in this section here can be found here [729].

- The risk to any healthy child of hospitalisation or death from covid is (and was) essentially zero [1][2][3][4]. For example, in the entire main period of the covid pandemic Feb 2020 – Dec 2022, just three people under the age of 20 in England and Wales died with COVID-19 as the only cause mentioned on the death certificate and even for these three no autopsy was conducted to confirm they were genuine 'covid deaths' [5]. In Jan 2022 the rare 'covid death' of a 7-year-old girl, Cassidy Baracka, in the USA [6] was used as a warning to urge parents to vaccinate their children; but the death was not from covid at all – it was the direct result of a covid vaccination [7] [8].
- The known risks of the vaccines have not been properly communicated to vaccine recipients. Doctors tasked with vaccination found blank information sheets

inserted [9]. The first product monographs (these sheets) were only provided and approved for distribution in America and Canada as electronic downloads on 16 Sept 2021 (around 10 months AFTER the rollout began - so doctors were in fact, and legally, flying blind up until that point) and the heavily modified current version links on both the FDA and Health Canada websites are both dated 21 March 2023. [10] The UK monograph approach was simply to re-publish the American one.

- Studies claiming vaccine efficacy against covid are systemically flawed [11] [12] [13] (a catalogue of the studies and their flaws is provided in [14]). Moreover, contrary to the efficacy claims widely made, the vaccinated are more likely to repeatedly test positive for covid (and hence be classified as a 'covid case') than those unvaccinated [15]. The Office for National Statistics data - that many have used against the Statistics Regulator's advice as the basis for claims of efficacy [16][17] – are systemically flawed and biased [18]. Indeed, in contrast to the ONS data, the UKHSA data was consistently showing higher covid case rates in the vaccinated than the unvaccinated [19] until its surveillance reports stopped providing this information in March 2022; that was when, bizarrely, a footnote was added to Table 14 stating "Comparing case rates among vaccinated and unvaccinated populations should not be used to estimate vaccine effectiveness against covid-19 infection" [20].

- Studies claiming vaccine efficacy against hospitalisation and death from covid are systemically flawed and biased [14] [21]. Responses to FOIs requesting hospitalisation by vaccination status data inevitably reveal disproportionately higher rates among the vaccinated. For example, in 2022 Public Health Wales confirmed that 6.4% of hospitalised patients aged 60+ were unvaccinated compared with 90.8% double vaccinated [22].

- Multiple extremely concerning safety signals for the vaccines were known before Feb 2022 but were generally suppressed from the public [23] [24] [25][26]. For example, the MHRA did not release the information on multiple adverse reactions recorded between Jan and June 2021 in its redacted 'not for publication report' [27] sent by the MHRA to the Pharmacovigilance Expert Advisory Group (PEAG) for advice. which was only released following an FOI request in 2023 [28]. This report showed that among the 26,000 people who had registered for the MHRA Yellow Card Vaccine Monitor (YCVM) at the beginning of 2021, 53% reported at least one adverse reaction by 30 June 2021 [27] (the MHRA have released no further update since then and appear to have abandoned the monitoring scheme shortly after this report).

- Multiple deaths confirmed by coroners have resulted directly from the covid vaccinations [29][30] [31] [32] [33] [34] [35] [36] with those under the age of 40 disproportionately affected [37] [38]. EMA and the European Parliament in April 2023 recognise 11,448 deaths following covid vaccination, and that there were 50,648 deaths attributed to the Covid vaccines in the Eudravigilance database

[39]. But coroner confirmed deaths are known to be just a tiny proportion of the true number. As of 28 July 2023 there were 35,726 deaths and 207,211 hospital visits reported in the VAERS system resulting from the covid vaccinations; the number of deaths reported for the covid vaccines in less than 2 years was almost four times the total number of deaths reported for all other vaccines combined in the 32 years of VAERS recording [40]. Despite claims to the contrary, a forensic analysis of a large sample of VAERS death reports in 2021 showed that most reports were submitted by health service employees and in only 14% of the cases could vaccine reaction be ruled out as a contributing factor in their death [25]; a forensic analysis of a random sample of 57 death reports in the UK's Yellow Card scheme pre-covid showed that 40 were true positives (77%) while none of the remaining 17 could be proved to be false positives [41]. Moreover, it has always been widely accepted that less than 10% of all vaccine adverse reactions are reported to systems like VAERS [42]. Taking these factors into account it was estimated that, based on the Yellow Card scheme up to 29 Sept 2022 there had already been almost 16,000 deaths in the UK directly caused by the covid vaccines [43].

- Even using data from the ONS that we have shown to be highly biased and flawed in favour of vaccine safety and efficacy, it now certain that all-cause mortality in those under 50 is higher in those vaccinated than those unvaccinated meaning that, in the simplest and most objective way possible, the risks of the vaccine outweigh any benefits [18] [44]. There have also been multiple studies showing (at an international level) increased all-cause mortality in the vaccinated [45].

- There has been significant variability in the lethality of the vaccines by vaccine maker and batch number [46] [47] [48] [49] including some so bad that UK recipients were banned from travelling to the EU with them [50]. There have also been major problems with contamination especially affecting the AZ vaccines (which although manufactured in the USA were never approved for use by the FDA) [51] and confirmed deaths from contaminated Moderna batches [52]. The AZ batch PV46664 that caused the rapid deterioration in my own wife's frontotemporal dementia is now known to have been the second most lethal batch with 6648 adverse reactions and 17 deaths reported to the Yellow card system [53]).

- The standard procedure of 'aspiration' for intramuscular injections was generally stopped for the covid vaccines (although some countries like Denmark reverted to the practice after serious adverse reactions were caused by lack of aspiration) [54] and therefore it is likely that approximately 2% of vaccinations went straight into the blood, potentially explaining why a small proportion of vaccine recipients suffered far worse than most [55].

- Masks were ineffective against covid [56] [57] [58] and even the largest study that claimed to show some efficacy was fundamentally flawed and misleading [59]. There is no evidence that masks are effective for children [60]; rather, masks have been shown to be harmful to children and pregnant women [61] while [56] found "a profound number" of participants "reported adverse reactions to prolonged mask use during COVID-19."

- The covid case numbers were continually inflated due to mass PCR testing of asymptomatic people because the vast majority of asymptomatic people testing positive did not have the virus, i.e. the vast majority were false positives [62] [63].

- None of the studies promoted to support vaccination of pregnant women is valid - they all suffer systemic biases and flaws which, if properly adjusted for, indicate the oppositive conclusion [64][65][66][67].

19.4. An explosive discussion with ex-CDC scientist

30 October 2023

Dr Norman Pieniazek is a molecular biologist, geneticist, epidemiologist with 147 publications [730] in virology and parasitology. Before he retired, he spent 24 years working at the Center for Disease Control (CDC) in the USA. He has also spent time abroad including time working in Spain and Poland.

We met up with Norman for what was planned to be a short meeting to introduce ourselves and informally discuss common interests around covid. However, this turned into a two-hour long, wide-ranging and fascinating discussion that touched on a huge number of topics.

Early in the meeting Norman made the wise suggestion that we record and share the discussion. So, he hit the record button on Skype, and we started again. The video, accessible here [731], is approximately two hours long. Be aware that, given it wasn't planned as an 'interview' or for broadcast, it is largely unstructured. However, for those short of time here is a synopsis of the discussion with a focus on what Norman said.

19.4.1. Pneumonia and early treatments

- The bacterial pneumonia hypothesis [732] suggests that early treatment - hydroxychloroquine, ivermectin and antibiotics address bacterial infection. Norman confirmed bacteria are everywhere in our bodies including in the lungs, creating an ever-present potentially hazardous predisposition that, given the right circumstances, might cause a deadly bacterial pneumonia infection.

- Well-understood remedies such as the stockpile of antibiotics, as recommended by Fauci, were cast aside in 2020. Bacterial infection can cause sepsis hence we need antibiotics. A Cytokine storm is caused by bacterial infection in the lungs, filling them with fluid; this lowers the oxygen level in the blood because of poor lung function.

- In-person diagnosis by a physician based on physical symptoms was largely replaced by the PCR test, and with the rise in tele-health visits, social distancing etc physicians stopped using stethoscopes to listen to a patient's chest. This is an essential diagnostic tool to enable a doctor to audibly tell whether a patient has crossed the line into a bacterial infection which will then require antibiotics.

19.4.2. NPIs and discarded organisational memory

- Norman knew Donald Henderson who co-authored a classic work on how to best respond to a flu epidemic. Henderson and colleagues did not recommend any of the NPIs that were followed during covid because of the obvious severe health, social and economic costs. (As an aside this work was co-authored by Prof. Thomas Inglesby at John Hopkins who attended Event 201 and, oddly, recommended NPIs be used for covid [733] - the very same ones he had rejected previously [734]).

- Orthodox immunology was ignored - herd immunity is a fiction given there is a 'soup' of constantly mutating coronaviruses.

- Why didn't scientists at the CDC question things early in 2020? Work from home restrictions meant that people at CDC couldn't communicate and coordinate to overturn the madness being imposed from the 'sixth floor' top brass. You could not isolate CDC from the HSS (Health and Human Services), and it was HSS that were calling the shots.

19.4.3. Wuhan, bronchial lavage and PCR

- The Wuhan scientists [735] were on a routine 'fishing expedition' for coronaviruses and unusual pneumonias. Why was this work being done in Wuhan? It is easier to do in China because it is legal and because there are lots of hospitals, in a concentrated area, where the population is in relatively poor health. Also, it is easier to get permission to perform a painful bronchial lavage [736] procedure on patients to obtain pathogens in China; this is much harder to do in the USA. This procedure is done in the lower respiratory tract and guarantees higher quality samples than can be obtained using swabs, which really just measure the quality of the air that has entered your upper respiratory tract.

- To determine what pathogen is causing lower respiratory tract symptoms you should not use swabs and PCR. Why not? CDC acknowledges the inability of swabs to collect causative agents as reported by the EPIC study in these 2015 NEJM articles (one done on adults [737] and one on children [738]). Hence a positive result gained from a sample taken from the upper throat or the nose does not mean an infection is caused by the detected pathogen.

- In 2002-2004 SARS-COV was not subject to mass PCR testing, yet SARS-COV-2 was. PCR was used for SARS-COV but only on samples taken using bronchial lavage, but NOT from swab samples taken from the nose or upper throat

19.4.4. Virus origins - from labs or bats or neither?

- Wu et al [739] discovered WH-Human-1 using samples collected by bronchial lavage, and next generation sequencing of the collected genetic samples, and ultimately reported it in GenBank.

- Before reporting on GenBank they published a preprint identifying the genetic sequences, which was appropriated and found its way into the hands of Corman and Drosten, who then decided to exploit it for personal gain (via commercial PCR testing), fabricating a story about validating it against SARS-1. It was subsequently renamed SARS-COV-2. (For a proposed timeline of events see here).

- Norman thinks SARS-COV-2 is simply a beta coronavirus (a cold), one of the many thousands of cold viruses that had remained undiscovered until 2020, but which have always been ever present in nature.

- SARS-COV-2 cannot be a novel virus created in a lab or by natural zoonotic mutation. It is simply novel to detection. As soon as the EUA approved PCR tests started to be used the virus was simultaneously discovered in a number of disparate geographical regions. There was no evidence of sudden spread.

- In effect the results of any test are as much determined by the choice of test to apply as by the presence/absence of viruses. Norman says, "you will find whatever you want to find". Hence people will be symptomless yet will have a lot of, whatever viruses happen to be around in their nose or throat.

- The established taxonomy [739] of viruses is unusable simply because there are so many unknown viruses circulating in the wild.

19.4.5. Vaccines

- The mRNA vaccine technology ended in a 'garbage heap', because it is extremely toxic, and was rendered obsolete by protein subunit vaccines by 2019. So, the mRNA vaccines were doomed from the start. Subunit (protein-based) vaccines have been known since the late 1970s, but Moderna, Pfizer and BioNTech needed a way to realise a return on their vast investments in mRNA. Hence the pandemic.

- Novavax is a protein subunit vaccine, based on the spike protein, which was available in August 2020 but did not get approval from the FDA. Although it is protein based it will stay in the deltoid muscle injection site. It was however approved in Canada. It may not be very good for you (and ineffective against coronaviruses), but it is less dangerous than the mRNA vaccines.

- mRNA vaccines were found to be too dangerous for animals. Also, arguments that they are a safe basis for cancer drugs are based on lies. There is a competing technology called humanised monoclonal antibodies that cured President Carter from a melanoma that had migrated to his brain and there are now 500 versions of these drugs currently available.

- Norman was told that the patent on the flu vaccines, grown in eggs, expired in 2020. Hence, there was little ROI in continuing with this technology.

- Viruses are in your respiratory tract and antibodies, responding to vaccines, are in your blood. These two things do not match well because the antibodies in the blood do not get into the lungs. The immune system 'stays away' from the complex respiratory system that deals with the thousands of pathogens we breathe in with every breath.

19.4.6. Antibody and antigen testing

- Are serology studies a pointless exercise? Because of wide variation between individual's antibody measurement only makes sense by studying change in any single individual over time.

- Testing for antibodies means nothing because antibodies in the blood cannot travel to the lungs to react.

- Testing for antigens is a cheaper and less sensitive version of the PCR test with the same limitation.

19.4.7. Infectious clones and bioweapons

- Norman is very sceptical of a number of covid virus theories including those by Walter Chesnut [740] and JJCoey's infectious clone theory, though they weren't discussed in any great detail and were probably not characterised fully (or maybe even fairly).

- The issue with 'infectious clones' is that 'you do not know what to create' because there are millions of sequences of coronavirus so there is no 'clonality' and each one has 30 thousand nucleotides and there are combinatorically infinite changes you could potentially need to consider when creating a coronavirus[5]. It therefore isn't possible to know what to change, via Gain of Function (GoF), to make the virus behave in more dangerous ways.

- As part of the 'partnership for peace' programme in 1994 Norman hired two ex-Soviet bioweapons scientists and asked them 'how come you worked for 20 years and didn't create any new deadly viruses?'

- They can create thousands of virus combinations, but the problem is how to test these creations. There is no way to test the billions and billions of possible changes to a virus and identify which changes to the sequence are 'bad'. You need the phenotype, and you cannot deduce the phenotype from the genotype. So how would GoF researchers - E.g., EcoHealth alliance - know exactly what to create?

- The claim that Saddam Hussian had biological weapons was groundless and this was confirmed to Norman by Donald Henderson who was involved at the time and who said it was not possible.

- Thus, GoF claims that changes to spike protein and furin cleavage sites make a virus more deadly are fiction. It isn't possible and there is no proof they can produce deadly bioweapons. Those advocating this position and making these claims - EcoHealth alliance (Fauci, Baric and Duszak) should get fired by their bosses for producing "not a tiger but a kitty".

- We discussed Gulf War syndrome. Norman said people imagine anthrax is dangerous, but the ex-Soviet bioweapons researchers said to attack New York with anthrax would need 20,000 Boeing 747s flying over the city, dropping millions of tons of anthrax spores from a low height then people spreading it with shovels. The only way to infect people with anthrax is by direct means via an oxygen line or a direct injection.

- Norman said the Tokyo gas attack [741] was successful in Japan because the terrorist used sarin, a nerve agent. The biological agents used, botulinum and anthrax, fortunately failed.

19.4.8. Fauci - the 'mean midget'

- Within the CDC Fauci was called the 'mean midget' and during the AIDS epidemic he sunk Robert Gallo by inventing the story that Gallo had stolen the HIV virus from Luc Montagnier, thus destroying Gallo's chances of being awarded the Nobel prize (he was also denied a patent).

- Fauci is "not stupid, he is mean". Fauci wanted to get a Nobel prize, but he didn't get a Nobel prize for AIDS, so he wanted it for the Wuhan virus. In January 2023 knowing that he wasn't going to get the Nobel prize he "pulled the plug" and published this paper [742] saying new types of vaccines are needed for respiratory infections, as an act of spite.

We learned a lot from Norman and are very grateful to him for giving us his valuable time. You will notice that we briefly discussed the vaccines, but you will be very pleased to hear that Norman has agreed to follow up with another meeting in early December to share his thoughts on this important topic (see here [743] for a sneak peek).

Chapter 20. Was Covid-19 novel and deadly?

20.1. 'Spikeopathy' does not explain Covid-19's 'novel' symptoms

21 December 2023

20.1.1. Introduction

"There is nothing more deceptive than an obvious fact."

— Arthur Conan Doyle, The Boscombe Valley Mystery - a Sherlock Holmes Short Story

---

In Chapter 17 we investigated the 'bacterial pneumonia hypothesis': that a proportion of Covid-19 deaths, those with associated respiratory symptoms (rather than deaths coded as Covid-19 because of a positive PCR test, that are absent symptoms), were caused by bacterial pneumonia, and that bacterial pneumonia was the primary, not the secondary, infection. We concluded that it was and believe this evidence contradicts the idea that SARS-CoV-2 was both 'novel and deadly', and hence there was no 'pandemic'.

Fauci et al [744] believe that the 1918 'pandemic' was largely caused by pneumonia, and in 2020 the number of influenza and pneumonia deaths in the UK and USA were relatively unchanged from historical patterns, at a time when 'flu' was said to have disappeared (see here [745] for details). This suggests that the mortality risk presented by these respiratory conditions had not changed in 2020 despite it supposedly being a 'pandemic' caused by a competing novel pathogen.

In this article we begin by chronicling and summarising the evidence provided by Dr Kory and Dr Stone who firmly believe that the world saw a novel pathogen in 2020, and that this pathogen was SARS-CoV-2. They attribute the symptoms of Covid-19 to 'spikeopathy', associated with the spike protein of the SARS-CoV-2 virus. We review the medical literature to look for supporting evidence about the symptoms and conclude that these symptoms cannot be explained by the single over-arching cause of a novel spikeopathy mechanism associated with SARS-CoV-2. We then consider alternative explanations.

The full version of this chapter is based on this article with relevant screenshots here [746], and our response in the debate with Dr Pierre Kory can be found here [747].

20.1.2. Evidence from Dr Stone and Dr Kory

Dr Stone's evidence (note that throughout CT stands for *computed tomography*).

1. It is not possible that this was a flu virus. It was not only a respiratory virus. It was transmissible and could enter through the gut and respiratory tract and could first present as diarrhoea, or flu, or fever, or unstable blood sugar. It was a disease of the endothelium and nothing else I have seen causes the clotting I saw.
2. Fear does not cause low saturation, chest X-ray and CT chest findings, and raised D Dimers and CRPs of over 200, or raised LDH and very low lymphocytes which were among the myriad of novel and objective findings seen.
3. Those who were "spiked" responded in a myriad of ways depending on the state of their immune system.
4. We treated for bacterial pneumonia in the first half of 2020, and they still died. Bacterial pneumonia complicated some patients, and the neutrophil count responded to IV antibiotics.
5. They only stopped dying when we added Ivermectin and the most noticeable and objective findings were the increase in sats, the increase in D Dimer with clot breakdown and the restoration of a good pulse waveform on the monitors, suggesting reperfusion. I have countless photos that I have presented on this. Ivermectin stopped coagulation, and clinically, patients survived hypoxia because of its effects on the mitochondria.

Dr Kory's evidence:

1. My paper shows extremely high incidence of organizing, pneumonia on CAT scans, and my early paper shows extremely high incidence of wickedly severe clotting.
2. Extremely high rates of anosmia, and ageusia.
3. I wholeheartedly agree that "they" use viral spikeopathy to blame everything on the virus and not the vax, my practice specializes in treating patients with Long Covid and Long Vax
4. They found that the predominant finding was an "organizing pneumonia" pattern. Yes, this pattern has been associated with viruses before, but never to such a high incidence and so reproducibly - I suddenly was rounding in an ICU where everyone's chest x-ray and CT scan were identical, oxygen requirements and vent settings maximal, it was impossible to remember the patients' names as so little differentiated their disease.
5. Organising pneumonia - ground glass is non-specific as a general finding on CT scans, but pneumonia is not typically bilateral, and the ground glass is not typically seen in an "organizing" pattern of lung injury, but is more typically seen in patchy or consolidative or micronodular patterns - organizing pneumonia (oddly well demarcated with a peripheral, subpleural predominance) is a somewhat rare disease, and suddenly we had ICU wards full of patients with organizing pneumonia patterns of lung injury.
6. Bacterial pneumonias requiring hospitalisation do not present with "happy hypoxia" (a puzzling finding to many doctors that was widely discussed even in newspapers), reason being is that the lungs are typically "heavy" with accumulated fluid/pus, they are not "dry" as they were with Covid. My partner Paul Marik, using a sophisticated device, measured the "extravascular lung water"

(EVLW) in like the first 5 Covid patients he admitted on vents to the ICU. They had zero EVLW.

7. Secondly, in ICUs most ICU docs have a hair trigger for empiric antibiotics with either a fever, raised white counts, increasing phlegm or unilateral or asymmetric consolidations. I saw a lot of antibiotics being used in patients in my NYC ICU in the spring - didn't help. However, reading your article, you do make a strong case for Patient zero having a bacterial pneumonia based on his CT scan finding.
8. The Covid patients were crashing on vents with organizing pneumonia as the inciting cause (organizing pneumonia is not associated with bacteria).
9. None were suggestive of a bacterial process (typically unilateral abnormalities) preceding the viral syndrome (typically bilateral). Also, they had dry lungs and happy hypoxia - i.e. not bacterial.
10. Now the 2nd aspect you analysed, whether lots of secondary bacterial pneumonia or VAP as we call it in the ICU went unrecognized and contributed to the mortality rates, that certainly maybe true......as it has always been true. VAP is and has always been a shitshow of a topic in ICU medicine.
11. Happy Hypoxia does not refer to a specific level of saturation, rather it refers to someone who evidences low to very low blood oxygen saturations, but the low saturations are not accompanied by a significant increase in the "work of breathing,", i.e. they look oddly and discordantly comfortable. Most patients with an acute lung injury or infection which leads to low oxygen saturation will be struggling to breathe (especially bacterial pneumonia leading to hypoxia). These Covid patients (on presentation only as with time they did eventually develop respiratory distress, just not on arrival to the ER or in the first days) were not overtly struggling to breathe initially, thus the term "happy hypoxia".
12. Covid has two phases, the first is a viral syndrome, typical as any other, except the high incidence of severe anosmia (which then persisted beyond the acute phase) but then on like day 6-10, a minority of patients went into what I call the "pulmonary phase" where the lungs would get inflamed with ground glass opacities in an organizing pattern, their sats would drop, they would come to hospital, often relatively comfortable, but then, without treatment (i.e. corticosteroids), they would then start the slow steady Covid trajectory towards worsening oxygenation, increased shortness of breath, high flow oxygen devices or non-invasive ventilators and then would get intubated. But again, it was the latter pulmonary phase, which was so unique, not the earlier acute viral syndrome phase - that one, as you guys point out, was relatively indistinguishable from other acute viral illness (with the exception of severe and more frequent anosmia/ageusia in some). Otherwise, yes, the acute phase was relatively indistinguishable, but the later hospital phase was not - i.e. the organizing pneumonia, happy hypoxia, the microclotting etc.
13. Also, obviously, I cannot describe hospital phase Covid occurring in other places, I can only describe what I saw in ICU's in Madison, NYC, Milwaukee, South Carolina, and Central Wisconsin - they were all similar/identical, but the incidence of severe clotting waned over time during that first year and a half.

Dr Stone and Dr Kory approved of the following summary of their views on the signs and symptoms associated with Covid-19 and for us to include it in a public article:

- Happy hypoxia (saturating between 51% and 90%)
- First present as diarrhoea, or flu, or fever, or unstable blood sugar.
- Raised D Dimers (blood clot marker) and CRPs of over 200 (marker of inflammation)
- Raised LDH (sign of tissue damage) and very low lymphocytes.
- Anosmia, and ageusia (loss of taste and smell)
- CT scans – Acute fibrous organising, bilateral pneumonia with ground glass opacities
- CT scans - Evidence of peripheral, subpleural predominance
- CT scans - Diffuse alveolar damage (DAD) (indicative of alveolar haemorrhage)
- Lungs were dry - They had zero EVLW "extravascular lung water".
- Micro clotting severe but waned over course of the 'pandemic'.

This article does not address treatments, which were a fast-moving and controversial topic early in the 'pandemic'. Illustrative of this is Dr Kory's testimony [748] to the Homeland Security & Governmental Affairs senate committee meeting in May 2020, where he recommended that the 'life threatening' ventilator shortage be addressed, that medicines like remdesivir or hydroxychloroquine be administered at home to keep patients away from hospital and that corticosteroids, which he says were lifesaving in prior 'pandemics', should be given to anyone beyond mild illness. Currently the FLCCC (Front Line COVID-19 Critical Care Alliance [749]), of which Dr Kory is the President and Chief Medical Officer, recommends a panoply of treatments, including ivermectin and the FLCCC have published a factsheet [750] on remdesivir suggesting its use is now known to result in a higher risk of sickness and death.

20.1.3. Evidential support for 'novel' Covid-19 signs and symptoms

We are sceptical as to whether these signs and symptoms are caused exclusively by SARS-COV-2 and will investigate a subset of them, looking at contradictory and confirmatory evidence, as well as alternative explanations for what may have caused disease in 2020, but which was then (wrongly, in our view) associated with the deadly and novel virus.

Initial reporting of the signs and symptoms of Covid-19 from Wuhan, in the form of the study of 1,099 patients by Guan et al [751] appeared in the NEJM in April 2020 and was very widely reported (17,901 citations). They say:

> "The median age of the patients was 47 years; 41.9% of the patients were female. The primary composite end point occurred in 67 patients (6.1%), including 5.0% who were admitted to the ICU, 2.3% who underwent invasive mechanical ventilation, and 1.4% who died. Only 1.9% of the patients had a history of direct contact with wildlife. Among nonresidents of Wuhan, 72.3% had contact with residents of Wuhan, including 31.3% who had visited the city. The most common symptoms were fever (43.8% on admission and 88.7% during hospitalisation) and cough (67.8%). Diarrhoea was uncommon (3.8%). The median incubation period

was 4 days (interquartile range, 2 to 7). On admission, ground-glass opacity was the most common radiologic finding on chest computed tomography (CT) (56.4%). No radiographic or CT abnormality was found in 157 of 877 patients (17.9%) with nonsevere disease and in 5 of 173 patients (2.9%) with severe disease. Lymphocytopenia was present in 83.2% of the patients on admission.

During the first 2 months of the current outbreak, Covid-19 spread rapidly throughout China and caused varying degrees of illness. Patients often presented without fever, and many did not have abnormal radiologic findings. (Funded by the National Health Commission of China and others.)"

It surely says something about the suspension of normal critical faculties within the scientific community that this paper became so widely cited and, apparently, played a major role in the propagation of the 'pandemic' narrative, given that:

- The median age of the subjects was 47 – dramatically lower than that observed elsewhere.
- Within 3 weeks of the "sequence" for the novel virus being identified, they were able to find more than 1000 patients infected by it across 552 hospitals.
- They assume all these hospitals were capable of a reliable diagnosis of Covid-19 in so short a period from its 'discovery' to the implementation of diagnostic tests.

It should be noted that diarrhoea was uncommon, and the most common CT findings were ground glass opacities (GGO [752] - this can be a manifestation of a wide variety of clinical features, including malignancies and benign conditions, such as focal interstitial fibrosis, inflammation, and haemorrhage). In the appendixes to their paper, they present a case fatality rate (CFR) comparable to the lower end of that reported for seasonal influenzas. Likewise, the CT scan reports do not differentiate from flu or bacterial pneumonia. It does not report dry throat or happy hypoxia as unusual symptoms, nor are either microvascular thrombosis (micro clotting) or alveolar haemorrhage reported at all.

In their July 2020 paper Kory and Kane [753], identify a set of Computed Tomography (CT) imaging descriptors that they claim are diagnostic of Covid-19 in the six patients they examined: an acute bilateral fibrinous and organising pneumonia. The paper mentions a rapidly progressive course exhibiting imaging findings similar to diffuse alveolar damage (DAD). Note also that in Dr Kory's testimony he mentions the presence of subpleural predominance – "oddly well demarcated with a peripheral, subpleural predominance" - but the paper says, "which can extend to the subpleural regions", which we assume to be equivalent.

In April 2020 Kory's co-author Kanne [754] identified the CT imaging descriptors that correlated with Covid-19. He recorded the usual ground glass opacities, consolidation, bilateral and peripheral distribution, but no pleural effusion or other findings related to the pleural cavity. Kanne says:

"The long-term imaging features of 2019-nCoV are not yet known but presumably will resemble those of other causes of acute lung injury."

In October 2021 Zarei et al [755] compared chest CT imaging descriptors from influenza pneumonia (H1N1) and Covid-19 patients and conducted an interobserver agreement study of radiologists to determine whether they could consistently differentiate between one disease or the other from the scan alone. They found that:

> "The most frequent clinical symptom in patients with COVID-19 and H1N1 pneumonia were dyspnoea (96.6%) and cough (62.5%), respectively. The CT findings showed that the COVID-19 group was characterized by GGO (88.1%), while the influenza group had features such as GGO (68.4%) and consolidation (66.7%). Compared to the influenza group, the COVID-19 group was more likely to have GGO (88.1% vs. 68.4%, p = 0.032), subpleural sparing (69.0% vs. 7.7%, p <0.001) and subpleural band (50.0% vs. 20.5%, p = 0.006), but less likely to have pleural effusion (4.8% vs. 33.3%, p = 0.001). The agreement rate between the 3 radiologists was 65.8%."

They reported that radiologists found that the similarities of lung involvement in both diseases meant it was very hard to differentiate between them. Their statistical results show that ground glass opacities and consolidation are not useful to diagnostically distinguish the two conditions from each other, and the only features that shows on a CT scan that might practically assist in this regard are subpleural sparing, effusion and banding.

They did not mention any symptoms related to DAD (diffuse alveolar damage), microvascular thrombosis (micro clotting) or alveolar haemorrhage.

The March 2020 study by Fu et al [756] retrospectively analysed CT features in Covid-19 patients and confirmed that ground glass opacities and consolidation were common features. However, interestingly they did record that the age variable had a mean of 45 (range was 20-67), only 14.5% had shortness of breath and only 0.02% had diarrhoea. They also said 5% of patients had severe progression with "white lungs". They did also make these comments when comparing to other diseases:

> "Nevertheless, we found that COVID-19 pneumonia has many similar CT features to those reported with SARS and MERS thus, it is difficult to distinguish COVID-19 pneumonia from them. Our findings were in accordance with the present studies. It is not surprising since the responsible viruses of SARS and MERS are also coronaviruses and viruses in the same viral family have similar pathogenesis."

They reported this experience about CT scans for Covid-19:

> "The common CT features of COVID-19 pneumonia are multiple lung opacities, multiple types of the opacity (ground-glass, ground-glass and consolidation, and consolidation alone), and multiple lobes especially the lower lobe involved."

Note that they did not report any findings of happy hypoxia, subpleural sparing, subpleural band or pleural effusion nor did they mention any symptoms related to DAD (diffuse alveolar damage), microvascular thrombosis (micro clotting) or alveolar haemorrhage. They emphasised that their reported CT features of Covid-19 should be considered preliminary rather than definitive.

In April 2020 Hani et al [757] performed a systematic review on a large series of 1014 patients and reported a 97% sensitivity of chest CT for the diagnosis of Covid-19 but said nothing about specificity (meaning that nearly all Covid-19 patients had abnormal CT scans, but the question as to how many of those with abnormal CT scans had Covid-19 was left unanswered.) The common features for CT findings in Covid-19 cases reported were similar to the papers discussed above. All cases were verified by PCR test which was often repeated until they got a positive test result. They even say:

> "when the viral load is insufficient, RT-PCR can be falsely negative while chest CT shows suggestive abnormalities. RT-PCR remains needed for final confirmation, but its positivity can be delayed, with the need to repeat the test if the CT features are suggestive."

They did not mention any symptoms related to DAD (diffuse alveolar damage), microvascular thrombosis (micro clotting) or alveolar haemorrhage.

In May 2020 Yin et al [758] also performed a comparison study of H1N1 influenza patients versus Covid-19 patients (30 patients in each cohort) and found the CT scan results to be similar, except that plural effusion was more evident in influenza patients. They also found that time from symptom onset to CT was much higher with Covid-19 patients. They did not mention any symptoms related to DAD (diffuse alveolar damage), microvascular thrombosis (micro clotting) or alveolar haemorrhage.

Sharif et al, 2020 [759], performed a systematic review, on papers from December 2019 until April 2020, and did a meta-analysis, reporting that:

> "COVID-19 cases had a higher risk of having ground glass opacities, but there was no significant difference between the presence of pleural effusion, positive CT findings, and bilateral involvement in two groups. However, non-COVID-19 patients showed an increased risk of having consolidation".

> "CT results in patients with COVID-19 were comparable with those of people having pneumonia from other causes".

They did not mention any symptoms related to DAD (diffuse alveolar damage), microvascular thrombosis (micro clotting) or alveolar haemorrhage.

In the BMJ, from July 2020, Cleverly et al [760] reported (in a study referring to chest X-rays rather than CTs) that:

> "Covid-19 pneumonia can be classed as an atypical pneumonia because of the radiographic appearances of multifocal ground glass opacity, linear opacities, and consolidation. These changes are also seen in other atypical pneumonias, including other coronavirus infections (severe acute respiratory system, SARS, and Middle East respiratory syndrome, MERS)."

> "No single feature on chest radiography is diagnostic of Covid-19 pneumonia".

Unlike many of the previous reviews Cleverly et al reported that evidence suggests a high prevalence of thrombotic complications in Covid-19 patients.

A Dutch study by Klak et al [761] from patients in April 2020 reported a 31% incidence of thrombotic complications in ICU patients with proven COVID-19 infections, which they say is remarkably high. The mean age of patients was 64 years old.

In April 2020 Revel et al [762], from the European Society of Radiology (ESR) and the European Society of Thoracic Imaging (ESTI), describe typical findings in CT scans for early diagnosis of Covid-19 (* means presence is disconformity and suggests other infectious disease of superinfection):

- "Presence of (bilateral, diffuse, confluent, patchy) ground glass opacities with /a rounded morphology/a crazy paving pattern/a peripheral distribution without subpleural sparing &
- Presence of ground-glass opacities admixed with perilobular consolidations /linear consolidation &
- Presence*/Absence of tree-in-bud pattern/centrilobular nodules/endobronchial secretion/lobar or segmental consolidation &
- Presence*/Absence of adenopathy/significant pleural effusion"
- However, they say findings of diffuse alveolar damage (DAD) are nonspecific.

The only paper we could find on CT and bacterial pneumonia was published in 2001 by Franquet [763], which reported that consolidation was indicative of community acquired bacterial pneumonia.

In 2020 Dhont et al [764] investigated the pathophysiology of 'happy' hypoxia in Covid-19, noting that it occurred in around 20% of hospitalised patients, but the condition was also observed in patients with atelectasis, intrapulmonary shunt (i.e. arterio-venous malformations) or right-to-left intracardiac shunt.

In 2020 Laredo et al [765] failed to find any strong evidence of happy hypoxia:

> "The RR/SpO2 relationship before oxygen administration does not differ between patients with COVID-19 and those without COVID-19, except in elderly patients."

As did Plummer at al [766] in 2022:

> "Patients with COVID-19 display a more symptomatic phenotype in response to hypoxaemia than those with other causes of hypoxaemic respiratory failure, however individual patients exhibit a wide range of responses. As such although asymptomatic hypoxaemia may be a phenomenon in any individual patient with hypoxaemic respiratory failure, it is no more frequently observed in those with SARS-CoV-2 infection than without."
>
> "Our results therefore refute the notion of COVID-19 infected patients being any more "happy" with hypoxaemia than non-COVID-19 patients"
>
> "The mechanism of severe hypoxaemia in COVID-19 … remains poorly understood".

In 2023 Lardet et al [767] looked at Extravascular lung water (EVLW) and Covid-19 and found no correlation between this condition and Covid-19 patients experiencing acute respiratory distress:

> "our main objective was to investigate the relationship between extravascular lung water (EVLW) and/or pulmonary vascular permeability index (PVPI) and respiratory mechanic variables in patients with COVID-19-induced ARDS.
>
> We found no clinically relevant correlations between EVLW and the respiratory mechanics variables.....driving pressure...., respiratory system compliance... or positive end-expiratory pressure. Similarly, there were no relevant correlations between PVPI and these same respiratory mechanics variables".

It is worth pointing out that some doctors sometimes refer to imaging characteristics (e.g. 'ground glass opacities') without specifying whether they are referring to findings from x-rays or CT scans. The Cleverly study above talks about GGOs, but in x-rays. Yet the majority of papers refer to CT scan findings. In most places, plain x-rays are in much more frequent use, CT scans for suspected pneumonia being used infrequently.

We do not know if GGOs found on x-ray have the same significance as those found on CT. There are few papers suggesting concordance between x-rays and CT yet generally speaking doctors talk as if there is. In a 2015 review Claessens et al [768] found that CT scanning changed the diagnosis made after x-ray alone in 58% of cases, concluding that:

> "In CAP-suspected (community-acquired pneumonia) patients visiting the emergency unit, early CT scan findings complementary to chest radiograph markedly affect both diagnosis and clinical management."

A 2008 review by Hayden and Wrenn [769] also found that CT scans 'found' considerably more cases of pneumonia than x-rays alone.

One is left wondering firstly whether faulty assumptions made about the concordance of findings between these two technologies may have been significant, secondly whether the increased use of CT scans in some places may have affected perceptions about the novelty of Covid-19 and thirdly whether this, like PCR testing, is a further example of the increased reliance on expensive technologies in lieu of clinical acumen.

Some evidence about CT is hard to fathom. In April 2020 Rubin et al [770] reported that:

> ".... CT screening of 82 asymptomatic individuals with confirmed COVID-19 from the cruise ship "Diamond Princess" showed findings of pneumonia in 54% (11)."

So here we have asymptomatic patients showing findings of pneumonia. This suggests a higher false positive rate than practitioners might assume given we might conclude many of these were perfectly well. It is also possible that the increasing number of CT scans resulted in higher numbers of patients suspected of having Covid-19.

20.1.4. Discussion of the evidence

All studies have limitations, especially observational studies. However, it is worth noting a few significant issues in the papers in our literature review:

Many of the academic papers written about diagnosing Covid-19 disease use a positive PCR test as the definitive diagnosis of SARS-COV-2 infection. In at least one study these tests were repeated until a positive was found.

There are no standard terminology, definitions, or causal descriptors in CT. This introduces the potential for interpretation bias and variability in interpretation.

In many of the papers potentially confirmatory biopsies were not taken from the lungs. For instance, in the Kory and Kane [771] paper, the authors say they never took tissue biopsies ante mortem, and that the majority of autopsies were carried out after patients had died post ventilation, hence represent the most severely ill patients:

> "Ultimately, the exact sequence of progression is currently unknown due to the lack of early, antemortem tissue biopsy in patients with COVID-19 along with the inherent bias that results from classifying COVID-19 lung injury only among those most severely affected given that the majority of autopsies were performed in patients after prolonged mechanical ventilation which unsurprisingly demonstrated DAD. Thus, in the early phases of the disease, the radiological findings and clinical assessment should be weighed more heavily in determining the type of lung injury occurring. The exact prevalence of OP or AFOP will ultimately be determined over time as the body of postmortem (and potentially antemortem) pathological studies accumulate."

Setting aside issues with terminology, gold standard verification of Covid-19 and the lack of biopsies we can summarise what we know about the ability of CT findings for Covid-19 and the extent to which they are genuinely diagnostic of this disease in isolation of other tests and indications. Most CT imaging descriptors appeared to be shared with influenza and bacterial pneumonia, as meta-analysis shows, and most papers acknowledge how difficult it is to differentiate one from the other from CT scans.

The only imaging descriptor that appeared to differentiate between Covid-19 and influenza was subpleural sparing, subpleural effusion (contra-indicating) and subpleural banding. Only Zarei et al [772] and Revel et al [773] reported these as features of Covid-19.

We also have little evidence to support differences in oxygen saturation between influenza and Covid-19 patient groups. Happy hypoxia is not identified in any of the papers reviewed, except for Kane and Kory. Likewise, there are no reported high incidences of diarrhoea in Covid-19 patients subject to CT scans.

Symptoms related to DAD (diffuse alveolar damage), microvascular thrombosis (micro clotting), alveolar haemorrhage are not consistently reported, with only the one Dutch study and the Kory paper both citing it as a specific finding related to Covid-19.

'Dry lung' was also reported but this does not appear to be confirmed by the one study that looked for evidence of it.

We conclude that CT cannot differentiate between any of the respiratory diseases, and in the absence of objective confirmation can only ever be suggestive. Furthermore, objective confirmation cannot be obtained by PCR test because of the inability of swabs to reliably collect and identify causative agents (as reported by the CDC EPIC study in two 2015 NEJM articles - one done on adults [773] and one on children [775]). Hence, a positive result gained from a sample taken from the upper throat or the nose does not mean an infection in the lung is caused by the detected pathogen. So, just because a patient is PCR positive, we cannot conclude it is Covid-19 and this conclusion should be reinforced by the fact that patients have been repeatedly retested, most times at high CT values, to establish positivity.

In June 2024 The Naked Emperor [776] reported on a 2018 paper published by Navascués et al [777] to investigate the feasibility of detecting influenza and other respiratory viruses in recently deceased persons and of estimating the prevalence of infections in persons who died within an influenza epidemic period. The authors wanted to see what viruses were in the bodies of over 65-year-olds who had died of natural causes, regardless of the reported cause of death. Only 7% of the patients had received a diagnosis of infection with the detected virus before death. 18% tested positive for influenza whilst only 5% had the virus detected before death. They found that 12% of the participants tested positive for a coronavirus whilst none of them had this diagnosis before death.

Clearly if one wished to 'spin-up' a deadly pandemic they could do so by simply increasing testing, declaring asymptomatic spread, and misattributing deaths to the virus du jour.

20.1.5. Credible alternative explanations

"How often have I said to you that when you have eliminated the impossible, whatever remains, however improbable, must be the truth?"

— Arthur Conan Doyle, The Sign of Four

The evidence presented here strongly suggests that none of the symptoms discussed are necessarily wholly and easily explainable by a single cause, that of a novel spikeopathy mechanism associated with an infection from SARS-CoV-2.

So, where does this leave us? We speculate that there are several non-mutually exclusive, potentially interacting, explanations. There seem to be two or more sets of observed disease manifestations, with distinct groups of symptoms seen in some patients caused by one or more different pathogens entirely, where:

- Many/most Covid-19 cases would have been 'ordinary' influenza and bacterial pneumonia cases.
- Some were not viruses or diseases at all but caused by toxicological events.
- Each of these were misattributed to Covid-19 either deliberately or through a process of human error.

In our view the first explanation is the most likely, for most cases, especially given there was a panic over Covid-19 which would have created an overwhelming psychological pressure leading to confirmation bias.

However, the second possibility, a toxicological cause, is worth considering despite the medical literature being largely blind to the possibility. Such an explanation would potentially explain the dry lung, happy hypoxia and diarrhoea as well as the rarer CT scan result - subpleural sparing. It might also explain the haemorrhagic and vascular events. This is worth discussing in a little more detail.

An interesting review paper by Chong et al [778] on subpleural sparing was published in 2021 which reviews a number of causes of this CT identifier, including nonspecific interstitial pneumonia (NSIP), organizing pneumonia (OP), pulmonary alveolar proteinosis (PAP), diffuse alveolar haemorrhage (DAH), vaping-associated lung injury (EVALI/VALI), cracked lung, pulmonary oedema, pneumocystis jirovecii pneumonia (PJP), pulmonary contusion, and more recently, Coronavirus disease 2019. And inhalational lung injury, associated with vaping and cracked lung.

The symptoms related to VALI (vaping associated lung injury) are consolidation with subpleural sparing seen in a very high percentage of cases, accompanied by dyspnoea, a non-productive cough (dry), fever and severe hypoxic respiratory failure requiring mechanical ventilation.

In March 2020 Layden et al [779] reported in the NEJM that:

> "In July 2019, the Wisconsin Department of Health Services and the Illinois Department of Public Health received reports of lung injury associated with the use of e-cigarettes (also called vaping) and launched a coordinated public health investigation......There were 98 case patients, 79% of whom were male; the median age of the patients was 21 years. The majority of patients presented with respiratory symptoms (97%), gastrointestinal symptoms (77%), and constitutional symptoms (100%). All case patients had bilateral infiltrates on chest imaging. A total of 95% of the patients were hospitalised, 26% underwent intubation and mechanical ventilation, and two deaths were reported. A total of 89% of the patients reported having used tetrahydrocannabinol products in e-cigarette devices, although a wide variety of products and devices was reported. Syndromic surveillance data from Illinois showed that the mean monthly rate of visits related to severe respiratory illness in June through August of 2019 was twice the rate that was observed in the same months in 2018."

Clearly many of the symptoms of VALI appear to be shared by a subset of Covid-19 patients, including GGO, and perhaps those in Spring 2020 more than others. Might it be possible that these 'Covid-19 events' were toxicological in nature and not caused by a viral or bacterial pathogen at all?

In an interview in the NEJM Christiani [780] points out that the ingredients in vapes are largely unknown and unregulated:

> "Since the industry has not been required by regulatory agencies to report all ingredients (nor their pyrolysis products), it would be imprudent to assume that patients with EVALI who report only nicotine vaping are underreporting THC use. Our default position as physicians is to believe our patients. The burden should be on the nicotine vaping companies to prove that their vaping fluids do not contain pulmonary toxicants capable of producing acute and chronic lung disorders. We need to heed the lesson from environmental public health regarding the precautionary principle that holds when a new product is developed that may have the potential for harm: it should be tested carefully for toxicity before being marketed widely."

Xantus [781] reports on the situation around VALI up to November 2019. This report identifies a new syndrome characterised by respiratory distress with bilateral (sometimes haemorrhagic):

> "Vast majority (98%) of the patients presented with respiratory symptoms; however, most (81%) had gastrointestinal (diarrhoea and vomiting) problems as well. Almost one-third progressed rapidly to respiratory distress needing intubation and mechanical (mostly positive pressure) ventilation. Imaging often revealed bilateral infiltration; however, the pathology was very diverse, varied from chemical pneumonitis (with one case of lipoid pneumonia) to certain degree of acute respiratory distress syndrome with bilateral infiltrates (sometimes haemorrhage)"

Specifically, it also mentions:

> "An investigation commissioned by National Broadcasting Company analysed 18 legal and illegal samples were analysed. The samples were analysed by CannaSafe Analytics LLC, the world first accredited cannabis laboratory. At least 10 samples had unacceptable level of pesticides and myclobutanil. Latter is a fungicide, which turns into the hydrogen cyanide and hydrogen chloride when heated: both compounds may result in lung damage if inhaled."

Rossana Segreto (a former DRASTIC [782] contributor) produced this paper [783] in 2022 comparing VALI and SARS-CoV-2, concluding that there is evidence to support the hypothesis that VALI cases were actually early manifestations of infections caused by early circulating SARS-COV-2. However, one commentator [784] noted that:

> "People with EVALI were presenting to the ED...chest x-ray and chest CT bore a striking resemblance to what was claimed to be CoV-2. They either get documented as 'suspected covid' or tested positive only a hypersensitive PCR. Boom! EVALI gets categorised as CoV-2."

As well as pesticides and fungicides illegal vapes have also included solvents which may have acted as effective super-warfarins leading to alveolar haemorrhage (and might show as DAD on CT).

Note that VALI patients are typically younger. Might this explain some of the young patients in New York and elsewhere – they were suffering from vaping lung injuries, and this was being misattributed to Covid-19? And the rest of the elderly patients may have been succumbing to untreated bacterial pneumonia?

Perhaps Segreto and frontline doctors got things the wrong way around? Perhaps VALI cases were being wrongly attributed to Covid-19, and physicians were mistakenly believing that the symptoms of VALI were symptoms of SARS-CoV-2 infection, also believing that since VALI occurred predominately in the young that Covid-19 was 'deadly' for the young as well as the elderly?

20.1.6. A more speculative hypothesis

Another more conspiratorial, hypothesis is that similar toxins to those found in illegal vapes or e-cigarettes might have been accidentally, or otherwise, spread as aerosols in crowds of people in enclosed spaces.

How might such toxicological events manifest themselves? A lot has been written about the transmission of SARS-COV-2 as an aerosol, such as this article written by Dr Pierre Kory in the USA Today [785]:

> "However, it has recently been determined that a major mode of transmission of SARS-CoV-2 is via aerosol droplets, exhaled by presymptomatic, asymptomatic or symptomatic persons. These small aerosol particles remain airborne indoors for extended periods and can infect those nearby who inhale them into their lungs."

The article argues for masks but in very special circumstances – in 'at risk environments':

> "The key point is that, for standard masks to be effective, there needs to be near universal wearing of these masks by all persons when in any poorly ventilated, air-recirculated, confined indoor, or highly congested outdoor environment."

These at-risk environments are 'indoors'. The article also goes onto describe super-spreader events at choir practice, in nightclubs, at karaoke, in ships and aircraft carriers and meat-packing plants. Although still extremely unlikely we cannot dismiss the possibility that super-spreader events in indoor spaces attributed to SARS-CoV-2 in 2020 were the result of a pathogen released to mimic a respiratory disease.

20.2. The debate – dissecting Dr Kory's response

16 January 2024

Dr Kory agreed to write a response to that article and has now done so here [786]. As there are no scientific papers cited to substantiate his assertions, we believe they cannot be corroborated.

In our article we covered a lot of papers on CT findings which challenged the presumption that you could find uniquely diagnostic CT findings for Covid-19. Kory responded with these statements:

> "Further, I would also then write "bacterial pneumonia is less favored given bilateral findings vs. unilateral, lack of consolidation on CT…..

> There was a pervasive "bilateral organizing pneumonia" on CT scan (OP is an uncommon finding in general and "organizing" patterns are quite differentiating amongst diseases…
>
> Often rapid progression to fibrosis on CT scans - this was novel to me, I had never seen such rapidly fibrosing lung findings on CT scans in ICU patients (again, not unique as there is a rare, rapidly fibrosing lung disease called AIP (acute interstitial pneumonia)"

Kory says there are unique signs of Covid-19 on CT. Yet, a few paragraphs later when addressing our conclusion that radiologic findings cannot reliably differentiate between Covid-19, influenza like illnesses, and bacterial pneumonia, he responds:

> "….despite the papers showing relatively equal incidences of various radiographic abnormalities overall - you are overlooking timing and stage of disease where radiography is a much better differentiator than those papers suggest)"

However, there is no substantiated evidence either that Kory cited or that we could find to support the belief that evidence of progression and timing of symptoms diagnostically discriminates for/against Covid-19. If this is such a strong diagnostic criterion then we should expect him and others to have been very careful to document it, 'in detail', in scientific papers, and for other medical scientists to confirm the findings.

Kory relies on his expertise in pattern recognition developed over many years:

> "….might be better explained as "intuition", it is almost an unconscious process when it occurs but I have been successfully relying on my pattern recognition skills to differentiate among causes of acute respiratory failure for 20 years."

It is difficult to understand how this can be reliably applied to a supposedly novel pathogen with a wickedly complex set of signs and symptom. Also, during the Spring 'outbreak' in NYC Kory had mere weeks to cut this Gordian knot.

Kory lists am overwhelming cacophony of what he believes are the indisputable signs and symptoms of spikeopathy. Again, he makes no attempt to compare what he 'sees' with those symptoms reported by other physicians in the academic medical literature.

Kory favours personal anecdotes to support the claim that Covid-19 can be reliably diagnosed, such as the following:

> "like my oldest and best friend who simply got nauseous, started projectile vomiting, went to hospital and was eventually diagnosed with adult-onset multi-system inflammatory syndrome related to Covid (note he was Covid positive on admission). But know that he never had a preceding upper respiratory symptom however all the other findings were consistent with the new rarer syndrome of MISC-A.. So, atypical presentation, but his eventual A-MISC syndrome has criteria for diagnosis and he met all of them" [*Note from this we don't not know whether the friend was tested for any other pathogen!]*

> "One other troublingly unique aspect was that in the first wave in NY, doctors and nurses were dying on the front lines. One of the first to die was an absolute giant of my specialty, he died in Seattle right after their first influx of patients. I have NEVER lost a colleague to the same disease we were treating.. ever. And I knew of at least 3 who died in the first wave of Covid. And that's just me."

Kory reports healthcare workers were dying on the frontlines. We assume he means they experienced symptoms and complications of some kind and died within days or weeks, not that colleagues were falling down dead in hospitals. There were several media reports about doctors, nurses, other hospital staff, and EMTs being killed by Covid during the New York death event. That the nature and intensity of these stories was not replicated elsewhere or after spring 2020, as far as we know, is strongly suggestive that whatever is responsible for those deaths is not likely to be a flu-like illness.

Also, cases which are atypical of Covid-19 are still typical of Covid-19:

> "I have also seen, on few occasions, other presentations that were atypical, i.e. more GI predominant than respiratory but the response to treatment was the same."

Despite us pointing out that the myriad of Covid-19 studies that did not report happy hypoxia, Kory defaults to his unique expertise:

> "Often presenting with "happy hypoxia" which is a clinical (i.e. observational) diagnosis not a defined mathematical one. In my career diagnosing and treating causes of acute respiratory failure/hypoxia, most patients with severe hypoxia evidence visibly obvious increased work of breathing"

Kory reports on 'blood issues':

> "Lots of deep venous thromboses and pulmonary emboli on admission or soon after admission."

We found little evidence of this reported in other papers; again, Kory's report is based on personal evidence. He cites one of his own papers [787] covering the symptoms from ten patients. However, his paper starts with the conclusion that Covid-19 was the culprit, based on a positive PCR test result. Since no results from tests for other pathogens were reported the paper is of little value in this debate.

Kory also refers to factors related to transmission, none of which appear in any of his papers or in any other academic papers. For example:

> "illness beginning after a holiday party where a number of others also subsequently fell ill,..."

> "obvious contagiousness as per history etc..."

> "High transmissibility with clear evidence of aerosol spread - I have never seen a disease which spread so rapidly and widely, with numerous super-spreader events, well described in the media and the CDC."

> "The contagiousness within families and after group events despite social distancing and masks were consistent and reproducible (even my own household saw such spreads, multiple times)"

In our view, such statements are speculation. If we have a novel disease and risk-additive pathogen, suspicions about its transmissibility should be carefully documented and subject to scientific scrutiny rather than rely on personal experience of life at home. Instead, they are taken as givens. How would we know it wasn't another respiratory ILI (influenza like illness)?

Note that, while Kory and other frontline physicians can diagnose Covid-19, we are cautioned to be aware that there are different evolving levels of severity of Covid-19:

> "In terms of how deadly it was, this also gets complicated because the disease changed over the past few years."

Despite this temporal change in what Covid-19 symptoms are, Kory claims :

> "the "pattern" of presentation of Covid was unique and easily discernible and distinct from other viral syndromes to a seasoned clinician."

These statements seem contradictory. Kory tells us why it was not bacterial pneumonia:

> "Why was it not bacterial pneumonia? Well, from the features above, bacterial pneumonias are not associated with OP, are generally unilateral (the vast majority of Covid was bilateral), most often consolidative rather than with ground glass."

Yet, we documented substantial evidence from many scientific papers that completely contradict his statement.

On bacterial pneumonia he says:

> "….bacterial pneumonias are random, relatively rare events in most people's lives, and instead mostly tend to affect the elderly"

We reject this assertion because it is well known that bacterial pneumonias are not random and are common in the elderly, the very cohort most affected by Covid-19.

Kory also rejects bacterial pneumonia because:

> "Also, outside of TB, bacterial pneumonias do not exhibit human to human transmission so cannot explain all the transmission and dying unless someone was to argue that widespread immunosuppression developed making most of the population uniquely susceptible to bacterial pneumonia in their environment all of a sudden."

It is unclear how he would reliably know about transmission at the point of diagnosis. It can merely be presumptive. We, and others, have covered explanations for this in the form of community-acquired bacterial pneumonia, caused by antibiotics being withdrawn, and the elevated rate of ventilator-associated pneumonias in vented patients misdiagnosed as Covid-19. We made no arguments about widespread spontaneous immunosuppression in our article.

Turning to the young and healthy he says:

> "In the young and healthy, they are very rare events. I had too many young and healthy (relatively) on vents suddenly - why/how would a bacterial pneumonia suddenly do this unless it was a new superbug"

We did not argue that young healthy people were presenting with bacterial pneumonia. We argued that the young and healthy people whose symptoms best matched those that Kory thinks are uniquely diagnostic of Covid-19 are consistent with those reported for younger people who have been injured by illicit vapes (containing fungicides and pesticides *inter alia*). Yet, despite this close match, Kory says this about vapes:

> "Vaping can be ruled out by history-taking. The vast majority of patients were not vapers. Smokers and vapers make up less than 20% of the population. This syndrome spared no segment of the population, and I am unaware of data showing a massive increase in the sales of vapes at that time."

This is a misrepresentation of our argument. We presented numerous papers supporting the possibility that vaping-associated lung injury (VALI) and Covid-19 have coincident pathology, as reported by Kory himself.

By way of a conclusion, Kory says that there is new mystery virus whose transmission characteristics are unknown, and which is sometimes deadly in one place but sometimes not in others:

> "….there are still things we don't know about how and why the virus spread the way it did and why it behaved so deadly in some spots at certain times and not others. One possible clue might be this paper finding that all variants were created in a lab."

Despite this almost unbounded level of complexity and variety it seems implausible that Kory and others, can reliably diagnose "it".

In finishing his article Kory says:

> "That's all I got. I am not sure if I "squared the circle" in terms of making coherent sense of all the data and viewpoints and I think that is because there are still things we don't know about how and why the virus spread the way it did and why it behaved so deadly in some spots at certain times and not others. One possible clue might be this paper finding that all? variants were created in a lab. Their concluding sentence: "The analysis showed that Omicron variants were formed by an entirely new mechanism that cannot be explained by previous biology and knowing how the SARS-CoV-2 variants were formed prompts a reconsideration of the SARS-CoV-2 pandemic."

This suggests Kory had a strong prior presumptive belief that a novel deadly pathogen was circulating (a bioweapon?) and that a positive test for this pathogen confirmed this as a fact, and it was this sole explanation, to the exclusion of all others, that accounted for the symptoms experienced by patients in his care. We believe confirmation bias of this kind was not restricted to Kory and was shared throughout the medical profession.

20.3. Differential diagnosis

Kory makes clear that diagnosis of complex diseases is notoriously difficult. We agree. There are well established methods for performing diagnoses that provide a framework to minimise errors in diagnosis and to, conversely, maximise the likelihood that the diagnosis made is the correct one. These methods are routinely taught to doctors at all levels. One such method is called differential diagnosis, which involves a process of elimination.

The Cleveland clinic defines differential diagnosis [788] this way:

> "Your healthcare provider will compile a differential diagnosis, which is a list of conditions that share the same symptoms to help make a final diagnosis. The differential diagnosis will direct your healthcare provider to offer tests to rule out conditions and lead them to find the cause of your symptoms.
>
> ......they will begin a process to diagnose your condition. Since there are a lot of different conditions that often share similar symptoms, your provider will create a differential diagnosis, which is a list of possible conditions that could cause your symptoms. A differential diagnosis is not your official diagnosis, but a step before determining what could cause your symptoms."

The character called 'House' in the very popular TV medical drama of the same name applies this method:

> "House often clashes with his fellow physicians, including his own diagnostic team, because many of his hypotheses about patients' illnesses are based on subtle or controversial insights."

As a drama it is written to entertain but it is based on what a doctor actually (should) do. Clearly a doctor should rule out the simplest or most common explanations before considering the most novel or complex. Hence, Covid-19 should have been considered at the end of the diagnostic process, after already well understood conditions had been eliminated, and not at the start.

Despite being portrayed as a real-life Dr House [789], based on his response to us Kory may not have followed this method. He does not refer to a list of possible alternative or competing diagnoses. Likewise, Kory does not show how these have been 'whittled down' using differential diagnosis. As a result, the competing conditions, that by necessity, must be considered during the process of arriving at a conclusive diagnosis are completely hidden from view: what we see is the conclusion only.

Unfortunately, this flaw is repeated in virtually all of the papers reporting symptoms of Covid-19 and shows how vulnerable medicine is to epistemic capture.

This paper [790], by Fryman and Mayo in 2020 is a very nice illustration of the problem of associating observed symptoms with a positive covid test and neatly sums up how the actual cause of symptoms might be obscured by the test result or the intervention.

The case is summarised thus:

> "A 52-year-old man sought treatment for nonproductive cough, fever, and worsening shortness of breath. On admission, he was in respiratory distress with oxygen saturation at 73% on room air. The patient was admitted with coronavirus disease 2019 (COVID-19) pneumonia, which was confirmed by PCR antigen testing. Four days after admission, the patient required endotracheal intubation for progressive hypoxemic and hypercapneic respiratory failure.
>
> On day 10 of medical ICU (MICU) care, the patient developed right anterior chest wall and neck subcutaneous emphysema with severe oxygen desaturation and hypotension requiring escalating doses of vasopressors. Concurrent with these events, the patient developed severe abdominal distention with a bladder pressure of 25 mm Hg.
>
> The abdominal ultrasound findings are consistent with the presence of a large pneumoperitoneum (free air). The absence of gut sliding and the inability to visualize any underlying structures within the abdomen suggest that free air is interposed between the ultrasound probe and the peritoneal space. Given the patient's shock state, elevation of plateau pressure, and intraabdominal hypertension, the MICU team established a diagnosis of abdominal compartment syndrome. This was managed by insertion of an ultrasound-guided catheter into the air-filled peritoneal space."

We asked an independent radiologist for their view of this case, and they said:

> "before 2020, this is a person that had ARDS and suffered a complication of too forceful/prolonged intubation."

Chapter 21. From horror fiction to cross reactivity in PCR testing

21.1. A New Years Eve Horror Story

31 December 2023

Things were getting depressing, so we published some 'light-hearted' fiction....

Imagine a fake pandemic sweeps the globe, perceived to be threatening enough to persuade almost everyone to get vaccinated but which spawns an effective antivaxx rebel movement, but who themselves don't realise the pandemic was faked. The leaders of the antivaxx rebel movement are themselves so convinced of the virus threat that they also get vaccinated despite all of their followers remaining unvaxxed.

Imagine the antivaxx rebel movement persists in maintaining the fiction there was a pandemic and that a new pandemic is just around the corner and that any lone wolf can create a deadly novel virus, in their garage, and this will cause the next 'big one'.

Imagine the vaccine developed to fight this pandemic transpires to be so dangerous it effectively destroys your immune system, causing you to become progressively more vulnerable to any and all infections no matter the source: man-made or natural.

Imagine this dysfunction is inheritable.

Imagine your government admitting that you had indeed been injected with this vaccine. They say it was a terrible mistake. They claim it was done with the best of intentions. To protect you. But it went wrong. They tried their best.

Imagine such a government being overthrown by the vaccinated and unvaccinated alike in a grand coalition.

The rebels take control. But they have a problem....

Imagine what the population will demand of this new rebel government.

Protection. Safety. From vaccines and viruses.

The people and the rebel leaders are terrified by the perpetual, deadly threat from any and every virus, man-made or natural. The vaccinated are vulnerable. Their offspring are vulnerable. They are vaxxed and their descendants will be indirectly vaxxed.

Imagine what such protection would look like in this new hyper-vulnerable world?

Safe cities sealed off from potentially infectious nature. Safe spaces separated from other infectious humans. Safe food supplies untainted by animal viruses. Biosecurity and digital ID everywhere and always. Implants to monitor your health and alert the authorities if you are infected. Eugenics to breed out the genetic changes caused by the vaccine. Euthanasia to eliminate the sickest who cannot be saved.

A New World Order.

But the irony is that it would be one ushered in by the rebels themselves.

The twist in the tale......

Imagine however that the vaccine, whilst being dangerous, does not actually cause the immune dysfunction to the extent claimed. And it isn't inheritable.

That narrative is also faked. And used to fool everyone that they are vulnerable.

A double bluff. First, bluff with the virus. Then, bluff with the vaccine.

21.2. Unacceptably high cross reactivity in PCR testing

Does it mean there was no pandemic? (23 February 2024)

The full version of this article with relevant screenshots is here [791].

Arguments that there was a genuine pandemic caused by the novel SARS-CoV-2 viral pathogen have largely relied on data from PCR testing used for diagnosis and transmission surveillance. Without PCR testing data, published official statistics about infection, hospitalisation, and death rates would not be reliably attributable to the novel virus. However, if this attribution is doubtful, partial or false we need to look to other explanations for the pandemic.

There has been a recent resurgence in interest in the role of PCR testing in establishing whether or not a pandemic can truly be said to have occurred. A prominent expert in PCR testing Kevin McKernan [792], has argued that PCR testing validated people's covid morbidity experiences (they got ill) and given this they would never be dissuaded from the belief there was a pandemic – and it was counterproductive to try to do so. Likewise, the online mouse character JikkyLeaks has stated that the PCR tests were 'not all fake' [793] (but makes the unfortunate conflation that any belief that they are fake must come with a belief that 'viruses don't exist', despite these not being logically conjoint propositions).

Much of our discussion so far on PCR testing for SARS-CoV has been statistical, but we have also uncovered scandals about 'asymptomatic covid' and the use of single gene testing. These articles and others relating to PCR testing can all be found here [794].

However, apart from one article about the 'smoking man' emails [795] we have not dug too deeply into the triggers and causes of false positives and asked: how might these false positives occur? Discussing this issue might appear like we are trawling over old coals, but it is crucial in addressing the question as to whether there was indeed a novel virus, whether PCR testing was honestly detecting it and whether there was a genuine pandemic.

While there are many possible causes of false positives, such as operational reliability and cross contamination within labs, the lack of standardised testing etc, here we will focus on one central aspect of PCR testing which has been given scant attention: cross reactivity.

Cross reactivity or (crosstalk) occurs when other viruses, such as those causing common colds, flu or flu-like illnesses etc. might trigger a positive PCR result for SARS-CoV-2. The extent to which cross reactivity was occurring is fundamental to the performance of the PCR test, but no one really talks about it.

The notion of cross reactivity is fundamental to the performance of the PCR test, as is identifying the ways in which PCR might fail. We can segregate many categories of false positive but the two categories we are going to examine here are:

- False positives in the *absence* of competing pathogens *FPR-Absence* : This is where the SARS-CoV-2 virus is known to be absent, but the test result is positive indicating its presence, despite the fact all other competing viruses or bacterial pathogens are also known to be absent in the sample. Typically, the substance being tested might be water, serum, or human lysate.

- False positives in the *presence* of competing pathogens *FPR-Presence*: This is where the SARS-CoV-2 virus is known to be absent from the sample, but the test result is positive for its presence, but where one or more competing viruses or bacterial pathogens are known to be present in the sample. Normally only one pathogen is presumed present, and the pathogens are normally competing causes of ILI (influenza like illnesses), such as other coronaviruses.

Here we are interested in observational experiments where laboratory tests are conducted using blind samples in idealised conditions, where the substance being tested is supposedly not known to the laboratory undertaking the testing (aka 'mystery shopper' tests).

At this point it is worth reminding readers that in relation to the discussion which follows about "false positive rates" (FPRs), quite small apparent FPRs (say 5%, which might mistakenly be regarded as acceptable) during a period when viral prevalence is low (say, 1%) are not simply a minor aberration. For statistical reasons, as we have explained elsewhere, such a scenario would mean that in practice nearly all the positive results obtained would be false positives.

21.2.1. Cross reactivity studies

The notorious Eurosurveillance paper by Corman and Drosten et al [796], published in January 2020 was supposed to determine whether their PCR could detect the '2019 novel coronavirus' and also assessed its specificity by measuring the rate of cross reaction when exposed to other coronaviruses, including HCoVs 229E, NL63, OC43, HKU1 and MERS-CoV. Identification of the novel 2019 novel coronavirus was based on testing for the E and RdRp gene assays. Their results were:

> "Using the E and RdRp gene assays, we tested a total of 297 clinical samples from patients with respiratory disease from the biobanks of five laboratories that provide diagnostic services (one in Germany, two in the Netherlands, one in Hong Kong, one in the UK). We selected 198 samples from three university medical centres where patients from general and intensive care wards as well as mainly paediatric outpatient departments are seen (Germany, the Netherlands, Hong Kong). The remaining samples were contributed by national public health services performing surveillance studies (RIVM, PHE), with samples mainly submitted by practitioners. The samples contained the broadest range of respiratory agents possible and

> reflected the general spectrum of virus concentrations encountered in diagnostic laboratories in these countries (Table 2). In total, this testing yielded no false positive outcomes. In four individual test reactions, weak initial reactivity was seen but they were negative upon retesting with the same assay."

Note that they claim 100% accuracy and zero cross reactivity.

However, in four individual test reactions "weak initial reactivity was seen". These were re-tested and found to be negative. They revealed their contorted reasoning by stating that:

> "These signals were not associated with any particular virus, and for each virus with which initial positive reactivity occurred, there were other samples that contained the same virus at a higher concentration but did not test positive."

Just retesting the samples which showed initial reactivity is a scientifically and statistically illiterate approach, constituting extreme selection bias; they have not ruled out whether some samples, which showed no initial reactivity, would have shown some cross reactivity had they also retested them. So, in practical terms this means there were four false positives.

In April/May 2020 Drosten was involved in another validation trial reported in Matheeussen et al [797] involving hundreds of participating laboratories worldwide and hundreds of tests. Rather than 100% accuracy they reported the following cross reactivity rates:

- FPR-Absence – 2.7%
- FPR-Presence (HCoV-NL63) – 3.1%
- FPR-Presence (HCoV-OC43) – 2.9%

Compared to the Eurosurveillance paper this paper may be considered to reflect more realistic rates of cross reaction.

The 'smoking man' emails [795] revealed statistics from the Instand report [798] suggesting a false positive (cross reactive) rate of 9.34% (calculated by simply totalling frequencies of false positives for single genes), given the primers used (E gene, N gene and ORF1ab), using samples of HCoV-OC43, HCoV-229E and human lysate tested in laboratories worldwide. A statistical analysis of the cross-reactivity rates, assuming any two from three genes must be positive for a PCR positive, and assuming statistical independence, yields numbers significantly less than 9.34%:

- FPR-Absence – 0.07%
- FPR-Presence (HCoV-229E) – 2.9 %
- FPR-Presence (HCoV-OC43) – 0.3%

Note that in both 'Drosten studies' the cycle thresholds used to detect competing pathogens were not revealed.

In the UK, single gene testing was used extensively to generate high positivity rates, as reported here [799]. If we consider the false positive rates for the Instand report and 'relax' the overall PCR positive criteria to one gene from three (E gene, N gene and ORF1ab), instead of two from three (in breach of WHO guidelines), we get significantly higher results for cross reactivity (again assuming the gene variables are statistically independent):

- FPR-Absence – 3.4%
- FPR-Presence (HCoV-229E) – 22.9 %
- FPR-Presence (HCoV-OC43) – 9.7%

Hence, based on this data we might be able to safely assume that there is evidence to support the contention there was a wave of false positive covid tests in the UK in winter 2020/21, likely partly caused by common colds (and in the UK these should have been officially recognised as false positives).

21.2.2. Australian PCR cross reactivity study

In correspondence from March 2023 Kevin McKernan discussed the smoking man emails (one name redacted):

> **Martin**: Hi Kevin, back to this old chestnut again! I published this the other day on our Substack and I'm wondering if you had seen it and what your thoughts are. Non-specific and cross-reactive PCR testing was known to be a thing right from the start Drosten even told us so. Am I getting this wrong? What do you think of "The Cleric's" email from 2020?
>
> **Kevin**: Good read. I posted it the other day. Hard to track what they actually did as there was so much PCR kit heterogeneity out there, but this is evident in the ring testing in Australia CT. Late cross talk in other viruses. Tran et al [800].
>
> **Martin**: Shows specificity in non-reference lab of 93.8% and I guess this is in somewhat idealised operational conditions. Yes? And these are below CT thresholds.
>
> **Kevin**: And Australia is used as the model for why they are perfect as they had a long stretch of 1:10 K positivity off season. XXXX won't answer question about the FP rate once 10% of the samples are true positive on season. Cross contamination goes up geometrically during on season very dishonest PCR schill.

The report Kevin is referring to is written by the Doherty institute in Australia by Tran et al. They tested the use of the Beijing Genomics Institute (BGI) PCR test at three laboratories in June 2020 looking to determine cross reactivity and found that the first laboratory was 100% specific with zero cross reactions found (no surprises here - it was the Doherty Institute laboratory). The two other laboratories had specificities reported as 99.1% and 97.5% respectively (and a cross reactivity of 0.9% and 2.5% respectively), as shown in Figure 70.

These numbers look reassuring small until you consider that of the 115 'negative' samples only 24 contained competing viruses: HCoV-OC43, RSV, Rhinovirus, Parainfluenza etc. These were presented for test mixed with either human saliva or VTM (virus transport media). The other 91 samples were inactivated cell-culture-grown SARS-CoV-2 (not water, serum or human lysate).

Table 4. Summary of specificity of each laboratory testing platform for the detection of SARS-CoV-2 (n=115).

	Laboratory 1[a]	Laboratory 2[b]	Laboratory 3[c]
False positives	0/115	1/115	3/115
Specificity	100%	99.1%	97.5%

[a] Doherty Institute. [b] Laboratory 2. [c] Laboratory 3.
Specificity rate was calculated from the number of negative detections divided by the 115 total true negative sample size.

Figure 70 Specificity of each laboratory testing specificity of SARS-CoV-2

Notice that the total number of samples was 115 across the three laboratories, so to compute FPR-Presence we need to use a denominator of 24 and for FPR-Absence we should use 91. The choice of denominator is therefore crucial in reporting the false positive rate and by including many non-pathogenic samples in the test suite the combined false positive rate can be suppressed. Hence, when we consider the FPR-Presence rate from laboratory 2 and divide by 24, rather than 115, we get FPR-Presence rate of 8%. For laboratory 3 the FPR-Presence rate is the same – 2 false positives from 24 samples also resulting in 8%. These are much higher values than that reported.

Furthermore, four samples from laboratory three were discounted because they breached cycle threshold cutoffs, that only applied to these tests. Here is the extract from the report describing this:

> "All samples were negative for SARS-CoV-2 by Laboratory 1. For Laboratory 2, sample 253 (influenza virus A in saliva matrix) and sample 260 (coronavirus-229E in saliva matrix), were excluded from analysis after returning invalid results (internal reference target Ct > 32 or not detected). The remaining 22 samples were negative for SARS-CoV-2 by Laboratory 2. For Laboratory 3, sample 259 (coronavirus-OC43 in saliva matrix) and sample 260 (coronavirus 229E in saliva matrix) were excluded from analysis due to their internal reference target having a Ct>32. The remaining 22 samples were negative for SARS-CoV-2 by Laboratory 3. Of note were 4 samples from laboratory 3: sample 236 (parainfluenza type-1 in saliva matrix), sample 246 (adenovirus type-5 in saliva matrix, sample 181 (rhinovirus in VTM matrix) and sample 191 (influenza virus A in VTM matrix) that generated a Ct value above 38 for SARS-CoV-2. These were interpreted as not SARS-CoV-2 positive as per manufacturer's IFU."

From the test report we have no idea what an internal reference control target is but, taken at face value, it presents itself as a convenient way to re-categorise false positives as true negatives, and thus improve test performance by subterfuge. When these discounted false positives are included the FPR-Presence, for laboratory 2, rises to 6 false positives from 24 samples – a whopping 25%.

This discounting of false positive samples with high CT values is not matched in the sensitivity analysis branch of the study where SARS-CoV-2 positives were found at CT values as high as 44. These were judged to be false negatives for SARS-CoV-2 because they had CT values > 38, but were subject to confirmatory retesting, whereas false positives were not subject to this retesting.

Kevin McKernan is therefore correct to point out that there was clear crosstalk between competing viruses and the SARS-CoV-2 PCR test at high CT levels. This Tran et al study is by far the most detailed and revealing of the surprisingly small number of public studies done into false positivity. It reveals systematic bias in the choice of denominators, leading to hugely inflated specificity rates for the PCR test evaluated, shows how cycle thresholds can be manipulated to reject inconvenient results and how confirmatory retesting might be preferentially done to unfairly boost performance.

McKernan also said:

> "And Australia is used as the model for why they are perfect as they had a long stretch of 1:10K positivity off season."

Given that respiratory viruses are seasonal pathogens this statement is very revealing. Our analysis clearly shows that the absence of false positives 'off season', in summer, proves little to nothing about cross reactivity, because competing respiratory pathogens will be largely absent and hence overall PCR specificity can be made to 'look good', with a false positive rate close to zero, by simply conducting PCR testing on people uninfected by any virus in summer (in the UK confirmatory testing was only performed was when very few people were ill and few were being tested). Of course, this situation is not equivalent to 'in season' testing when competing pathogens are all in circulation.

21.2.3. Limits to diagnosability and the myth of vanishing flu

The effect of the cross reactive false positive rate on any estimation of the prevalence rate for SARS-CoV-2 is highly significant. Let's take some of the statistics we have discovered thus far and look at the probability that someone is infected with SARS-CoV-2 given a positive PCR test result.

First, for example, we assume SARS-CoV-2 is circulating in 1% of the population and all other competing respiratory viruses are circulating at a combined 10% rate: hence 89% of people are virus free. We can use Bayes Theorem to calculate the chance of someone being infected with SARS-CoV-2 when they have a positive PCR test. Let's further assume a high sensitivity for the PCR test, 99%, with an FPR-Presence of 25% (as per Instand report), and FPR-Absence of 0.07% (as per Tran et al study) so those with a competing ILI will have a 25% chance of showing a false positive and 0.07% of people uninfected, with either, will also show a false positive (this balances the propensity of testing to generate cross reactive false positives on season and off). Using Bayes' the calculated result is only a 28% chance that the person tested actually has SARS-CoV-2. Note that these calculations ignore symptoms and do so because the studies we cite are based solely on samples and not people, hence even with positive tests people might be asymptomatic or post symptomatic or might never develop a reaction to the virus.

In this example a SARS-CoV-2 PCR positive test result might only be considered 'reasonably' diagnostic in the most favourable circumstances where, if and only if, we assume competing ILIs have almost completely disappeared. For example, if we flip the prevalence of ILIs with SARS-CoV-2 where competing respiratory viruses are circulating at a combined rate of 1% and SARS-CoV-2 is circulating with a prevalence rate of 10% then, again using Bayes' the calculated result would be a 97% chance that the person tested has SARS-CoV-2.

In Bayesian terms, to be near certain in the diagnosis of SARS-CoV-2 infection you would have to hold the prior belief that ILIs had all but vanished and that SARS-CoV-2 was exclusively dominant. However, we have argued elsewhere [802] that there is no reason to believe that, caused by the supposed circulation of SARS-CoV-2, other competing ILIs simply disappeared during 2020 and 2021.

The reported global downward trend in competing bacterial and viral infections during spring 2020 is exemplified by a chart, published by the BioFire syndromic trends reporting system, showing the percentage detection rate of pathogens in the USA from 2019 through to 2021. We have argued here that the proposed hypothesis of viral interference between SARS-CoV-2 and influenza or other viruses to explain why these competing viruses simply disappeared only to reappear a few years later is just not credible, with changes in testing being a much more likely explanation.

Finally, in the absence of an available and deployed gold standard, these arguments are circular because the supposed downward trend in the prevalence of competing ILIs are themselves dependent on the same PCR testing technology. If this technology is deployed in a systematically biased way the results will be misleading. One example of this is the startling revelation, by RemnantMD [803], that for one popular PCR multiplex test [804] which claimed to be able to differentiate between influenza A/B and SARS-CoV-2, a negative SARS-CoV-2 result means then any accompanying negative tests for influenza should be considered presumptive. This was explained in their documentation.

So, if a sample that is tested is positive for SARS-CoV-2, it is assumed to be negative for Influenza.

The reader should note that there are related important issues [805] that would also suppress the signal from influenza such as the timing and availability of influenza testing, the role of quarantines and confirmation biased baked into the influenzas testing protocol.

21.2.4. 100 percent false positive rates and contamination

In 2020 Etievant et al [806] published a paper analysing the performance of WHO referral laboratories in testing PCR assays for SARS-CoV-2. The laboratories evaluated included Charité (Germany), HKU (Hong Kong), China CDC (China), US CDC (United States), and Institut Pasteur, Paris (France). These assays included several PCRs targeting two or three different SARS-CoV-2 gene regions, including RdRp, N (nucleocapsid protein), E (envelope protein), ORF1ab nsp10, and ORF1b nsp14.

They performed specificity testing for other respiratory viruses: human coronaviruses 229E, OC43, HKU1, and NL63, human influenza A and B viruses, rhinovirus, respiratory syncytial virus, parainfluenza virus, adenovirus, metapneumovirus, and picornavirus.

No false-positive results were obtained on clinical samples that tested negative for SARS-CoV-2 and/or positive for other viruses than SARS-CoV-2, except for gene E Charité and gene N2 for the US CDC, which were positive for ***all*** specimens and replicates, including negative samples and controls (including water).

And note that these are false positives from (supposedly) the best laboratories in the world!

It is puzzling that he authors of the paper explained away the results as caused by 'contamination' without evidence nor justification.

Note that at the time these tests were rolling-out a number of stories broke about contamination, including this article by Mögling et al [807] from August 2020. They report that ten laboratories from 8 countries in Europe reported PCR template contamination in commercially ordered primer and probe batches, which led to SARS-CoV-2 PCR signals in their no-template controls and provided detailed information. Five additional laboratories (including the addition of a ninth affected country) indicated that they received contaminated material but did not provide details. The contamination issues concerned primer and probe batches for the E and the RNA-dependent RNA polymerase gene targets, as well as batches for nonrelated targets. The authors note that the massive laboratory response in early 2020, with few established protocols, would have had 'consequences' but fail to spell out what these were.

21.2.5. Drosten's warning

In a podcast interview [809] on March 18 2020 Christian Drosten, head of virology at Berlin Charité, discussed the risk to the population of SARS-CoV-2, concluding that it was currently high. He also said (in translation):

> "Well, this new coronavirus is now coming to us as a pandemic. That means there will be a wave of infections if we don't do anything. **And this wave of infection is the simultaneous occurrence of many coronavirus infections.** And even if these coronavirus infections with the new coronavirus were just as harmless as those with the four well-known human coronaviruses, that would be worrying."

This is an oddly contradictory thing to say, is it not? He is explicitly saying that the 2020 Spring wave is, in aggregate, a simultaneous combination of infection caused by many coronaviruses, and not just SARS-CoV-2 alone. Yet only supposed infections caused by SARS-CoV-2 were being monitored and reported, as if all other coronaviruses had disappeared from circulation. He also admits that even if SARS-CoV-2 was not risk-additive then it would still be worrying, despite the risk level being set at 'high'.

To our minds this statement is tantamount to an admission that what is being tested for and reported as Covid-19 is the presence of many seasonal viruses, including coronaviruses, and not solely SARS-CoV-2. The evidence on cross-reactivity of PCR testing supports this conclusion and no other.

21.2.6. Historical precedents

The problem of false positives is not local to SARS-CoV-2. This study [808] from 2015 on the use of PCR for HCoV-MERS reveals that over 8% of laboratories produced false positive results where there was a cross reaction against HCoV-NL63, HCoV-229E and HCoV-HKU1.

This study [810] from 2003 reported that care home residents and staff with respiratory infections tested positive for SARS-CoV yet subsequent testing showed that they had been infected by HCoV-OC43. Eight residents died, six of pneumonia. They reported that the SARS-CoV PCR test had cross-reacted with the N protein from OC43.

Finally, there is the famous case from 2006 where a whooping cough outbreak spread through the Dartmouth-Hitchcock Medical Center 'like wildfire'. The New York Times [811] reported that:

> "Not a single case of whooping cough was confirmed with the definitive test, growing the bacterium, Bordetella pertussis, in the laboratory. Instead, it appears the health care workers probably were afflicted with ordinary respiratory diseases like the common cold.
>
> … specialists say the problem was that they placed too much faith in a quick and highly sensitive molecular test that led them astray … At Dartmouth the decision was to use a test, P.C.R., for polymerase chain reaction … their sensitivity makes false positives likely, and when hundreds or thousands of people are tested, as occurred at Dartmouth, false positives can make it seem like there is an epidemic.
>
> There are no national data on pseudo-epidemics caused by an overreliance on such molecular tests, said Dr. Trish M. Perl … but, she said, pseudo-epidemics happen all the time. The Dartmouth case may have been one the largest, but it was by no means an exception, she said. There was a similar whooping cough scare at Children's Hospital in Boston last fall that involved 36 adults and 2 children. Definitive tests, though, did not find pertussis.
>
> "Because we had cases we thought were pertussis and because we had vulnerable patients at the hospital, we lowered our threshold," she said.
>
> "If we had stopped there, I think we all would have agreed that we had had an outbreak of whooping cough and that we had controlled it," Dr. Kirkland said.
>
> "It's a problem; we know it's a problem," Dr. Perl said. "My guess is that what happened at Dartmouth is going to become more common."

21.2.7. Discussion

We analysed the very few studies that used blind colds or flu samples to undertake 'mystery shopper' testing. In these studies, we found strong evidence for cross reactivity between other competing viruses and the PCR tests sampled, rising to up to 25% for other circulating pathogens. In fact, 25% might be considered a gross underestimate given that German and US laboratories were reported as 100% false positive for a wide number of common viruses, based on single gene tests (E-gene and N-gene). We also found that there was strong evidence of contamination of primers and probes giving rise to false positives independent of the sample under test!

We identified many systematic weaknesses in these studies, finding that numerous implicit tricks had been used to supress evidence of cross reactivity, thus misleading the public into believing PCR tests are reliable. We found that the only circumstance in which a positive PCR test for SARS-CoV-2 might be considered strongly diagnostic of infection is where there is an unfeasibly strong prior assumption that competing viruses, such as influenzas and coronaviruses, had virtually vanished. As well as acting as a strong and unsupported prior disposition this assumption is circular and is based on test results collected using the same faulty PCR technology.

The argument that there was a genuine pandemic caused by the novel SARS-CoV-2 viral pathogen has largely relied on data from PCR testing. Given that we have shown such data are highly inaccurate and unreliable, this line of argument is not tenable.

There are other issues we have not touched on here relating to genetic sequencing etc. We have also not commented on the fact that the sample sizes used in these studies is shockingly small. If we took this into account and computed confidence intervals and performed confidence tests our results would likely be even worse, leading to an inevitable conclusion that PCR testing is not particularly specific and suffers from irreducible cross reactivity and false positive inaccuracies.

It might be tempting to argue that even if PCR testing was a failure, then the available alternative, in the form of lateral flow testing (LFT), clearly showed a pandemic was taking place. But this is a moot point because LFTs were not available during much of 2020, and this initial phase of the pandemic was entirely driven by PCR testing. By the end of 2020 when LFTs were being widely used the accuracy gap between PCR and LTF positivity was significant. With PCR at 18% versus 4% positivity for LFTs, in week 53 of 2020 in England, it was clear PCR was over inflating the positivity results (see our article here [812]).

Our evidence presented here about PCR's ability to identify a novel deadly virus needs to be considered in combination with more recent revelations made about supposed uniqueness of symptoms about 'spikeopathy'. A pivotal point we made in that article is just as relevant here: objective confirmation cannot be obtained by the PCR test because of the inability of swabs to reliably collect and identify causative agents (as reported by the CDC EPIC study in two 2015 NEJM articles). Hence, a positive result gained from a sample taken from the upper throat or the nose does not mean an infection in the lung is caused by the detected pathogen. This evidence brings into question all arguments about the relevance of PCR.

Kevin McKernan has recently espoused the view that that PCR testing validated people's covid morbidity experiences. He may be correct about current public opinion, but its relevance is questionable here given that, in 2023, he was scientifically correct when he said there is 'late crosstalk with other viruses', and his statement is relevant to all PCR testing undertaken up to and including that year.

Without PCR testing data, published official statistics about infection, hospitalisation, and death rates would not be attributable to the novel virus. This, and our other analyses have questioned this attribution and there must therefore be other explanations for the 'pandemic'. Such explanations need not include the conclusion there was 'no virus'.

21.3. The Australian respiratory season puzzle

2020 respiratory mortality season (March 2024)

An article [813] by Arkmedic published in October 2023 provided an excellent and comprehensive analysis of multiple aspects of the Covid-19 pandemic which supports many of the arguments we have been making in the last three years on this substack.

However, we challenge one of Arkmedic's claims - that PCR testing was reliable enough to prove that there was a novel virus that caused deaths. Specifically, Arkmedic uses official statistics in Australia that purport to show that influenza had disappeared in 2020 and that, despite an initial outbreak in Victoria state, Covid-19 largely disappeared too. Arkmedic claimed that the absence of influenza, coupled with the increased surge in influenza PCR testing, proves that the PCR test for SARS-CoV-2 was reliable.

21.3.1. PCR specificity and supposedly novel symptoms

Arkmedic claims that PCR is 'really' specific, and that the specificity rate published for some PCR manufacturers can be trusted (Roche is quoted at 99.8%). However, if you read it closely you will find that nowhere in the Roche documentation is there any description of the cross-reactivity tests undertaken that might support this low value. In a recent article [814] we showed that failure to account for cross-reactivity systemically overestimated the specificity of PCR testing.

Arkmedic makes the correct point that the false positive rate is partly driven by prevalence, but then splits the population of those tested into those with symptomatic covid and those without (i.e. asymptomatic) and assigns to each of these a different prevalence rate. Strictly speaking, this is a mistake because prevalence means the proportion of people in the whole community, not prevalence in particular subsets of individuals with or without symptoms.

Logically a patient known to have an infection has a prevalence for the infection with probability value one (certainty), and a patient known not to have it has a prevalence with probability value zero (impossibility). But we are dealing with uncertainty about the infection in the population *before* we take account of the evidence we have about a particular patient. Hence, it is wrong to twist the definition of prevalence and define it based on symptoms.

We do not believe that an asymptomatic PCR test positive provides strong evidential support for a SARS-CoV-2 diagnosis (see, for example, this article [815]). Objective confirmation cannot be obtained by PCR test because of the inability of swabs and PCR to reliably collect and identify causative agents (as reported by the CDC EPIC study in two 2015 NEJM articles - one done on adults [816] and one on children [817]). Hence, a positive result gained from a sample taken from the upper throat or the nose does not automatically mean an infection in the lung or elsewhere is caused by the detected pathogen. Therefore, it is not currently possible to differentiate between

- someone who has viral fragments in their upper respiratory system, detected by PCR, and who is and will remain 'uninfected' and will never show symptoms; and
- someone who might go on to develop an infection in the lower respiratory tract, or elsewhere, and show symptoms.

Hence, we cannot neatly separate a given population into asymptomatic and symptomatic groups and estimate the prevalence of a virus in each. All we can do is estimate and diagnose using probabilities over a single population.

To deal with symptoms properly we should therefore make them conditional on population infection prevalence in the same way we did with the PCR test. Both 'signs and symptoms' and the PCR test result are observable consequence of these various competing latent pathogens. Hence, the direction of causality is: infection causes the PCR test result and also causes the signs and symptoms.

Critically, the signs and symptoms for 'covid' are no different, or hugely overlapping, from the signs and symptoms for other Influenza-like-illnesses (ILIs). Here is a quote on differentiating between RSV (respiratory syncytial virus) and Covid-19 from the advisory committee on immunization practices (ACIP) [818] at the Center for Disease Control (CDC):

> "...RSV is a well-recognized respiratory pathogen of infants and a common cause of respiratory disease in older adults. In adults, RSV can be difficult to differentiate from COVID-19 and influenza based on symptoms alone — and is frequently overlooked as a diagnosis for a viral respiratory disease in adults."

Likewise, Figure 71 is a screenshot of the UK NHS advice on the similarity of Covid-19 symptoms with colds and flu.

Hence, observing these in a person does not discriminate between these competing causes but does make both more likely than 'no infection'. Likewise, if a person is asymptomatic (no signs and symptoms) then the likelihood for either ILI or SARS-CoV-2 decreases in tandem to the same degree.

There is no differential diagnosis based on symptoms, except where it differentiates between no infection and any infection (logical but useless from a decision-making perspective).

21.3.2. Australia 2020 PCR testing

Arkmedic goes onto claim that the maximum false positive rate was 0.2% for New South Wales in Australia during the 'covid lull', the period from September 2020 to July 2021, and that because this matched the Roche false positive rate, one confirms the other as an accurate measure of specificity. Hence, there was no SARS-CoV-2 circulating at that time and no competing pathogens that might trigger false positives. This later point is backed up (according to Arkmedic) by the fact there was a high rate of influenza PCR testing done and that the test positive rate dropped to 0.1%.

Symptoms of COVID-19

COVID-19 symptoms can include:

- a high temperature or shivering (chills) – a high temperature means you feel hot to touch on your chest or back (you do not need to measure your temperature)
- a new, continuous cough – this means coughing a lot for more than an hour, or 3 or more coughing episodes in 24 hours
- a loss or change to your sense of smell or taste
- shortness of breath
- feeling tired or exhausted
- an aching body
- a headache
- a sore throat
- a blocked or runny nose
- loss of appetite
- diarrhoea
- feeling sick or being sick

The symptoms are very similar to symptoms of other illnesses, such as colds and flu.

Figure 71 UK NHS symptoms of Covid-19

So, if we accept these arguments we are left with two possible explanations:

- That the flu and SARS-CoV-2, as well as all other competing pathogens, genuinely (almost) disappeared from Australia, or
- The PCR kits being used were producing results that were manipulated, but manipulated in ways that differed from the way PCR was used elsewhere globally.

The first explanation is not credible given that Victoria state in Australia suffered a covid peak in July - August 2020, yet the state next door, New South Wales, did not. For this to make sense we would have to believe viruses stop at borders or that the lockdowns and border restrictions are dramatically effective. Evidence to date is overwhelming that neither of these can be true. Where did this highly infectious virus go after 'landing' in Victoria in 2020?

On the second of the possible explanations Arkmedic thinks Australia is the exception that proves the rule about PCR testing, but there are several points worth bearing in mind:

- There were no transparent, public, independent evaluations of PCR testing throughout the pandemic, except for those discussed here [819] and it is abundantly clear that the false positive rate is high in the presence of competing pathogens.
- New multiplex array test kits were being introduced to test for both flu and SARS-CoV2 and we know of at least one test [820] which exhibited 'interference'

between flu and SARS-CoV-2. Likewise, the rate of test positives for all Biofire test kits dropped and did so for all competing pathogens in 2020 - it defies belief that this was a purely biological phenomenon.

- Some hospitals were not culturing flu viruses [821] in the same way as before, so the gold standard had changed just as the pandemic began, with a switch over to the multiplex array PCR. It is conceivable that this change may have occurred globally.

- It is possible that, during the 'covid lull' period, confirmatory PCR testing was happening. As explained in this article [822] this has the effect of drastically - but artificially - reducing the false positive rate.

There is ample evidence that the influenza surveillance systems had been altered. Here is a report from an Australian GP in our substack comment thread:

> "Great news with the general decreasing influenza illness trends for the year but not sure about the eye-catching headline statistic …
>
> 1. GPs were specifically told not to test for influenza and indeed some labs were actually not running the test at all for a period of time. It is therefore difficult to make an accurate comparison between years given access to testing was very different. I am surprised there is no mention of this in the article.
> 2. Additionally, 2019 was a big influenza year compared to other previous years on the graph. Comparing to any previous year on the graph or an aggregate of the years, there is still a reduction but not the astonishing '99%'…"

This first-hand report does not match the official influenza sentinel surveillance data [823].

However, looking closely at official mortality for Australia in 2020, we find something quite puzzling. The data for the ICD-10 influenza and pneumonia (J09-J18) deaths were similar in 2019 and 2020, as reported by the Australian Bureau of Statistics [824]. Influenza and pneumonia deaths in 2020 were 60% of the 2019 deaths (it varies considerably year by year; in 2018 there were 3102 deaths).

These mortality rates are similar to those reported for the USA and the UK in 2020 as described here [825]. This shows there was no significant change in respiratory mortality and hence no pandemic. But 70% of the deaths in 2019 are categorised as pneumonia 'organism unspecified' (J18), compared to 94% in 2020. What can we conclude from this? That, despite the supposed absence of influenza and absence of SARS-CoV-2, the pneumonia death rates remained largely unchanged, while coincidentally the rate of 'unknown' causes of pneumonia death rose from an already significant proportion, 70%, to 94%!

Also, at this time people in Australia were searching the internet for the flu, as we reported here [826], and in Chapter 90, Figure 1 despite the fact that there was, according to the Flunet reports no flu.

To a jaundiced, untutored, eye Australia had a normal respiratory mortality season in 2020 and that the only thing that varied was PCR testing rates, technology, and results. The facts on the ground remained the same and we can only assume the PCR testing done was highly suspect.

21.4. PCR positives using single genes as the rule

Was declaring PCR positives using single genes the rule and not the exception? (27 Feb 2024)

A friend of Martin's took a PCR test after arriving home from holiday abroad on 5th October 2021. At that time the government required a PCR test be undertaken upon returning and if you were positive you had to quarantine for 10 days.

A screenshot of his PCR test result from Randox Laboratories, using their PCR test [827], launched on 26 January 2020 can be seen here [828]. He was found to be positive for the coronavirus. The report contains a table with the following information:

Target Name	Result	CT Value
ORF tab	Positive	33.57
E-gene	Negative	Undetermined

So, two genes were tested: the "ORF1ab-gene" and "E-gene", and one of the genes was positive, with a CT value of 33.57. The E-gene result was undetermined.

Seven months before, in March 2021, we exposed that the UK lighthouse laboratories breached WHO EUA and violated manufacturer instructions for use because they were calling positives on single genes rather the 'two from three' genes' required by the WHO. This was being done throughout winter 2020/21 in the UK clearly creating a 'casedemic'. See here [829] for details.

Not only did the Randox PCR only test for two genes but, as with the UK lighthouse laboratories, it declared a positive on one only, thus also breaching WHO guidelines. Either that or an indeterminate result on the other gene was judged to be equivalent to a positive (just to be safe?).

In their defence at least Randox were open enough to acknowledge that their test was essentially useless (this statement remains on their website). Dr Peter FitzGerald, Managing Director of Randox Laboratories, commented:

> "Current technologies for the diagnosis of coronavirus are designed simply to detect the presence of lack of COVI-19 and therefore neglect to differentiate between this strain and other respiratory infections."

Out of curiosity Martin's friend then dutifully self-monitored the progress of his 'illness', using LFTs, for 10 days from the 5th October to end of his self-imposed quarantine on the 15th October. The LFT results were all negative as shown in the photograph here [830]. Clearly, he was not infected with SARS-CoV-2.

What this proves is that single gene testing was common practice not only within the NHS lighthouse laboratories but also in private laboratories and this went on throughout 2020 and late into 2021.

Obviously one motive was to maintain the perception of a pandemic. My friend also suspects another motive was at play. At the time he was single-shot-vaccinated and had refused all other offers of the second and subsequent or booster vaccines. Hence, he was unvaccinated (or even ant-vaxx?) in official eyes. A quick check of his NHS record would reveal this status.

His suspicion is that his positive result and the application of a single gene test was intentionally set as a lower bar to ensure that the unvaccinated were more likely to be labelled as infected than those vaccinated. This covid positive status would then act as means to punish the unvaccinated (quarantine and loss of earnings etc) and would help boost the casedemic numbers.

As an aside it is worth noting that at that time a positive PCR test required voluntary self-isolation upon returning from abroad. However, there was no explicit mention in government guidelines about what to do if the PCR test result was 'unclear' or indeterminate. Commercial testing companies advised people to retest or quarantine but this differed from government guidelines, and they were in essence advising people to follow policies that did not exist.

So, the smart thing to do to avoid quarantine was to simply run your PCR test swab under the tap and then submit that in the hope of an unclear result (or simply ignore the nonsense altogether).

Chapter 22. Virus origins and gain (claim) of function research

30 May 2024

22.1. There is nothing novel about a novel virus

This chapter is based on an article with relevant screenshots which can be found here [831]).

"Fields Virology" is cited as one of the most authoritative references in virology, including virus biology as well as replication and medical aspects of specific virus families. Chapter 28 [832] of Volume 1 of this book [833] was written by Masters and Perlman and provides some fascinating insights into our knowledge of coronaviruses which are considered to infect humans, including:

- HCoV-NL63 and HCoV-HKU1 were only discovered recently, in the post-SARS era (2002), even though each is prevalent globally and has been in circulation for a long time.
- Four known coronaviruses—HCoV-OC43, HCoV-229E, HCoV-NL63, and HCoV-HKU1—are endemic in human populations. The first two of these are thought to cause up to 30% of all upper respiratory tract infections.
- HCoV-NL63 and HCoV-HKU1 can be found worldwide, causing up to 10% of respiratory tract infections.
- Initial reports following its "discovery" suggested that HCoV-NL63 was associated with severe respiratory disease; however, subsequent population-based studies showed that most patients developed mild disease, similar to those infected with HCoV-229E or HCoV-OC43.
- Also, HECV-4408 [834] coronavirus was first detected in Germany in 1988 and is associated with acute diarrhoea in humans, and is (likely) related to bovine coronaviruses. However, the literature on this virus is incredibly sparse and there seems to be no active research interest in this virus at all.

Pyrc et al [835] report that HCoV-OC43 and HCoV-229E were discovered in the mid-1960s and since have been found to be prevalent worldwide. Though it isn't quite clear how prevalence was established, it seem the assumption was that they were already endemic rather than novel, either created in a laboratory or by zoonosis. HCoV-NL63 and HCoV-HKU1 were coronaviruses that were unknown to science until relatively recently, despite causing a high proportion of respiratory infections worldwide and probably having done so for centuries, if not since the dawn of time (as described later). A full one quarter of coronavirus infections were attributable to these coronaviruses that were hitherto completely unknown to science. Also, as we explain later, upon discovery, one of these was associated with severe respiratory disease, yet subsequently careful population-level analysis proved this to be false.

There are striking similarities between the histories of HCoV-NL63 and HCoV-HKU1 coronavirus and SARS-CoV-2. They were all novel to detection, two were associated with severe disease and the severity of two of these was significantly downgraded once the population data were analysed.

Yet as regards the origin of SARS-CoV-2, we are presented with a choice between two competing stories: either it was the product of a lab-leak, or it leapt into existence by zoonotic transmission from animals to humans, and in both cases, this happened shortly before its first detection. The third possibility – pre-existing endemicity - is hardly discussed as a possibility. An analogue of this situation would be turning on the high-resolution Hubble telescope and declaring that the newly detected exoplanets (planets revolving around stars other than our sun) sprang into existence at, or just before, the moment the telescope was turned on rather than consider they had already been there for aeons past.

Why are some newly discovered coronaviruses (HCoV-NL63 and HCoV-HKU1) assumed to be already endemic, whereas others are assumed, upon discovery, to be entirely novel and capable of starting a pandemic? This should be an important scientific question, but it is one which few have bothered to ask, let alone attempt to answer.

An article [836] discussing the discovery of a new virus, Redondoviridae, from 2019 asks: how do you find a virus that is completely unknown? They point out that:

> "Viruses, the most abundant biological entities on earth, are a scourge on humanity, causing both chronic infections and global pandemics that can kill millions. Yet, the true extent of viruses that infect humans remains completely unknown. Some newly discovered viruses are recognized because of the sudden appearance of a new disease, such as SARS in 2003, or even HIV/AIDS in the early 1980s. New techniques now enable scientists to identify viruses by directly studying RNA or DNA sequences in genetic material associated with humans, enabling detection of whole populations of viruses — termed the virome — including those that may not cause acutely recognizable disease. However, identifying novel types of viruses is difficult as their genetic sequences may have little in common with already known viral genomes that are available in reference databases."

They also report that researchers at the University of Pennsylvania identified a previously unknown viral family, which turns is the second-most common DNA virus in human lung and mouth specimens, where it is associated with severe critical illness and gum disease!

So, are novel viruses really that novel? As we have seen, since the 1980s there have been at least six "novel" new coronaviruses detected (MERS-CoV, SARS, SARS-CoV-2, HCoV-NL63, HCoV-HKU1 and HECV-4408), an average of one every seven years. How can we rule out the possibility that, had they doubled their efforts to find these apparently novel viruses, they wouldn't have found twice as many?

22.2. MERS-CoV and SARS and the fallacy of a single cause

In a 2014 paper MacIntyre [837] recorded that the Middle East respiratory syndrome coronavirus (MERS-CoV) was a newly emerged infection affecting humans in the Arabian

Peninsula, Europe, and North Africa. Most MERS-CoV cases have been associated with hospital outbreaks in Jordan, KSA, UAE and France. These clusters have been somewhat variable in clinical features, with the first outbreak in Jordan notably featuring renal failure, which does not feature as much, or at all, in other clusters, and would be an unusual feature of an illness caused by a respiratory virus.

A single infectious agent should not manifest in such varied ways. Under an old-fashioned disease model MERS-CoV would be categorised as separate illnesses, and it is only because of the new-fangled way of looking at sequences and the fact that a sequence is detected (or suspected as present), that it is assumed there must be a single cause – "the virus". However, this example of the 'fallacy of the single cause' and has no clinical validity; it is an artifice.

The source and persistence of the infection in humans remains unknown, despite having infected 681 people and killed 204 over a 2-year period. Cases were concentrated in the Middle East, and it appears not to have spread much beyond that region. The author says:

> "When the observed data were fitted to different disease patterns, the features of MERS-CoV fit better with a sporadic pattern, with evidence for either deliberate release or an animal source. There are many discrepancies in the observed epidemiology of MERS-CoV, which better fit a sporadic than an epidemic pattern."

Although the virus had been found in bats and in camels, it was speculated that most humans contracted the virus asymptomatically. Camels were believed to be the most likely source despite no particularly compelling evidence of transmission to humans from camels, except it had been found in some camels. Larger outbreaks have occurred in South Korea in 2015 [838] and in Saudi Arabia in 2018 [839].

Gardener and MacIntyre [840] dispute that the pattern for MERS-CoV should even be considered sporadic never mind epidemic because even though it was in circulation during the Hajj and Umrah pilgrimages to Saudi Arabia, supposedly perfect conditions for an epidemic, it did not visibly spread. They also say MERS-CoV was primarily a nosocomial infection (hospital acquired) associated with people already in hospital. They say that SARS was also predominantly a nosocomial infection.

In a comparison between SARS-CoV-2 and MERS-CoV Khalid et al [841] report that postintubation was similar between MERS and Covid-19 patients, with each group receiving prolonged mechanical ventilation with all that entails.

Abid et al [842] confirmed that MERS-CoV cases were complicated by bacterial and fungal infections. Half of patients had oxygen saturations less than 90%, and the majority who died did so after a prolonged period of ventilation. Antibiotics were given on admission to hospital (which may be too late, here [843]).

SARS was discovered in 2002 with the first known cases and was said to have caused the 2002-2004 outbreak, mainly in China (Andersen et al [844]). Wikipedia [845] provides a good overview of what is known about SARS, the most interesting difference to MERS-CoV being that the WHO declared that SARS disappeared as an acute respiratory syndrome in 2003 because of containment (attributed to public health measures). However, the virus failed to spread in 2003 and 2004 despite four laboratory accidents and it is claimed to be persistent as a zoonotic threat. Sound familiar?

- The assumption is that there is infection, and it might spread worldwide, even though the patterns of spread defy currently authoritative epidemiological mechanisms.
- Infection is mainly acquired in hospital, yet the only assumption worthy of consideration is that a new virus has just recently emerged from nature or are speculated to be manmade – the possibility of pre-existing endemicity is ignored.
- The perceived high fatality rate, in already hospitalised cases, is assumed to be caused by the virus not the underlying medical conditions of the patients.
- The possibility of asymptomatic spread is simply assumed, yet no evidence for this is offered. This hypes the possibility of a pandemic despite the alternative and simple conclusion being that if it was spreading invisibly, it therefore could not be that deadly.
- Symptoms for both MERS-CoV and SARS are nonspecific, causing flu like illness. Nothing was diagnostic. Radiographic evidence was also said to be diagnostic of SARS but, as we found in our article on spikeopathy, no radiological signs could distinguish between this and any other respiratory viral illness.
- It is acknowledged they can both lead to bacterial pneumonia.
- Wikipedia [847] says that 72% of people required mechanical ventilation for MERS-CoV and ventilation was used for treatment of SARS.
- Antibiotic treatment for both SARS and MERS-CoV was discouraged, as per WHO guidelines [848].
- Both were diagnosed by PCR, but diagnosis on mere suspicion was encouraged by the WHO and CDC [849] (a mere cluster of unexplained pneumonia would be enough).

Again, we see the fallacy of the single cause at play and are presented with these highly speculative single explanations about the diseases supposedly caused by these past epidemics are being caused by viruses and viruses alone.

The key thing here is that the mortality and morbidity of SARS and MERS-CoV are likely hugely overestimated, and this is due to the confounding effects of inappropriate medical treatments and diagnoses based on presumptions of high prevalence and travel history. Hence, the apparent virulence and pathogenicity of newly discovered viruses appears to be regularly hugely overestimated soon after their discovery, only to be either massively downgraded later (HCoV-NL63) or the fiction of their severity to remain unchallenged (SARS-CoV-2, SARS, MERS-CoV). This playbook gets repeated again and again, such as more recently with H5N1 (here [850]).

22.3. Would we recognise a novel virus when we see it?

If we are told to accept SARS-CoV-2 as novel, such acceptance should be conditional on how robust the process was for appending the label 'novel' to the virus. In this regard it is useful to examine the decision-making process underpinning this decision (Engler [851]).

In February 2020 the Coronavirus Study Group (CSG) International Committee on Taxonomy of Viruses (ICTV-CSG), which is responsible for developing the official classification of viruses and taxa naming (taxonomy) of the *Coronaviridae* family, assessed the novelty of the human pathogen tentatively named 2019-nCoV (pre-print on biorxiv Gorbalenya et al, [852] Perlman and Drosten are co-authors).The virus was temporarily named 2019 novel coronavirus, 2019-nCoV and renamed SARS-CoV-2 based on the CSG's recommendations. This is how they expressed the challenges in deciding novelty:

> "The term "novel" may refer to the disease (or spectrum of clinical manifestations) that is caused in humans infected by this particular virus, which, however, is only emerging and requires further studies. The term "novel" in the name of 2019-nCoV may also refer to an incomplete match between the genomes of this and other (previously known) coronaviruses, if the latter was considered an appropriate criterion for defining "novelty". However, virologists agree that neither the disease nor the host range can be used to reliably ascertain virus novelty (or identity), since few genome changes may attenuate a deadly virus or cause a host switch.
>
> Likewise, we know that **RNA viruses persist as a swarm of co-evolving closely related entities**..., known as quasi-species. Their genome sequence is a consensus snapshot of a constantly evolving cooperative population *in vivo* and may vary within a single infected person and over time in an outbreak.
>
> If the strict match criterion of novelty was to be applied to RNA viruses, it would have qualified every virus with a sequenced genome as a novel virus, which makes this criterion poorly informative. To get around the potential problem, virologists instead may regard two viruses with non-identical but similar genome sequences as variants of the same virus; this immediately poses the question of how much difference is large enough to recognize the candidate virus as novel or distinct?"

So, novelty depends on a genome sequence which is a mere snapshot of a continually evolving dynamic swarm of co-evolving related entities, and thus the decision of what constitutes novelty is complex, owing more to judgement than objective analysis. It also depends on both the disease or clinical manifestations and the completeness or incompleteness of matches against other viruses. This presents a smorgasbord of confounding and confusion of cause with effect, and in no way defines a 'thing' in and of itself.

If the strict match criterion of novelty was to be applied to RNA viruses, it would have qualified every virus with a sequenced genome as a novel virus. Therefore, they cannot be considered as isolated singletons with unique attributes, but rather as mutually overlapping families of individuals with shared attributes, making the idea of novelty, in an absolute sense, redundant. Thus, the ICTV apply a taxonomy to viruses that recognizes five hierarchically arranged ranks: order, family, subfamily, genus, and species (in ascending order of inter-virus similarity). Critics of this approach argue that genetic diversity can only be reliably expressed, mathematically [853], as pairwise distances between them and probabilities of overlap in genetic divergence, or to put it another way there can be no taxonomy in a swarm.

By the time the paper was published in Nature microbiology [854] all reference to the difficulty and role of expert opinion in deciding the assignment of the name SARS-CoV-2 had been deleted, giving the impression that the decision was straightforward and uncontroversial. If the name had remained 2019-nCoV it would probably have been considered just another cold virus and nothing to worry about. In the pre-print the ICTV-CSG clearly label SARS-CoV-2 as **not** being a novel virus showing they came to a different decision to the WHO.

There is some evidence of possible disagreement between the ICTV-CSG and the WHO (this paragraph didn't make it into the paper published by Nature):

> "In contrast to SARS, the name SARS-CoV-2 has NOT been derived from the name of the SARS disease and in no way, it should be used to predefine the name of the disease (or spectrum of diseases) caused by SARS-CoV-2 in humans, which will be decided upon by the WHO. The available yet limited epidemiological and clinical data for SARS-CoV-2 suggest that the disease spectrum, and transmission modes of this virus and SARS may differ. Also, the diagnostic methods used to confirm SARS-CoV-2 infections are not identical to those of SARS. This is reflected by the specific recommendations for public health practitioners, healthcare workers and laboratory diagnostic staff for SARS-CoV-2/2019-nCoV (e.g. WHO guidelines [855]for 2019-nCoV). By uncoupling the naming conventions used for coronaviruses and the diseases they may cause in humans and animals, we wish to help the WHO with naming diseases in the most appropriate way (WHO guidelines [856] for disease naming)."

They also hint at the possibility that both SARS and SARS-CoV-2 have suspect origins:

> "Although SARS-CoV-2 is NOT a descendent of SARS and the introduction of each of these viruses into humans was likely **facilitated by unknown external factors**, the two viruses are genetically so close to each other that their evolutionary histories and characteristics are mutually informative."

And then confess that differences in opinion about novelty are themselves not novel:

> "Since the current sampling of viruses is small and highly biased toward viruses of significant medical and economic interest, the group composition varies tremendously among different viruses, making decisions on novelty group-specific and dependent on the choice of specific criteria selected by researchers. Practically, this means that definitive evidence for novelty in one group may not stand up to scrutiny in another."

The idea that there are distinct species that fall into neat mutually exclusive categories is questionable. In the animal kingdom, what are presupposed as novel species or subspecies turn out to overlap. Take for instance the Liger [857] – the hybrid offspring of Tigers and Lions. Similarly, different subspecies of bear interbreed quite easily. Life is on a continuum and if it isn't possible to categorise animals and neatly place them in a taxonomy, might we be overconfident with viruses, organisms which are not readily observed, and about which we know much less? We would suggest that the ICTV are aware of these limits to the science of virology, especially since debates about virus taxonomy have raged since its inception, with many prominent scientists within the discipline arguing that descending hierarchical divisions are based on arbitrary and monothetic assumptions (see Murphy et al [858] - introduction to the universal system of virus taxonomy).

Together the assignment of the word novel and the use of the name looks like the result of contentious political process or social construct, presented as a scientific one where all uncertainty, doubt and dispute have been stripped out.

22.4. Are spike proteins, inserts and furin cleavage sites dangerous or novel?

Much has been made of the fact that SARS-CoV-2 contains both a spike protein (the S protein) and furin cleavage site (FCS). This has caused much concern and controversy. Some claim that the spike protein is particularly dangerous and that the 'unique' furin cleavage site in this spike protein makes it responsible for high infectivity and transmissibility.

But are they dangerous and novel in and of themselves?

In Nature Xia et al [859] say:

> "The rapid spread of SARS-CoV-2 .....a novel lineage B betacoronavirus.., has caused a global pandemic of coronavirus disease (COVID-19). It has been speculated that RRAR, a unique furin-like cleavage site (FCS) in the spike protein (S), which is absent in other lineage B [betacoronavirus], such as SARS-CoV, is responsible for its high infectivity and transmissibility. ...
>
> Therefore, it has been speculated that this unique FCS may provide a gain-of-function, making SARS-CoV-2 easily enter into the host cell for infection, thus efficiently spreading throughout the human population, compared to other lineage B betacoronaviruses."

Speculative claims have been made that the FCS causes fibrosis [860].The supposed fragility [861] of the spike protein against antibodies raises questions about the origin.

This review by Liu et al [862] identifies:

> "....248 other CoVs with 86 diversified furin cleavage sites that have been detected in 24 animal hosts in 28 countries since 1954.
>
> ....Besides MERS-CoV and SARS-CoV-2, two of five other CoVs known to infect humans (HCoV-OC43 and HCoV-HKU1) also have furin cleavage sites. In addition, human enteric coronavirus (HECV-4408) has a furin cleavage site...."

The paper by Ambati et al [863] makes the case that the composition of the SARS-CoV-2 FCS is very unusual, but 'unusual' means little without a comparison against the typical. They say:

> "...presence of the 19-nucleotide long RNA sequence including the FCS with 100% identity to the reverse complement of the MSH3 mRNA is highly unusual and requires further investigations."

They queried a database of 24,712 genomic sequences and calculated a coincidence probability of 3.21×10^{-11} for the SARS-CoV-2 furin cleavage sequence, concluding that the FCS was man made.

Dubuy and Lachuer [864] disputed this assertion by assessing the probability of coincidence that other viruses might exhibit these same features. Based on a careful probabilistic analysis, that considered that sequences are not independent, sequences are of different lengths and other factors, they found a coincidence probability of 0.0037 – orders of magnitude higher than that calculated by Ambati et al. This number itself might look small but if we express the odds of it being natural versus man-made, as a ratio, it is approximately one (a certainty).

Notice here that the key assumption in the work of Dubuy and Lachuer is that viruses might share the same features, perhaps because of parallel evolution but also because of co-evolution, whereby recombination takes place across species of virus, which is exactly what you might expect to take place in a viral swarm, as acknowledged by the ICTV.

Therefore, the FCS could have been created naturally and was perhaps simply a newly discovered virus that was already prevalent within the environment. Hence there may be nothing much that is truly novel about either the spike protein or the FCS. Masters and Perlman point out that in many beta and gamma coronaviruses, the S protein is partially or completely cleaved by a furin-like host cell protease into two polypeptides. Currently available structural and biochemical evidence accords well with an early proposal that S (spike) is functionally analogous to the influenza HA protein.

Likewise, much is made of the fact that the spike binds to human ACE2 receptors. Again, turning to Masters and Perlman:

> "The receptor for SARS —angiotensin-converting enzyme 2 (ACE2)—was discovered with notable rapidity following the isolation of the virus.
>
> ACE2 also serves as the receptor for the alphacoronavirus HCoV-NL63 and the corresponding structural complex for that virus reveals that the HCoV-NL63 RBD (receptor-binding domain) and the SARS RBD bind to the same motifs."

So here we have another coronavirus, which was previously pronounced as being 'deadly' that also uses the ACE2 receptor, but which caused (in the main) mild respiratory disease.

It should be noted that ACE2 is expressed in less than 1% of human lung cells (here [865]), being most abundant in the alveolar type II cells, which themselves are only 5% of the alveolar surface area, the other 95% of the area being covered by squamous alveolar cells. Hence it is debatable whether human lung function is critically dependent on ACE2 (as it might be in mice specially bred to have human ACE2 receptors).

Much controversy has been attached to the pre-publication, and subsequent withdrawal of a paper by Pradham et al [866] claiming to have found a glycoprotein, called gp120, in the spike of the 2019-nCoV virus. This protein is thought to be specific to the HIV virus alone and given this, it suggests that the virus must be man-made. The 2008 Nobel prize winner Luc Antoine Montagnier replicated the finding.

Is gp120 unique to the HIV virus? Simian immunodeficiency virus (SIV [867]) has been identified as the progenitor to HIV, and in SIV it is present on the SIV spike protein. Given recombination events between HIV or SIV and coronaviruses are not beyond the world of possibility, that SIV is the source for the presence of gp120 in the SARS-CoV-2 spike protein cannot be discounted. We have no idea how much HIV and SIV are 'out there', and this notion has received zero attention, but surely the absence of evidence cannot therefore be assumed to be evidence of absence (note that asymptomatic HIV infection can last more than 10 years and the latency of SIV infection is largely unstudied).

We can conclude that spikes on coronaviruses are nothing special and spike proteins are similar or common to proteins in other viruses, including influenza. FCSs are common. But the vast majority of the 248 identified (so far) have not been studied anywhere near as closely as SARS-CoV-2. ACE-2 receptors are used by one other coronavirus, HCoV-NL63, that is not considered deadly. Arguments that 'unusual inserts' must be man-made might be contradicted by parallel evolution or co-evolution between viruses 'in the swarm'.

Hence, we see no reason to believe that the spike protein or FCS should be a source of special and unique concern in SARS-CoV-2. Even those 'unusual inserts' that supposedly make the virus remarkable may indeed be unremarkable, given it appears much more likely that other viruses might contain the same features by natural co-evolution between viruses.

22.5. Novelty of the SARS-CoV-2 furin cleavage site

Much of the argument about the origin hypothesis for SARS-CoV-2 revolves around the novelty of specific features of the virus and whether these resemble viruses known to be extant in nature or which are man-made (and are coincident with submitted research proposals).

The lab theory is partly based on the evidence that no bat colonies have been found to be infected by the exact virus, hence the virus had never previously existed in the natural world. The implication it was man-made was then supported by the revelation, obtained by FOIA, [868] of the existence of the DEFUSE project proposal, an application to DARPA (a Pentagon research agency) for a grant to enhance SARS-like bat viruses (we will see later that this was not a unique ambition).

The idea of a lab leak is presented as shocking, but Nass [869] has documented 309 lab acquired infections and 16 escapes between the years 2000 and 2021, including some which caused several deaths. Yet caused no pandemics.

The pre-print paper from Bruttel et al [870] argued that SARS-CoV-2 is man-made because of the 'endonuclease fingerprint' (endonuclease recognition sites *Bsm*BI/*Bsa*I) found in SARS-CoV-2. *Bsm*BI/*Bsa*I are commonly used for molecular cloning.

The proposal presented here is that DEFUSE, and the Wuhan lab engaged in Gain-of-Function research, where the genome of a known virus is amended to create some additional desired functionality such as enhanced transmissibility, pathogenicity (*enhanced* is the important word here – creating equivalent pathogenicity or transmissibility to an existing virus isn't the goal, the goal is to 'gain' this new functionality).

The fundamental assumption underlying GoF research is that any phenotype (trait or function) can be identified and directly matched to a one or more specific genotypes that together create that effect in the target species, and that by amending or replacing these genotypes in a special way, a desired functional phenotype can be created. A virus created by GoF could then be used as bioweapon or to be one step ahead by creating anticipatory treatments for potential future bioweapons or pandemic viruses.

22.6. Is engineering of more lethal viruses possible?

A counter argument to this has been presented by Wu [871] who analysed 1316 betacoronavirus and 1378 alphacoronavirus genomes collected before 2020 and found that a significant subset of these had the same unusual endonuclease fingerprint characteristics (*Bsm*BI/*Bsa*I) associated with SARS-CoV-2. Hence, it might not be that unusual after all, and of Bruttel et al he said:

> "...the pattern of BsamBI/*Bsa*I restriction enzyme recognition sites in alphacoronavirus and betacoronavirus is very diverse, and SARS-CoV-2 is not the only outlier in terms of the number and position of the two endonuclease sites."

Hence it looks like these fingerprints are not unique to SARS-CoV-2 and are not necessarily associated with man-made interference.

Additionally, in a very interesting analysis, Wu examined the feasibility of man-made development of SARS-CoV-2, focusing on Gain-of-Function insertions (reverse genetics) and serial passage (the process of growing bacteria or a virus in iterations):

> "The challenge of engineering a new virus is not about the approach or tool for genome assembly but is generating a sizable mutant library and developing an efficient high-throughput screening system to identify the most infectious clones.

Wu estimated the costs of creating a Gain-of-Function virus by comparing the endeavour to the number of steps in the natural evolution of SARS-CoV-2 alpha to the omicron variant; Wu extrapolated this to the evolution from the bat virus RaTG13 (Bat-origin RaTG13 is currently the most phylogenetically related virus to SARS-CoV-2.) to SARS-CoV-2 (using the number of people infected by each variant worldwide and the timescales involved):

> ".....it is reasonable to believe that it needs at least (80-250 million) experimental iterations to generate a new virus like SARS-CoV-2 from RaTG13....the laboratory consumable cost for a ~250 million screening and testing experiment would easily exceed 10 billion dollars.... the cost of creating a SARS-CoV-2 would require the Wuhan Institute of Virology's institute's full investment for at least 100 years."

On the implications of conducting serial passage:

> "One infection cycle in cell culture is typically 1–3 days depending on the inoculated viral MOI (multiplicity of infection). So, to generate directed mutations on those 1182 nucleotides in RaTG13, we would need at least 121,230 days (332 years) by serial cell passaging. The challenge for animal-based serial passaging should be higher than the cell culture-based approach because of the longer viral incubation time and workload related to animal care. Thus, it is unlikely to obtain SARS-CoV-2 from serial passaging."

By Wu's reasoning it would be impossible for anyone to engineer a new viable virus that met a pre-prepared set of GoF requirements. Not only would the DEFUSE project have had to have been very lucky to discover a virus that could be reliably cultured and had all required properties, but they would also have had to test whether it was viable for human transmission and increased pathogenicity.

A fascinating article [872], in the Bulletin of Atomic Scientists, explored Gain-of-Function research and reported that:

> "Across biology, gene background is important. The same mutation can yield different results in different strains. This indicates that the impact of some of these mutations cannot be easily extrapolated. In turn, this suggests the pool of mutations that could make a virus a pandemic threat could be large, a problem for both gain-of-function research and alternative approaches. There are a host [873] of other highly detailed virological arguments [874] about why pandemic prediction is virtually impossible.
>
> The gain-of-function thesis has been characterized by a belief that virology is akin to engineering; just define the (obviously small) numbers of permutations of mutations allowing a virus to cross over and transmit between humans, and "we'll figure it out." Biology and evolution were forgotten.

As we discuss later, we find that experiments undertaken to investigate 'wild' SARS-CoV-2 have amended the FCS and created new viruses. These experiments can and have been conducted, but that doesn't mean the experiments are necessarily successful since no one knows whether the viruses produced are themselves going to be viable and can be made such that they meet the 'transmissible and deadly' (or any other) functional requirement. Ultimately, if the requirements are for a virus pathogenic to humans, challenge studies will be required, not on mice but on humans. Ralph Baric [875] said:

> "When you adapt a coronavirus to another species …just putting a human receptor in and using a mouse model is not predictable of human transmissibility".

As far as we know they have not been performed, and in any case all the challenge studies done on wild SARS-CoV-2 have failed (here [876]), and rather ignominiously so. Thus, any claims about functional viability might be partially validated in vitro, or in animal models, but cannot be fully validated in humans or in society at large. All we know is that viruses can be produced but you cannot guarantee that these will 'go viral' or be 'deadly'. Wu's analysis suggests the whole endeavour is doomed to ruinous failure, if not simply impossible.

Is there any evidence that a viable virus has ever been engineered to match some pre-prepared functional specification and which could cause a pandemic? To our knowledge there are no end-to-end unambiguous successes. For instance, Masters and Perlman cite a case of Feline enteric coronavirus (FeCoV) where reverse genetics was used to swap S proteins from (presumably) virulent and avirulent strains, but the effect of this on pathogenesis is acknowledged to be unknown since experiments were done in vitro only.

An earlier controversy in 2014 surrounded GoF research centred on three forced-evolution experiments conducted on ferrets infected with H5N1 & H7N1 'bird flu' viruses (documented here [877], here [878], and here [879]). The first two GoF experiments on ferrets demonstrated that transmissibility might be enhanced (but may not be predictive for humans). However, the GoF variants produced were found to be insufficiently replication competent.

In the third of the studies cited above (by Sutton et al), researchers directly infected four ferrets, conducted serial passage experiments on these and then tried to infect naïve ferrets. They reported that a highly pathogenic avian influenza virus of the H7N1 subtype, with no history of mammalian adaptation, become capable of airborne transmission in the ferret model of influenza virus. This looks alarming and much might be made of the fact that all four of the directly infected ferrets were euthanised because they showed signs of severe disease. However, these ferrets were subject to serial passage numerous times rather than a single time as is the convention. Therefore, an alternative probable explanation for these animals being euthanised was not necessarily increased pathogenicity but that their immune system was simply overwhelmed by repeated reinfections. The authors reported a successful adaptation of bird flu to become capable of airborne transmission in ferrets but concluded that the GoF enhanced virus created may not have acquired the transmission efficiency required to cause a pandemic. Given the small sample sizes involved the question of increased pathogenicity in ferrets infected by the GoF variant was inconclusive, but the balance of evidence suggests that the GoF virus was less pathogenetic, in the lungs and bronchi etc., than the wild-type virus (as one might expect). Infected ferrets were reported as having lesions showing moderate meningitis and encephalitis with lymphocytes in the thalamus, compared to animals who were infected with the wild virus. However, no tests were done for bacterial meningitis hence this evidence, coupled with the small sample size is very weak.

Given that Loss-of-Function (LoF) experiments, involving the removal of features of a virus, are commonplace, and are akin to developing attenuated virus vaccines, another nail in the coffin is this paper [881] from Fauci himself, which admits that vaccine development is fraught with difficulty for respiratory viruses simply because of inherent rapid viral replication, error rate during mutation and antigenic drift. He says this (after the launch and injection of the Covid-19 vaccines into billions of people!):

> "Durably protective vaccines against non-systemic mucosal respiratory viruses with high mortality rates have thus far eluded vaccine development efforts."

If these features make vaccine development for respiratory viruses difficult if not impossible then they also make virus development via Gain-of-Function equally, if not more, challenging (well, maybe actually just as impossible).

In mathematics this is called *the curse of dimensionality*. In many problems where each variable (protein, genomes, cells, virions) can take on several values, taking the variables together, a huge number of combinations of values must be considered, leading to a combinatorial explosion. This results in an exponential set of possibilities each of which must be considered and evaluated. In the biological domain things are even more challenging because of non-monotonicity – any phenotype (trait or function) cannot be directly matched to a single specific genotype; hence the problem is not reducible and there exists no algorithm that can feasibly search the space of possibilities and identify the single genotype sequence that delivers the phenotype required. RNA viruses are mutation machines with the potential to adapt to a new host hence, even if a stable virus function is isolated, it will quickly mutate and lose this newly gained functionality (Wain-Hobson [882]).

Therefore, to create a genuinely pandemic-causing coronavirus would probably involve the re-engineering of one or more coronaviruses and would simply not be possible using GoF. Only the timescale of natural evolution could deliver the time and space needed to create both viable and non-viable combinations in a way that man cannot. Evolution (or God) is needed to defeat the curse of dimensionality.

22.7. Gain (or loss) of function experiments

Research on SARS-CoV-2 naturally involves using the tools of the trade, including applying reverse genetics to engineer variations in the virus. Such variations might include amendments to the furin cleavage site and the spike protein.

In January 2021 Johnson et al [883] carried out a LoF experiment using reverse genetics, observing that four hamsters infected with wild virus lost weight and showed some signs of infection compared to the LoF arm. They also found that the LoF virus was replicated more efficiently, defying expectations. When they repeated the experiment with transgenic mice, they found no differences in viral burden but based on the totality of evidence they concluded the LoF mutant produced reduced disease and replication at early times after infection, as compared to wild-type virus. They also used transgenic mice with hACE2 receptors (12 per arm) to examine pathogenicity, claiming there was evidence that the wild virus caused more weight loss, but with no differences in viral burden in the lungs or brain. To determine the functional effects on the lung, mice were mechanically ventilated to measure biophysical parameters, with the wild type mice showing more damage. Histopathology confirmed this.

In July 2021 Davidson et al [884] cloned WT (wild type) SARS-CoV-2 and produced variants with GoF enhancements by engineering spike variants. Laboratory results showed LoF, specifically the deletion of the furin cleavage site, did cause higher infection rates of human endothelial cells (airways), and when they tested viral transmission on eight ferrets, they found 2 of the 4 ferrets, cohoused with ferrets intentionally pre- infected with WT, showed signs of infection. And 0 of the 4 ferrets, cohoused with ferrets intentionally pre-infected with the GoF variant, showed signs of infection. They say:

> "We show that, in contrast with WT SARS-CoV-2, a virus with a deleted furin CS did not replicate to high titres in the upper respiratory tract of ferrets and did

not transmit to cohoused sentinel animals, in agreement with similar experiments using hamsters".

This study uses such a small sample size that the results are not significant, and we don't know whether infection had any effect on pathogenicity. No ferrets from either experiment showed appreciable fever or weight loss. When they used a 'competitive' 70% WT and 30% LoF mutant mix the results were not clear at all. In some ferrets the lost function mutant dominated in those inoculated with the mixture, and of the four co-housed ferrets only one was infected by transmission. This makes the results difficult to interpret.

In a similar study [885], in February 2021, Zhu et al, used naïve hamsters co-housed with a single infected hamster, examining changes to the furin cleavage site using six hamsters in each arm (wild type and LoF arm). Despite heroic applications of statistical skill on such a small sample size the results are, not surprisingly, poor and unconvincing. The hamsters infected with the wild type virus did show around a 10% weight loss, whilst the hamsters infected with the LoF variant put on weight; there seems no reason why weight should increase, suggesting experimental confounding. The other results were no more persuasive, unsurprising given the small sample sizes.

In 2024 Valleriani et al [886] conducted a much larger study using 150 transgenic mice expressing the hACE2 receptor, on the assumption these are permissive of SARS-CoV-2 infection and believed capable of developing severe disease (hence they are vulnerable to spike). Again, the comparison was carried out using a LoF arm. They say the LoF infected mice exhibited reduced shedding, lower virulence at the lung level, and milder pulmonary lesions. The mice in the LoF arm had a slightly higher survival rate and lower clinical scores than the wild type of virus.

If we take these experimental results at face value, they suggest that the LoF variant had higher transmissibility but lower pathogenicity, and the GoF variant had lower transmissibility and higher pathogenicity, thus illustrating the inherent trade-off in these functional characteristics: you cannot have both a highly transmissible virus and one that is highly deadly. This might confirm the challenges in overcoming the curse of dimensionality – it being near impossible to make changes that can deliver both functions.

Note that in all these experiments there were no controls using other coronaviruses or influenzas viruses for comparison with SARS-CoV-2. We just don't know how these LoF or wild virus results compare with common colds or influenzas. We also do not know what might happen if we removed FCS, or other genes, from these other coronaviruses. Would they become more pathogenic or transmissible? Are they already more pathogenic or less? Also, there were no tests to rule out bacterial pneumonia or other competing pathogens, which may have confounded the experiments.

There has been some discussion of pathogenesis associated with spike in many other coronaviruses, such as that by Millet and Whitaker [887] published in 2014; however the correlation between pathogenesis and the spikes of particular coronaviruses are biased, simply because they are based on heavily confounded observation data (E.g. the spike for MERS-CoV is assumed to be more dangerous because it is associated with a 'pandemic', whilst those from coronaviruses that don't have that associated are not). This is an important point – if the mortality data from previous pandemics is biassed by treatment protocols and medical negligence, how do we know the spike, or some other feature, is genuinely the driver of mortality?

The vast differences in symptoms for SARS-CoV-2 reported in different countries, for patients supposedly infected with the same virus, should raise alarm bells, since it suggests that reported symptoms were being confounded by location and test results (Neil et al [888]). It is an inversion of reality to claim that the same virus causes different symptoms, occurring in different geographical locations, when historically different viruses (especially those associated with respiratory illnesses) have caused the same symptoms world-wide.

Published GoF and LoF experiments are unpersuasive on the point of our ability to engineer viruses to meet functional requirements. The absence of comparative controls is enough to confirm this, as are issues related to heterogeneity of symptoms from a supposedly engineered virus. It therefore remains an open question as to whether all coronavirus infections appear to be relatively non-pathogenic to humans, with or without the spike or FCS or any other inserts, man-made or natural, and that SARS-CoV-2 might be no different in this regard.

22.8. Contradictory evidence on zoonotic origins

Let's turn to animal reservoirs to examine estimates of the phylogenetic origins of the virus. Munnik et al [889] report that SARS-CoV-2 can infect domestic lions, tigers, cats, dogs, ferrets, hamsters, tree shrews, rabbits and even tigers in zoos. But not pigs or poultry (so far!)

They studied a zoonotic outbreak of infection of Dutch mink farms in 2020.

> "A high diversity was observed in the sequences from some mink farms, which is likely explained by multiple generations of viral infections in animals before the increase in mortality was detected....the investigation has failed to identify common factors that might explain farm-to-farm spread. This could mean that the virus was already circulating in mink farms for some time before it was identified."

Might it be possible the virus was already in the mink?

In 2020 Boni et al [890] investigated the evolutionary origins of SARS-CoV-2, and reported:

> "SARS-CoV-2 itself is not a recombinant of any sarbecoviruses detected to date, and its receptor-binding motif, important for specificity to human ACE2 receptors, appears to be an ancestral trait shared with bat viruses and not one acquired recently via recombination....
>
> Divergence dates between SARS-CoV-2 and the bat sarbecovirus reservoir were estimated as 1948 (95% highest posterior density (HPD): 1879-1999), 1969 (95% HPD: 1930-2000) and 1982 (95% HPD: 1948-2009), indicating that **the lineage giving rise to SARS-CoV-2 has been circulating unnoticed in bats for decades.**"

If it has been circulating unnoticed in bats for decades, why wouldn't it have been circulating in humans for decades also? And by decades we mean any point between 1879 and now?

This fascinating result has been much ignored. In 2024 Holmes [891] in his widely cited work on the emergence and evolution of SARS-CoV-2 barely mentions the paper and doesn't cite the conclusions.

Markov et al [892] also studied the evolution of SARS-CoV-2 examining:

> " ...the selective forces that likely drove the evolution of higher transmissibility and, in some cases, higher severity during the first year of the pandemic and the role of antigenic evolution during the second and third years."

They found:

> "After the emergence of SARS-CoV-2 in humans, for the first nearly 8 months the virus seemed to exhibit limited apparent evolution. This was partially due to the relatively small global virus population, while spread was still not ubiquitous, and later as a result of non-pharmaceutical interventions in many parts of the world, and partially an artefact of virus undersampling."
>
> It took 8 months for the first divergent SARS-CoV-2 lineages to appear...., marking a turning point in the pandemic from an evolutionary point of view. The first three such lineages, later termed VOCs Alpha, Beta and Gamma, emerged independently in different parts of the world and were the result of puzzling higher evolutionary rates. The sheer number of mutations involved in VOCs is particularly striking from an evolutionary point of view."

This suggests that at the start of the pandemic the virus was a standardised copy identical in every way, but by the end of 2020 there were many. However, on the mink farms in the Netherlands we find minks with a very high range of diversity in sampled sequences suggesting it was present in the animal reservoir well before 2020. How can the human population be infected by a standardised version of SARS-CoV-2 yet animals are found with variants, and still no bats are found with SARS-CoV-2 at all. And careful phylogenetic analysis suggests progenitors of the virus has been circulating unnoticed in bats for decades (maybe since 1879?).

Despres et al [893] looked at the wildlife in Vermont to see if they could detect SARS-CoV-2 and found none in the wildlife throughout the state, including deer, despite most published North American studies finding SARS-CoV-2 within their deer populations. They cited "environmental and anthropogenic factors" as the reason for this.

Kumar et al [894] conducted global sequencing of SARS-CoV-2, combined with computational methods, to identify the most recent common ancestor of the virus, suggesting that the Wuhan patient zero was not the index case, nor gave rise to all human infections. The inference then is that the progenitor of the virus was spreading worldwide months before the outbreak in Wuhan. They claimed to have identified the progenitor (root) genome of SARS-CoV-2 by measuring 'coronavirus diversity'.

A critical limitation of phylogenetic analysis is the assumption there is no recombination between species and sub-species of virus. Instead, it is assumed that variation occurs 'within' and not 'between' species, and that genetic sequences that occur in one or more viruses might share a common ancestor in another. Given this there is no validity to the concept of a 'root' to the tree. Likewise, these issues cast serious doubt on any assumption that there is a predictable molecular clock that can be inferred from similar coronaviruses, and which itself remains constant over time. The ICTV as much as admit to this.

Given this, it is perhaps optimistic to believe that the discovery of the existence of antibodies to SARS-CoV-2 in wastewater and other samples from 2019 (nicely summarised here [895]), could in any way be definitive. This is because antibodies cover epitopes shared between different viruses, allowing our immune system to mount a highly diverse attack to destroy different viruses and variants without exhausting itself (how else might it defeat the combinatorial complexity of a continually evolving viral swarm?) It is therefore possible, if not certain, that the supposedly specific antibodies to SARS-CoV-2 could have been developed to counter a progenitor to SARS-CoV-2, containing the same epitopes, or to other similar coronaviruses, rather than to SARS-CoV-2 itself.

There are too many contradictions here. Neither phylogenetic analysis or antibody studies can be fully trusted to provide the definitive origin and we have a much-ignored estimate of the evolutionary origins of SARS-CoV-2 going back to 1879. The possibility it may already have been endemic in the animal population for some time, as a result co-evolution of viruses in a swarm, therefore cannot be readily dismissed.

Is there any evidence for endemicity pre-pandemic? The presence of SARS-CoV-2 was reported in Barcelona wastewater samples in a pre-print published in by Chavarria-Miró et al [896] in June 2020. The wastewater samples were archived from December 2019 to May 2020, with positive samples reported from as early as March 2019, a full 12 months before Covid-19 was declared a pandemic. However, when their pre-print was finally published, here [897], there was no mention of the positive sample from March 2019 and the earliest sample reported was from January 2020. This article [898] reports failed attempts to discover the reasons for this volte face and also summarises numerous studies, mainly from Italy, where pre-pandemic SARS-CoV-2 positive samples were reported.

The hypothesis of zoonotic endemicity has therefore not been falsified (and to be fair it probably cannot be because the fundamentals are so poorly understood).

22.9. GoF research is routine and involves creating (infectious?) clones

Interestingly, the 2014 Millet and Whitaker paper (funded by the US NIH) ruminates on the potential for research on the FCS and is clearly advocating for GoF research focused there, thereby illustrating that it is a shared research theme in coronavirus research circles. They explicitly say:

> "Overall, it seems likely that modulation of either of two protease cleavage sites by coronaviruses can have a profound impact on disease outcome, depending on the individual coronavirus."

The FCS is an example of a protease cleavage site. This suggests that research on GoF/LoF focused on the FCS isn't particularly unique to the DEFUSE project, thus devaluing significantly the hypothesis that because the DEFUSE project was researching into this precise area, the properties of the 'novel' virus must mean that it was man-made.

Bruttel et al [899] says this about the routine use of reverse genetics to produce mutations (i.e. changing function):

> "Making a reverse genetic system from a wild type CoV requires breaking the 30 kb coronaviral genome into 5-8 fragments, each typically shorter than 8kb.... To design a reverse genetic system, researchers often modify their synthetic DNA constructs from the wildtype viral genomes by **introducing synonymous mutations** that alter restriction enzyme recognition sites without significantly impacting the fitness of the **resulting infectious clones**."

The first paper Almazán et al [900] describes the engineering of a full-length cDNA (complementary DNA) clone from SARS. A cDNA clone contains the entire viral genetic information necessary for replication, transcription, and translation. To put it another way they have the potential to be infectious, just like the original virus they cloned. They use it:

> ".....for the recovery of infectious virus and has been used for the generation of a large collection of deletion mutants of SARS-CoV"

A deletion mutant is a genetic anomaly in which a segment of a chromosome or DNA sequence is omitted during DNA replication, leading to the absence of specific nucleotides or entire chromosomal segments. This can result in altered gene function or expression. This is GoF.

Let's look at Becker et al [901] (Ralph Baric is a coauthor on this 2008 paper):

> "Here, we report the design, synthesis, and recovery of the largest synthetic replicating life form, a 29.7-kb bat severe acute respiratory syndrome (SARS)-like coronavirus (Bat-SCoV), a likely progenitor to the SARS-CoV epidemic. To test a possible route of emergence from the noncultivable Bat-SCoV to human SARS-CoV, we designed a consensus Bat-SCoV genome and replaced the Bat-SCoV Spike receptor-binding domain (RBD) with the SARS-CoV RBD (Bat-SRBD). Bat-SRBD was infectious in cell culture and in mice and was efficiently neutralized by antibodies specific for both bat and human CoV Spike proteins."

This is clearly GoF research and was published 12 years before the SARS-CoV-2 pandemic.

Here is the title of the paper from Cockrell et al (2018) [902]:

> "A spike-modified Middle East respiratory syndrome coronavirus (MERS-CoV) infectious clone elicits mild respiratory disease in infected rhesus macaques".

This is GoF research.

Likewise, note that the studies on LoF we have already discussed previously, in principle, are implicitly no different from GoF. Hence GoF research is ongoing.

Also, it should be obvious that cloning viruses is straightforward and even quite routine in virological research and development. For instance, the Bruttel paper says:

> "The BsaI/BsmBI map of SARS-CoV-2 is anomalous for a wild coronavirus and more likely to have **originated from an infectious clone designed** as an efficient reverse genetics system. The research goals and laboratory logistics of infectious clone technology can leave a previously unreported fingerprint in the genomes of infectious clones".

A moratorium announced by the Obama administration was lifted in 2017 after three years (2014 – 2017), and despite the moratorium the US government continued to assess and fund some GoF experiments (here [903]). So not a ban at all then.

It therefore appears to be the case that, like the DEFUSE proposal GoF research was and is still routine. Indeed, it looks like standard practice applied globally across many research groups studying coronaviruses.

22.10. If not lab leak or wet market, then how did 'it' arise?

On the animal origins of SARS-CoV-2 Wu had this to say:

> "Most recently, Wang et al discovered a high frequency of mammalian-associated viral co-infections and identified 12 viruses that are shared among different bat species by meta-transcriptomic analysis of 149 individual bat samples in Yunnan, China. The authors also found two coronaviruses closely related to SARS-CoV-2 (92%–93% genetic identities), with only five amino acid differences in the receptor-binding domain of one genome compared to the Wuhan-Hu-1 strain. These findings indicate that **viral co-infections and spillover are common in bats, which explains the high recombinant events in coronavirus and points to the origin of SARS-CoV-2 from recombinational exchanges among multiple related genomes**."

Of course, neither side of the argument can say how SARS-CoV-2 might have come to have been detected in humans, but it is not beyond possibility that it neither arose recently in nature, nor emerged from a laboratory but may instead have been with us for quite some time, lying low in the human population or in nature until it was discovered.

Let's consider the explanation of the single point zoonotic event, in the Huanan seafood (wet) market in Wuhan sometime between October to December 2019 (molecular epidemiology described here [904]). Does it seem unlikely that the virus arose spontaneously in the wet market at the same time GoF research was going on in Wuhan. What's the chance of nature creating a new virus at that exact place and time? The probability would be astronomically low, especially given it supposedly might include bats, humans, and pangolins.

The patchy pin-point pattern of spread of SARS-CoV-2 offers strong support to alternative explanations for the origin of SARS-CoV-2, with mortality rising in spring 2020 only after lockdowns were implemented and not before, and morbidity only revealing itself as attributable to a new virus with the roll out of PCR testing. (Rancourt [905], Engler [906], Pospichal [907]).

We can therefore speculate about alternative theories, two of which are pre-existing endemicity and virus clones, intentionally manufactured to create the impression of a pandemic. The first theory is one of pre-existing endemicity across the world (supported by existing T-cell immunity [908] and other things). The second is that lab manufacture was involved but not necessarily involving a leak from a laboratory in Wuhan, but 'something' was intentionally released first in Wuhan and then in multiple pinpoint locations worldwide. These theories need not be mutually exclusive but operationalizing these would require them to be coupled with a project involving high levels of mendacity and inventiveness.

Pre-existing endemicity:

> Imagine stealing a march on the science and discovering a coronavirus already endemic in humans but not in bats or camels (perhaps it spilled over zoonotically in the long distant past). You keep this secret because you realise this is an exploitable opportunity if you can successfully pull off a bait and switch. You apply for GoF research funding to engineer new viruses, for the benefit of humanity (vaccines etc.). You use the newly discovered virus in your research and maybe you might even toy around making some small changes. You feel confident enough to reveal these in the grant application because it might prove useful later. However, you know GoF is impossibly difficult (but you don't admit this to your sponsors or the public) and you therefore cannot make it any more lethal or transmissible than it current is (which is not much anyway given it has been in the background maybe for aeons). Next, you create a vaccine for this virus (which also doesn't work but that's another story). All that would be left to do would be to create a test for this virus so that it can now be discovered by the rest of humanity, giving the impression it has suddenly appeared, and given its endemicity create a fake pandemic to motive the sale of vaccines. Variants of the origin myth can then be used to create fear, to increase vaccine take-up, and the 'accidental' revelation of the secret GoF formula might be used to proclaim technological prowess (and potentially also to create future scapegoats and confusion if that is required).

Intentional spread of non-infectious clones:

> If we set aside pre-existing endemicity then all that is required is some functional amendments to some existing localised virus (from a bat, say), either known or newly discovered. Because it is from a bat GoF design of a human version would be impossible, hence, deadliness and transmissibility could not be 'designed in'. It won't 'go viral' because it isn't infectious and could not cause a pandemic. However, you could clone it so that it contains novel and deadly looking features, but you don't much care what its functional features are apart from that because the symptoms will be non-differentiable from other respiratory viruses. You would then simply need to distribute these clones artificially to make it look like a virus that spreads. Also, despite not being any more deadly than other coronaviruses it might still poison people and cause some morbidity. You would

then invent a vaccine and create a test designed to detect the DNA associated with the 'virus'. This, in summary form, is the hypothesis of JJ Couey (here [909]) We understand this hypothesis is partly inspired by the video lecture given by Dr James Giordano [910].

Relevant to both scenarios, but yet largely ignored as a factor in the events of the past few years, is the well-known and widely researched propensity of chronic stress to manifest as physical illness. The covid era was, after all, characterised by what was the most sustained and sophisticated and co-ordinated propaganda campaign ever imposed on human populations, specifically intended to increase fear and anxiety. In his video lecture, Giordano specifically invokes this aspect of how a pandemic could be manufactured (an essay containing a few interesting examples of this so-called 'nocebo' effect can be found here [911]).

Note that the 'non-infectious clone' theory would not create a self-sustaining global pandemic but might instead be considered to be akin to localised chemical attacks, where people would inhale an airborne pathogen but not transmit it.

Acknowledging the operational difficulty involved in continually manufacturing and distributing viral clones, in respect of JJ Couey's thesis, clones may only have been needed to have been deployed in hot spots (NYC and Bergamo Italy etc.) in 2020 to trigger a fake pandemic, and that subsequent positive SARS-CoV-2 cases, from then on, were a combination of PCR tests cross reacting with other viruses to cause false positives and/or natural endemic SARS-CoV-2 virus circulating at a low background rates.

There is a third explanation, elements of which overlap with the foregoing: that the characterisation of SARS-CoV-2 as a novel entity is entirely an artefact of virological testing and genomic sequencing methods. This is a hypothesis we will not be expanding upon here but are equally happy that others examine this possibility in further detail.

22.11. Discussion

"I would rather have questions that can't be answered than answers that can't be questioned." – Richard P. Feynman

The virus which has become known as SARS-CoV-2 doesn't appear to be that novel when looked at from several angles. Claims that something novel emerged in 2019 – whether or not through Gain-of-Function experimentation appear to be without foundation.

Firstly, it appears to be just another coronavirus, of which at least eight other similar such viruses have been detected since the 1980s. Furthermore, the lethality of the latest addition to the collection looks as if it is following a similar course to the others - overestimated soon after discovery only to be downgraded later. Attribution of virus lethality suffers from the fallacy of the single cause – the presence of the virus is presumed to be enough to explain death and illness independently of comorbidity and the medical treatments applied (or not).

Likewise, the clinical characteristics of illness associated with SARS-CoV-2 also appears to be largely indistinguishable from other coronaviruses and other viruses which, in any event, are often multiply present as coinfections.

Secondly, the much touted 'special' structural characteristics of SARS-CoV-2 do not – on deeper scrutiny – appear that unusual. Similar features having been identified in other apparently unremarkable viruses. Even the gp120 HIV inserts might have originated from wherever that sequence can be found elsewhere in nature and in man.

Thirdly, the complexity of the relationship between genotype and phenotype is too great and poorly understood to make the deliberate act of engineering the pathogenicity of viruses ever reliably achievable. Due to 'the curse of dimensionality', only the timescale of natural evolution could deliver the time and space needed for this. A review of so-called Gain-of-Function and Loss-of-Function experiments does not suggest that much practical and / or relevant progress has been made in overcoming this insurmountable barrier.

Fourthly, the possibility of long-standing – but hitherto unnoticed - endemicity of SARS-CoV-2 in various animal reservoirs at various times cannot be ruled out. Inherent limits to the dependability of phylogenetic analysis and antibody testing mean that we have, in Popperian terms, an unfalsifiable hypothesis that the virus, or its variants, were endemic and have been for some unknown time.

Fifthly, it appears that the engineering of clones carrying genetic material is and has been standard practice around the world for some time. Given the above, the creation and distribution of such clones seems a more likely explanation for the rapid spread of a particular sequence around the world than the natural spread of a novel pathogen from a class of viruses known to be highly mutable.

Given the above, we would suggest that Gain-of-Function should be more aptly known as Claim-of Function.

We are therefore left entertaining four competing hypotheses that might explain the viral 'signal': (i) pre-existing zoonotic endemicity; (ii) a natural zoonotic act that spontaneously created the virus at the right place in the right time in Wuhan; (iii) a Gain-of-Function lab leak; or (iv) the (intentional?) distribution of non-infectious clones producing a global viral signal. Given the results of our analysis we believe that the available virological and epidemiological evidence does not adequately support either the lab leak or the wet market theories for the origins of the virus.

Finally, none of the above is meant to excuse shortcomings in the discipline of virology (which seems to have lost its way over the past decades), nor express approval for Gain-of-Function research. Much research in the area looks to be neither ethical nor useful, and whilst we disagree that scientists can make viruses with pandemic potential, it is possible, or in fact even likely, that such experimentation may pose dangers locally (but not globally). Moreover, as we have seen, the constant hunting for viral sequences and frenzied analysis of those thought to be novel help lay the foundations for a constantly fearful humanity, empowering those who wish to impose 'pandemic preparedness' on the world, with its paraphernalia of control mechanisms and attendant loss of freedoms.

In this article, we are not intending to defend those who may have conducted such research, but nor do we think it is right to solely blame such research when the evidence for a spreading pathogen having caused a pandemic of a novel disease is so weak. It is perfectly possible to simultaneously believe (as we state above) that such research is unethical and that it did not (directly at least) cause the 'covid pandemic', which was an iatrogenic phenomenon. In this regard if there actually was a function gained by the virus it was the power to help trick humanity into a dramatic act of self-harm.

Chapter 23. Dodgy epidemiology and the ONS admit the cheap trick

23.1. Exaggerated estimates from epidemiological modelling

were growing exponentially during the 'pandemic' (8 May 2024)

23.1.1. Dashboards reflecting reality or manufacturing it?

Acting in 'journalist mode' Martin recently wrote an article [912] for the Conservative Woman online magazine, summarising an original article, The Dashboard that Ruled the World [914] written by Thomas Verduyn, about the John Hopkins University (JHU) Dashboard. This section is based on this article with relevant screenshots here [913]). The thrust of Verduyn's claim is that the Covid-19 dashboards were using epidemiological computer models as surrogates or as supplemental to actual case/death data.

Verduyn cites the data from New York City as proof that the output from these epidemiological models was used to simulate a pandemic, i.e. simulated death data were being used as if they were actual deaths 'on the ground'. This potentially explains why certain cities/regions experienced spikes in deaths whilst neighbouring cities/regions experienced nothing much at all (New York City and Bergamo, Italy for instance whilst neighbouring regions were unaffected).

This got us reflecting on what the epidemiological models were producing as output and how good the quality of the input data were. Verduyn cites an X/Twitter post by jockthedog [915] showing that JHU, dated January 29th, 2020, simulated (modelled) infection data for various countries on that date (one week after the dashboard went live). This is shown in column i) of the table below (Figure 72).

Dashboard Cases 29th January 2020					
	JHU Github (i) Infected cases	JHU Github (ii) Confirmed cases	ourworldindata (iii) Confirmed cases	ourworldindata (iv) Confirmed cases	ourworldindata (v) SEIR Modelled cases
China	6,970,300	7,678	1,985	266	49,722
Thailand	116,612	14	5	0	NA
South Korea	44,232	4	3	0	69
Singapore	20,164	10	4	0	NA
Japan	19,400	11	3	0	76
United States	14,292	12	7	1	NA
Australia	9,084	7	4	0	NA

(i) https://github.com/enshengdong/covid19/blob/master/nCoV_RR.ipynb

(ii) https://github.com/enshengdong/2019-nCoV-1/blob/master/current cases/cases 0129 9pm.csv

(iii) https://ourworldindata.org/explorers/coronavirus-data-explorer

(iv) https://ourworldindata.org/covid-models

(v) https://ourworldindata.org/covid-models#youyang-gu-yyg

Figure 72 Dashboard data

Notice that the estimated number of infected cases is huge, even for counties where the number of confirmed cases is tiny, as shown in column ii). So, for South Korea we have 4 confirmed cases and 44,232 estimated infected cases. This pattern is repeated for the other countries.

We can compare this with another dashboard, OurWorldInData's Covid-19 dashboard, which provided two measures of confirmed cases [916], columns (iii) and (iv), showing confirmed cases on the 29th January 2020 for the same countries (it probably won't surprise you that OurWorldInData actually have two sets of confirmed case numbers available in different parts of their website).

The table shows three different values for confirmed cases, two from OurWorldInData and one from JHU, reflecting a huge amount of uncertainty about these figures, suggesting chaotic differences in data definition, and data collection standards, which will be affected by administrative delays etc. A good article describing this problem in data collection was written by Justin Hart in April 2020 and can be found here [917].

So, for South Korea we either have 4, 3 or 0 confirmed cases. Yet JHU was estimating infections in column (i), from their computer model, at 44,232. The Australian confirmed cases were not much different at either 7, 4 or 0 yet the JHU estimated infections was one quarter the size at 9,084 (maybe the model considered differences in population density or some suchlike). But the key message here is the exaggerated scale of the predicted cases compared to the actual cases.

Clearly these epidemiological models appear to 'overshoot' reality. An analogy would be finding a wasp's nest in your attic and assuming that the nest size will grow doubling every hour, like bacteria in a petri dish, until it takes over every other room in the house. Plainly wasp's nests don't operate like that, and we can see that the Covid-19 pandemic also didn't.

These models are not only producing extremely large values but also values that are precise. Statisticians would expect to see confidence intervals here, to reflect inevitable uncertainties, but they are not provided. Furthermore, given the input data includes zero confirmed cases, such confidence intervals should include zero infections, but they do not. Hence, they have a predilection to exaggerate.

This problem can also be found in the computer models used by OurWorldInData. Column (v) shows the output from one of their computer models; they used three SEIR (Susceptible, Exposed, Infectious, Recovered) models - this column shows the output from one. Based on their confirmed case counts, 0 or 3, they estimated 69 infections in South Korea on 29th January 2020. So JHU estimated 44,232 and OurWorldInData estimated 69, which is a whopping difference. The question arises: If you worked in public health which one, would you pick to communicate to decision makers?

If we look back, the public were being told the pandemic was 'going exponential' at various stages throughout 2020, 2021 and 2022. The New York Times [918] even took special care to ensure the public knew what this meant. As usual with the media there was no attempt to caveat or question the exponential assumption; it was simply taken for granted.

As we said OurWorldInData use three epidemiological models. The above table contains the results from one model, estimated infection estimates produced by the YYG model. Figure 73 compares estimates from the other two of the OurWorldInData computer models

(IHME and ICL (Imperial)) from, on 31st December 2021. Notice how much they differ from each other and how much they inflate confirmed cases: by up to 25 times (5 million versus approx. 200k).

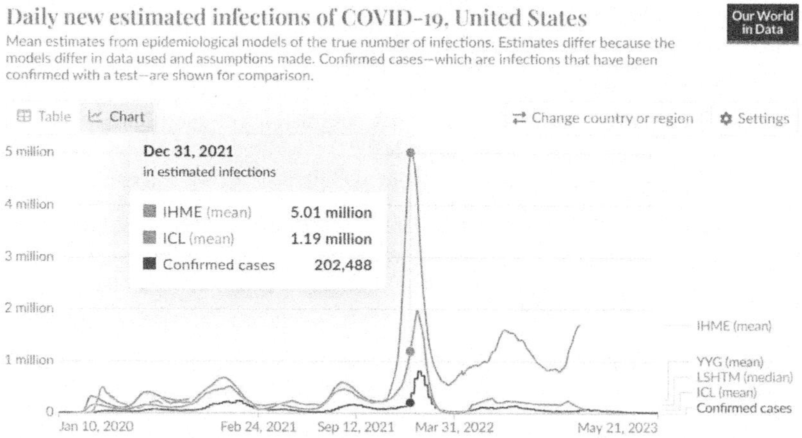

Figure 73 Highly variable model estimates

Clearly, the modelled estimates are of such variability to be not only unusable for prediction purposes but also of such poor quality they should never have been used as surrogates for the 'inevitable future' (and we are leaving aside ethical questions for another day).

Moreover, and it probably will not surprise readers, the accuracy of these models had not been previously established using data from past 'pandemics'. And what is more, there was no gold standard to determine if they could ever be trusted given the known issues with PCR testing and the myriads of unverified assumptions that such models rely on (social distance, size of social network, virus reproduction number, etc.).

It is worth reflecting on the fact that some people were suspicious of the dashboards right from the start in early 2020. Perhaps the earliest expression of concern is recorded in this article [919] again by Justin Hart. In it he quotes John Ioannidis, professor of disease prevention, Stanford University:

> "The data collected so far on how many people are infected and how the epidemic is evolving are utterly unreliable."

We couldn't have expressed the sentiment better ourselves.

Notice we chose to look at model predictions of infections before a pandemic had even been declared. These were huge exaggerations on 29th January 2020 but by March 2020 the exaggerations had themselves grown exponentially.

23.1.2. Ferguson's model- exponential growth in exaggerations

Imperial College's serial exaggerator Neil Ferguson, along with a bevy of coauthors, pulled out his now infamous 13+ year old software program for predicting infectious disease spread and cases and used it to model infections, hospitalisations and mortality from Covid-19. In this report [920] Ferguson et al predicted 510,000 deaths in the UK, and over 2.2 million in the USA, in eight weeks, based on an infection fatality ratio of 0.9%.

Ferguson's model was programmed with inputs that included an arbitrarily assumed virus reproduction number referenced to two prior works:

1. A paper [921] by two Swiss researchers that estimated the reproductive number in China using a simulation model, 'estimations of uncertainty' and a process of elimination using sparse available data, a 'wide range of parameter combinations' and the incredibly named variable 'comparison to past emergencies'; and

2. A paper [922] from Chinese researchers who acknowledge they lacked key epidemiological data but instead guesstimated several important variables, outputting a weakly estimated reproductive number and the only definitive conclusion of their paper - *that human-to-human transmission had occurred.*

Ferguson's model assumes values for reproduction number that are respectively 10% and 20% higher than those of either paper specifically cited for that value.

It was shocking to see the unfailingly doomsday predictions of Neil Ferguson being used yet again as a false premise [923] to direct important government health policy response. At the time Ferguson presented his now infamous Covid-19 report, that almost everyone now agrees was erroneous and exaggerated, despite his history of failures - having already delivered numerous wildly exaggerated predictions for disease transmission and death that were the cause of controversial and expensive UK policymaking (here [924], here [925], here [926], here [927], here [928], and here [929]).

On 26th March 2020 he confirmed on twitter – see Figure 74 - his doomsday predictions (without confidence intervals or any caveats of any kind!)

This was either an input to policy (or an output of policy if you are cynical and sceptically minded) and supposedly formed the basis for the 'flatten the curve' lockdown pushed by UK governmental advisor Dominic Cummings, which was supposed to reduce Covid-19 deaths by half.

With 500+ UK cases, Whitty says, many in No 10 still did not realise how fast things would move:

> "This was a lot of people really not getting what exponential growth was going to mean."

These policies lead to numerous presentations by scientific advisors and government officials where they exulted in the dangers of exponential growth. Here is the Guardian [930] waxing nostalgically about the 'best bits' from the 'pandemic'.

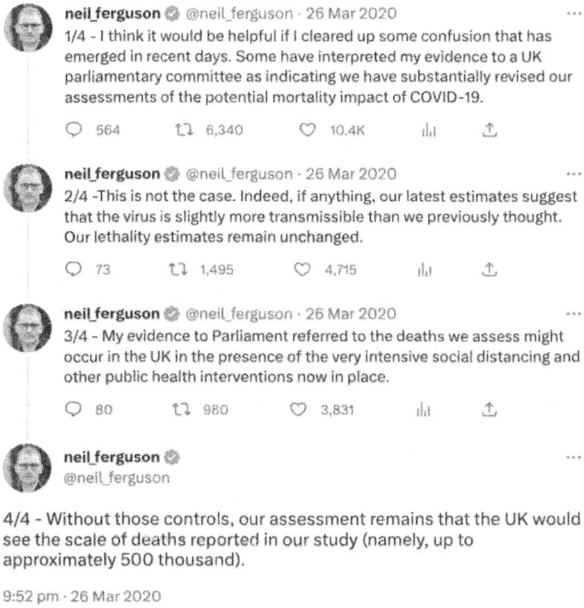
neil ferguson @neil_ferguson · 26 Mar 2020

1/4 - I think it would be helpful if I cleared up some confusion that has emerged in recent days. Some have interpreted my evidence to a UK parliamentary committee as indicating we have substantially revised our assessments of the potential mortality impact of COVID-19.

564 6,340 10.4K

neil ferguson @neil_ferguson · 26 Mar 2020

2/4 -This is not the case. Indeed, if anything, our latest estimates suggest that the virus is slightly more transmissible than we previously thought. Our lethality estimates remain unchanged.

73 1,495 4,715

neil ferguson @neil_ferguson · 26 Mar 2020

3/4 - My evidence to Parliament referred to the deaths we assess might occur in the UK in the presence of the very intensive social distancing and other public health interventions now in place.

80 980 3,831

neil ferguson
@neil_ferguson

4/4 - Without those controls, our assessment remains that the UK would see the scale of deaths reported in our study (namely, up to approximately 500 thousand).

9:52 pm · 26 Mar 2020

Figure 74 Ferguson tweet

23.1.3. How well did the models predict Covid-19 deaths?

When we examine the total number of Covid-19 deaths for 2020 (that is, not just for Ferguson's eight-week period but for the whole of March to December 2020) the variation and inaccuracies in the Covid-19 data that prominent researchers have previously identified several times (here [931], here [932], and here [933]) persisted.

No two UK government data sources agreed on any single figure. For Covid-19 deaths in 2020 the UK Govt Coronavirus Data [934] website reports 86,765. The ONS [935] reported 69,711 and the UKHSA [936] reports 72,178. And the number reported to OurWorldInData is even higher, peaking at 94,998.

In any event, every one of these numbers is only a fraction of the Ferguson prediction of 500,000 or of half of the figure given by Ferguson assuming the lockdowns were effective.

A close look at mortality data for 2020 makes it clear the UK has not had to face a pandemic any worse than that presented by any historical flu season. This is shown in Figure 75 where the age standardised mortality rate in 2020 was comparable to that in 2008. Compared to the 5 years preceding 2020 the excess mortality was circa 8%.

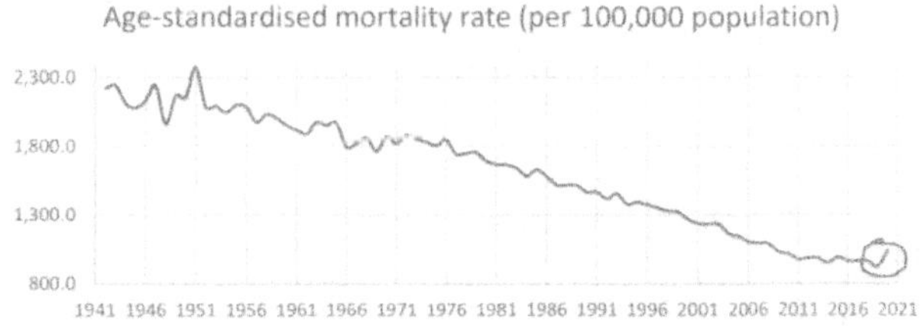

Figure 75 UK age standardised mortality from 1941 to 2020

The complete absence of exponential growth in deaths had already been revealed by April 19th by the Times of Israel [937] which showed that many countries, most notably Sweden, did not experience any exponential growth in cases or deaths despite not enacting major lockdowns (expect in care homes). This was also reported throughout the press, such as here [938], but government policy was immune to this refutation. See Figure 76.

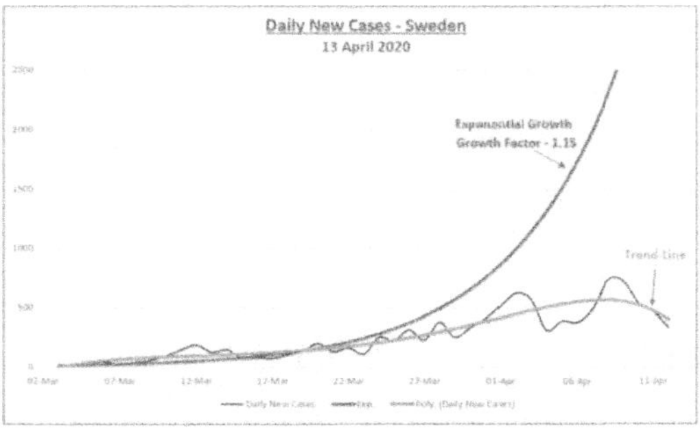

Figure 76 Daily cases in Sweden versus estimates

It is also notable that the Flaxman paper [939] coauthored with Ferguson, unashamedly stated that "our model relies on fixed estimates of some epidemiological parameters (such as the infection fatality rate)", despite the fact that these should have been treated as uncertain estimated values. When applied to Sweden this fixed fatality rate estimate would have resulted in 90,000 deaths by May 2020 when in fact there were only 4,350 deaths.

The FatEmperor compared Sweden's experience, managed by Anders Tegnell who used the WHO 2019 pandemic guidelines, and compared them with that predicted using of Ferguson's model and found that 'Sweden won' (here [940]).

The Spectator magazine produced its own dashboards for the UK SAGE group's modelling, accessible here [941]. Figure 77 shows the chart used by UK Chief Scientific Advisor Patrick Vallence's with his prediction of Covid-19 cases, 21st September 2020, showed just how wrong the exponential exaggerations can be.

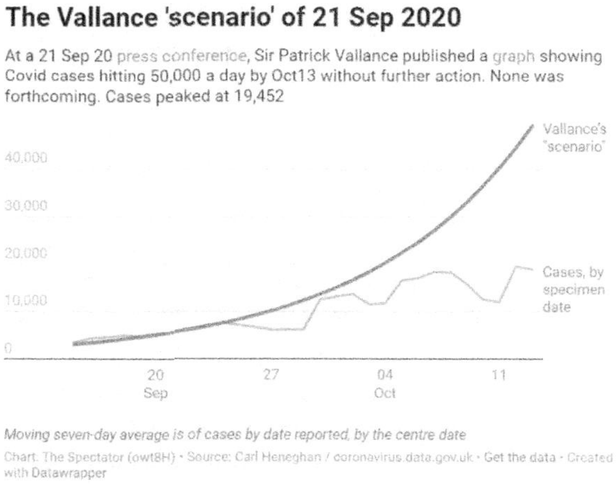

Figure 77 The Valance doomsday scenario

And here is the one for Covid-19 deaths in 2020 (and many of the actual deaths are themselves an exaggeration and not even due to a spreading virus), Figure 78:

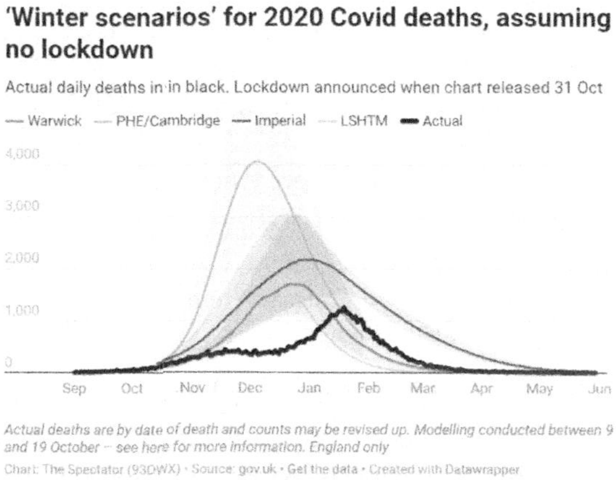

Figure 78 Actual Covid-19 deaths versus modelled

23.1.4. If the UK didn't go exponential could a ship?

So clearly the epidemiological models failed to predict the number of deaths in many countries, some of which were simply ignored (Sweden). If they couldn't predict what happened in a country could they do better in a more controlled, smaller and isolated environment, such as that presented by a cruise ship?

Luckily such a ship was available for study - The Diamond Princess.

Dr. Michael Levitt carefully examined events on the Diamond Princess cruise ship and used this to refute Ferguson's computer model estimates. The full report can be found here [942].

What he found was stunning. The cruise ship offered the perfect environment to model the spread of the virus and its impact on an elderly population in quarantine:

> "Cruise ships are ideal for studying characteristics of infectious disease, both in terms of population and environment. There are many features similar to a community taking place in small spaces with close contact: gambling rooms, theaters, performances, pools, and shared daily facilities like buffets, toilets, spas, elevators, and narrow hallways."

The 'epidemic' began when one passenger began having symptoms on 19 January 2020 and boarded the Diamond Princess the next day. From then all passengers were repeatedly exposed, and hence had a high contact rate and exposure.

He found that the actual Covid-19 deaths were a fraction of those that might be estimated using Ferguson's computer model, and that the mortality burden would only be approximately equal to an additional one month of normal mortality.

Levitt found that:

- Ferguson predicted 59 deaths when in fact there were 7.
- The deaths were 'with' Covid-19 not 'of' Covid-19.
- He had to tweak an unrevealed 'fudge factor' or the herd immunity threshold to get Fergusons model to match his published estimates for the USA, UK and Diamond Princess.
- The inaccuracy in Ferguson's model was calculated by dividing the actual deaths by the predicted deaths (actual were 12% of predicted).
- When applied to the UK the revised estimate was 61,310 deaths.

Levitt took these calculations to the UK SAGE group and Professor Sir David Spiegelhalter in March 2020, after Spiegelhalter had published an article [943] on Covid-19 mortality risk. Levitt claims Spiegelhalter's estimates also turned out to be exaggerations, but in any case, Levitt was simply ignored and warned off.

Levitt believed the reason the Ferguson (ICL-Ferguson) model was mainly wrong because:

> "Part of the reason ICL-Ferguson's estimates were so wrong may be that they used a CFR as an IFR. Despite accusations levelled at those who opposed lockdowns that they were confusing infections with cases, it was in fact Neil Ferguson and ICL themselves who appear to have confused or conflated the two. An IFR should be lower than a CFR, and as Dr. Levitt knew from his work on China, the ICL-Verity IFR was far too high. It is actually much closer to case fatality ratio, not an infection fatality ratio."

Additionally, the fact that it ignored asymptomatics, didn't properly account for different infection rates in different population age strata and miscalculated herd immunity also led to overestimates.

Despite these issues lessons were not learnt. The Ferguson (Imperial) model, and other models used by OurWorldInData, as demonstrated in the previous section, continued to massively differ and exaggerate the level of infections and deaths and did so beyond 2020.

No one thought to look back at what earlier estimates were being produced by such models. If we look again at the estimates form JHU, we had almost 7 million infected in China on 29th January 2020 and 116,000 in Thailand. Applying Ferguson's 1% infection fatality rate would predict over a thousand deaths in Thailand and 70,000 deaths in China. Yet Thailand would experience no deaths throughout 2020 and China peaked at just over 5,700 and did not reach that until 2023!

We think Levitt was being kind. But he was also over certain of his prognostications. After all, how is one supposed to know the exact parameter values needed to predict a pandemic right at the start of a pandemic? And how uncertain should they be assumed to be?

Also, how do you know you even have a pandemic on your hands? Levitt assumed the label 'Covid-19' was meaningful and independent of the PCR test and that the symptoms of Covid-19 were in some way differentiable from other respiratory illnesses. We now know this is not the case.

23.1.5. If a ship can't go exponential how about a single person?

If epidemiological models fail spectacularly in complex systems, such as those presented by countries and ships, surely, they could predict viral infection of a single person or between two people?

Jonathan Engler has written [944] about a SARS-CoV-2 virus challenge experiment, reported here [945], where they tried to give people 'Covid-19' and failed. This includes vaccinated and unvaccinated experimental volunteers, each of which were given the virus via nasal droplets. None developed symptoms (the paper says: "unable to induce sustained infection in any volunteers").

Unfortunately, this isn't new. Jonathan Engler points out that Rossenau could not force infection of influenza between people in 1918. Sure, there are studies that demonstrated flu shedding (here [946] and here [947]) but, critically, did not demonstrate transmission.

If infection cannot be forced in a controlled environment how can epidemiologists hope to model viral transmission dynamics in complex societies with mixed populations?

23.1.6. Neil and Fenton's epidemiological model

As an aside, it is worth mentioning that we ourselves attempted to estimate the infection prevalence and fatality rates for Covid-19 and reported our model in this article [948] published in the journal of risk research in May 2020. Our estimate of the infection fatality rate was 0.3%-0.5%, which wasn't 'too bad' and perhaps comparable to the flu. However, as we have discussed here [949], we were naïve and too trusting of the authorities, but also at that time we were blind to the iatrogenic healthcare effects and the issues with PCR testing. Additionally, from the estimated community prevalence rates in different countries and regions it was clear there was no evidence for exponential spread.

23.1.7. Conclusion

We are left with the conclusion that epidemiological models of respiratory pathogens produce hopelessly exaggerated estimates based on assumptions about parameters that are either unknowable or are so difficult to measure that their credibility is highly suspect.

Given it is likely there are many models as PhD qualified epidemiologists it difficult to imagine which model might be trusted a priori. Even 'averaging' the results of many models looks fruitless given the wide uncertainties in the inherent inaccuracy of outputs produced by each.

Moreover, the fundamental mechanism at play - infection and transmission - is something we know next to nothing about and for some inexplicable and odd reason looks to be subject to ongoing disinterest from virologists, epidemiologists and public health wonks. Likewise, as well as being blind to the harmful effects of the non-pharmaceutical interventions being modelled, they also neglected the impact of harmful medical interventions and policies.

Finally, these computer models are built on the assumption a pandemic has started. Unfortunately, this provides an inevitable hidden incentive to confirm the belief there is indeed a pandemic to be modelled and a reputation to be made.

23.2. We were right!

The UK ONS now admit that deaths in the vaccinated were categorised as unvaccinated in 2021 (23 May 23 2024).

In 2021 when the UK ONS (Office for National statistics) started releasing its vaccine by mortality status reports we exposed that there were large spikes in the *non-covid* death rates in the 'unvaccinated'. These spikes in mortality coincided with the first main vaccine rollout and did so for each age group (see this report [950]. for example).

We asserted that these obvious anomalies were a result of the standard ONS procedure of categorising anyone within 20 days of their first dose as 'unvaccinated'. However, in our own discussions with the ONS they maintained that, although that method ***was*** used for their efficacy calculations, it was ***not*** used when it came to mortality. They clearly said that a person dying any time after vaccination was correctly categorised, as a vaccinated death, in the mortality data they regularly released to the public and which formed the basis of a massive public communication campaign encouraging vaccination.

To 'explain' the spikes the ONS pushed the implicit assumption that there was a phenomenon called the 'healthy vaccinee' effect, whereby they claimed that people 'close to death' were not vaccinated. And they made this bold claim without any data to support it whatsoever.

Apart from the fact that this would have contradicted the NHS policy at the time we showed that, while a healthy vaccinee effect might have partly explained the longer term lower non-covid mortality rates in the vaccinated, it could not possibly have explained those spikes in mortality rates.

They could ***only*** be explained by categorising deaths shortly after vaccination as unvaccinated. Yet the ONS, along with many of the staunchest covid vaccine disciples, doubled down on their insistence that such miscategorisation did not occur. To them all the anomalies in the ONS data could only be explained by the hallowed 'healthy vaccinee effect'.

Later, the ONS did actually claim [951] that there was indeed an 'unhealthy vaccinee effect' but did so to explain other anomalies in the data. Clearly the ONS was so self-serving they did not see the contradictions between these claims and simply wanted to have their cake and eat it. As a result of a subject access request that Clare Craig submitted to the ONS we have now found out that we were correct after all!

Clare has posted on this twitter/X thread [952], an internal ONS email confirming that the NIMS database of vaccinated people, that the ONS relied upon, had excluded those people who had died before vaccine records had been sent back to the central system, as shown in Figure 79:

[redacted]

From: [redacted]
Sent: 28 March 2023 11:04
To: [redacted]
Subject: FW: New concerns regarding Deaths by vaccination status data

Hi all,

Any view on that? [redacted] Clare rightly pointed out in the past that te NIMS data were incomplete (eg excluding people who had died before vaccine records had been sent back to the central NIMS system).

[redacted]

Thanks
[redacted]

Figure 79 FOI email release

When we pointed out to the ONS exactly this possibility for miscategorisation in 2021 they continued to deny that it had happened (see Table 8 of our report here [953]).

Why is this so important? Because the ONS data - possibly more so than any other source of data in the world - was used to bolster the claim that the vaccines were highly effective and safe.

And, as we have always argued, and which is now certain, any claims of efficacy and safety based on their data were completely illusionary and subject to the cheap trick [954] of miscategorisation whereby even a placebo - or something even worse - could be 'shown' to be safe and effective.

They therefore lied and intentionally created and spread misinformation. We were accused of conspiracy thinking and our reputations were tarnished as a result.

But we were right!

Chapter 24. Conclusions and Recommendations

This book has presented our journey through the Covid-19 event in diary form based on our blog and substack articles starting March 2020. In doing so we have provided an honest chronological account of how our analyses, models, hypotheses, and conclusions changed as the 'pandemic' evolved. This is not a standalone book about events during the Covid-19 event. We make no claim of completeness. We therefore recommend that it be read alongside other work and contrasted and compared with a sceptical eye and careful balancing of arguments and data on all sides.

For several years prior to the Covid-19 event, we had already been sceptical of the mainstream media narrative on many important world events. Also, despite having senior academic posts at a leading research university, we were also quiet dissidents from the so-called progressive academic conformity, much of which was driving the mainstream media narrative on topics such as climate change and political science. Nevertheless, when the Covid-19 event first hit we were not aware of the extent to which academics, media and globalist organisations like the WHO and WEF would be prepared to create a narrative that was not based on serious evidence. So, given we had no direct clinical experience, when we first tried to make sense of what was happening, we relied on the assumption that a novel deadly virus was circulating the world, that the PCR test to diagnose the virus was reliable, and that the reported case and death data based on this diagnostic test were sufficiently accurate to be meaningful.

Before we discovered that none of those assumptions were correct, we were more concerned that governments around the world were basing lockdown decisions on mathematical simulation models of disease spread that we knew were wildly inaccurate. Therefore, we were concerned at the unprecedented decision to lockdown country after country, especially as there had been no attempt at cost-benefit analysis nor much of any debate about the ethical and constitutional basis for these unprecedented actions. Thus, even if lockdowns could genuinely stop or reduce the spread of "the virus", we did not believe that such draconian removal of civil liberties could ever be justified.

Our concerns were heightened by our knowledge that many of the academic members of the UK government's SAGE committee held extreme authoritarian views. Indeed, we were shocked that the academic on SAGE who was leading the advice on behavioural change, was a known Communist Party member. Therefore, it was not unsurprising that the government adopted the recommendation to 'increase the level of fear' in the population to ensure conformance to the new measures. That such recommendations were made and accepted in March 2020 – and on the day after the UK Advisory Committee on Dangerous Pathogens (ACDP) determined that Covid-19 should no longer be classified as a high consequence infectious disease, and hence there was no pandemic - is especially scandalous. It was also clear that many academics revelled in the first lockdown and were pushing the narrative that such lockdowns were also 'helping to combat climate change'.

Our concerns triggered us to look more deeply into the Covid-19 event. While the journey we have documented has taken many twists and turns in the four years since, we believe the key take-away conclusions, and brief recommendations, are as follows (grouped into appropriate categories).

24.1. Virus origins

- A thorough review of the available evidence suggests that the emergence of a novel engineered virus is the least likely explanation for the event known as the 'covid pandemic'.
- The discovery of 'novel' viruses is a function of how determined we are to find them - the more we look the more we find, suggesting that the attribution of novelty to a virus is as much the result of a politicized process rather than something based on an objective analysis of its properties.
- There is no good evidence that the many and complex hurdles in front of deliberately engineering viruses to become more pathogenic or transmissible in humans have been overcome.
- The theory that there was a long-standing but hitherto undetected virus endemic in animal (and possibly human) reservoirs is difficult if not impossible to falsify.
- There are other possible explanations for the sudden and rapid global appearance and spread of a specific sequence than the spread of a novel virus. The available virological and epidemiological evidence does not adequately support either the lab leak or the wet market theories for the origins of the virus.
- The idea that the virus escaped a laboratory, that created a deadly pathogen using Gain-of-Function research, or spontaneously appeared in wet market in Wuhan is incredible on its face. The most likely explanation is that of prior endemicity: the viral signal was long established in nature but novel to discovery.
- SARS-CoV-2 is simply one of thousands of viruses, the majority of which are undiscovered, belonging to a constantly co-evolving swarm, all of which cause near identical symptoms in humans. Or to put it another way, it is just another cold virus that prior to 2020 would be no big deal.
- We therefore suggest that it would be more apt to refer to 'Claim-of-Function' than 'Gain-of-Function' research.
- In this regard if there really was a function gained by the virus it was the power to help trick humanity into a dramatic act of self-harm.

24.2. Covid-19 lethality

- It is not possible to measure the lethality of a virus, or any disease, independently of the measures taken in response to it, including treatment. Despite this caveat it was clear from very early on that 'the virus' was much less deadly than was being claimed by government and public health sources. Indeed, it was certainly no more deadly than the seasonal flu.
- There was an absence of excess mortality or morbidity in many countries and cities that were supposedly suffering from a pandemic assault. It was a 'pinpoint'

pandemic that spared most of the globe's population including the elderly and vulnerable, who were supposedly at great risk.

- Where there were local peaks in mortality in Spring 2020 these were the result of the public health response to the pandemic rather than the virus. The decision of the authorities to withdraw antibiotics, to increase the use of palliative care opioid medication, coupled with DNR (do not resuscitate) orders, ventilation and social isolation all contributed to increased mortality in the elderly and vulnerable sub-populations.
- Those who were recorded as having died of Covid-19 were either wrongly labelled as having died *of* the virus rather than *with* the virus, or if they died of a respiratory disease their death was likely caused by untreated bacterial pneumonia infection or from other iatrogenic harms (or the data was manipulated).
- Many Covid-19 deaths were simply incidental because the changes to death certification ensured deaths from other causes were simply recategorised as caused by Covid-19.
- FOI responses show UK hospital ICUs were never overrun with Covid-19 cases. The special pandemic surge Nightingale hospitals never treated a single patient for the new disease.
- In the entire two-year period when the vast majority of Covid-19 classified deaths occurred in England (from Jan 2020 until Dec 2021) less than 5% of the (Covid-labelled) deaths in UK hospitals were people who did not have at least one major underlying comorbidity. And even most of those were not hospitalised because of Covid-19 but rather with it. Only 3 deaths in total of people under 20 were in people without at least one major underlying comorbidity. Evidence from the Diamond Princess cruise ship shows no elevated mortality and does so in the age group supposedly most at risk.
- Large differences in fatality and infection rates point to what occurred in some cities and regions being more similar to isolated mass casualty events than a pandemic.

24.3. PCR testing

- Anybody with a positive PCR test result was classified as a Covid-19 case irrespective of whether they had, or went on to develop, symptoms. Anybody hospitalised who had a PCR positive test within 14 days prior to hospitalisation or any time while hospitalised, was classified as a Covid-19 hospitalisation irrespective of the reason for hospitalisation. Anybody who died, of whatever cause, within 28 days of a positive PCR test was classified as a Covid-19 death. As millions of people without symptoms were tested regularly, these definitions were used to massively inflate the number of Covid-19 cases, hospitalisations and deaths.
- The claim that '1 in 3' have the virus but are unaware of it was massively exaggerated based on fabricated statistics and fraudulent PCR testing.
- The PCR test was never an accurate test. It could be easily manipulated in multiple ways and was not specific to the virus signal SARS-CoV-2. Indeed, the positive

results from a large proportion of PCR tests were likely caused by everyday human coronaviruses, influenza and other viruses and not the novel virus, or false positives due to cross-contamination.

- Most people testing positive (and hence classified as a Covid-19 case, hospitalisation or death) therefore did not have the SARS-CoV-2 virus, and even if they did have a respiratory infection, any presumptive causative link to the virus, would have been entirely misplaced.
- The perception of risk, amongst medical practitioners and the public (but not the politicians and health bureaucrats and academics) was driven by a casedemic of false positives produced by the overuse of unreliable PCR tests.
- Our view is that PCR tests may well have been adopted in the manner they were so that mass testing resulting in associated high Covid-19 positivity enhanced the public perception of a pandemic.
- WHO guidelines required at least two SARS-CoV-2 virus genes for a Covid-19 positive diagnosis – but at various times positive results were declared for single genes, thus breaching these guidelines.
- Argument around high cycle thresholds, either deliberately amplified or at the least actively tolerated, served to hide the fact that it wasn't low or degraded levels of SARS-CoV-2 that were triggering false positives, but it was rather the presence of cross-reactive pathogens.
- PCR tests might be designed to cross react with competing viruses to meet any required detection threshold. Published results show that the best research German and American research units developed PCR tests that were 100% cross reactive false positive.
- The only circumstance in which a positive PCR test for SARS-CoV-2 might be considered reasonably diagnostic of infection is where there is an unfeasibly strong prior assumption that competing viruses, such as influenzas and competing coronaviruses, had virtually vanished, and when the test is performed in someone with symptoms of a respiratory illness.
- There is also evidence of contamination of primer and probe batches. Quality control problems have already been reported in laboratories and the PCR kits are not standardised or subject to any form of meaningful and independent quality control.
- In the UK there was no correlation between people ill with symptoms, and contacting the emergency services, and those getting a single PCR positive test.
- The argument that there was a genuine pandemic caused by the novel SARS-CoV-2 viral pathogen has largely relied on data from highly inaccurate and unreliable PCR testing. PCR testing was the central tool in what can only be described as a 'casedemic'.
- By defining Covid-19 cases, hospitalisations and deaths based solely on a positive PCR test, and by mass testing of asymptomatic people, Governments around the world were able to easily control the narrative about the progression of the virus and its deadliness. This enabled them to provide false evidence of both the need for lockdowns and the effectiveness of interventions.

24.4. Lockdowns and other non-pharmaceutical interventions

- The epidemiological models from Imperial College, predicting mass deaths without interventions like full-scale lockdown, were based on the same flawed assumptions which proved completely wrong in previous 'pandemics'.
- The UK Government's SAGE committee recommended the lockdowns based on these models without any overall cost-benefit analysis. They then repeated the errors multiple times even when there was actual data on harms and effectiveness available allowing empirical analysis and testing of their models. Knowing the difficulty of implementing such unprecedented measures, behavioural psychologists on SAGE recommended the need for a psychological campaign to increase the level of fear among the population.
- The entire mainstream media was compelled by government to push the fear campaign and censor all dissent. There is no serious evidence that the lockdowns, masks and other social distancing measures stopped the spread of the virus or saved a single life. But there is overwhelming evidence it led to massive societal and economic harms.
- The only 'success' of the lockdowns was that it demonstrated to governments around the world that it was easily possible to get entire populations to surrender their freedom and liberties to government control in the event of a future declared 'emergency'. The Track and Trace programme introduced in the UK in 2020-21 to control the spread of the virus cost £40 billion. There is no evidence it saved a single life.
- The largest studies on masks provided no evidence that they were effective in stopping either infection or transmission.

24.5. Vanishing flu

- There is no compelling empirical evidence that proves SARS-CoV-2 interferes with the flu in a dominant way. Therefore, there is no support for the widespread assumption that SARS-CoV-2 prevents flu transmission or infection.
- Flu did not globally disappear since we know it was playing hide-and-seek in some far-flung places.
- Flu disappeared simultaneously just as SARS-CoV-2 appeared simultaneously across the globe. Flu then reappeared and did so simultaneously globally with no evidence of transmission from place to place. The sequence of these events does not concord with any notion of viral spread.
- Detection of all bacterial and viral pathogens except for SARS-CoV-2 decreased precipitously just when the pandemic was announced. This cannot be explained by viral or bacterial interference.
- If flu has vanished there would surely be reduced evidence of zoonotic transmission of flu in animals, or from animals to humans via animal virus reservoirs. There was no evidence of this.
- There is zero empirical or theoretical evidence to support the idea that non-pharmaceutical interventions, such as masks and social distance, eliminated the flu. Indeed, if they worked for the flu why did they not work to prevent the

transmission of SARS-CoV-2, given that the primary mechanism for both is said to be aerosol transmission?

- The fact that flu did return and co-existed with SARS-CoV-2 during the twindemics of 2021/22 and 2022/23 should be the nail in the coffin for the idea that flu disappeared because of viral interference from a novel interloper.
- The supposed disappearance of the flu and other viruses, including colds, was not because they were 'outcompeted' by the virus. Influenzas and colds did not disappear, but their reported disappearance was caused by manipulative changes to the influenza surveillance and 'influenza like illness' reporting systems coupled with the prioritisation of PCR testing for SARS-CoV-2 over other viruses.

24.6. Vanishing flu detection system

- The WHO changes to death certification guaranteed that influenza as a cause of death, or death cause by other viral pathogens, were displaced by Covid-19.
- Mandatory Covid-19 tests, run at high cycle thresholds and suffering from cross-reactivity with other pathogens, will have resulted in false positives for Covid-19, when the viral pathogen associated with such symptoms may have been flu.
- Quarantines would likely produce a false negative result for someone with flu, even if and when such tests were done (which was exceedingly rarely).
- In many countries testing for flu and other viruses simply ceased and changes to PCR testing guaranteed false positives in the presence of other influenza and coronaviruses. In the UK the flu testing system was effectively closed down and priority was given to testing for SARS-CoV-2.
- Compared to Covid-19, diagnosing flu 'out of season' and during a pandemic known to be caused by Covid-19 faced clinical and bureaucratic barriers, which served to depress the likelihood of reporting flu cases.
- There appears to have been a collective and systemic failure in flu surveillance and flu death reporting systems in the UK during 2020 and into 2021. This failure was not coincidental, and nor were the observed inconsistencies in changing patterns of flu surveillance and reporting.
- The UK FluDetector system reported that flu disappeared in 2020/21. This is contradicted by Google's own data and UKHSA reports, both of which report a clear signal for flu in the UK in 2020/21.
- With no justification the UK FluSurvey system abandoned flu tracking until January 2021 when they announced that the flu season had now restarted, after supposedly witnessing the near eradication of flu in the preceding year.
- Routine mortality reporting by the ONS switched almost entirely to Covid-19 deaths in 2020 and flu was only included in surveillance reports from 2021, thus giving the impression flu had disappeared in the preceding year.
- There were almost as many deaths involving flu as there were involving Covid-19 in the UK in early 2020, yet for only 5% of these flu deaths was flu recorded as the underlying cause of death.
- For the whole of 2020 there was no significant change in the number of deaths in the UK recorded as having been caused by flu, compared to previous years,

directly contradicting the ONS, which deliberately published no comprehensive data on flu. Similarly in the USA the CDC WONDER system reports flu deaths for 2020 at similar levels to those seen in 2015-2019.

- Despite these facts the WHO's international flu surveillance system, FluNet, shows no significant flu for 2020/21 in either the UK or USA.

24.7. The illusion of a pandemic and Covid-19 waves

- There never was a pandemic in the conventional sense, as understood by the public, that involved mass casualties or even the realistic threat of additional risk from a supposedly novel virus. If we had done nothing the world would not have noticed anything unusual.
- The 'massive second wave' in the UK starting autumn of 2020 was driven entirely by the mass testing of asymptomatics which was deemed necessary following the end of the first lockdown. Independent NHS data on people with genuine Covid-19 symptoms shows that there was no such second wave. Yet this wave was used to justify both the second major lockdown and the urgent need for the mass vaccination programme as the 'only way out'.
- Neither was it a mis-managed pandemic as many claim. There was a manufactured illusion of a medical emergency. Our fear of viruses has been artificially manufactured over a long period making the populations of many Western and other countries vulnerable to manipulation and exploitation.
- Governments and public health authorities used mass psychological manipulation to terrify the public with the threat of a novel deadly, highly transmissible 'sci-fi' virus that was typically caused by the common cold or a flu or, if caused by the newly discovered but already endemic SARS-CoV-2 virus, of equivalent (low) risk to the cold or flu.
- The mass casualty events reported in places like Wuhan, Bergamo (Italy) Madrid (Spain) New York City, and even London are inconsistent with what could be expected from a viral outbreak
- While there was a spike in excess deaths in March-April 2020, most of these excess deaths that were attributed to Covid-19 were the result of the inappropriate response to the virus rather than the virus itself (or data manipulation).
- Humanity caused the Covid-19 event – it was pseudo-pandemic or might also be dubbed a 'man-demic'.

24.8. Virus symptom novelty, spread and risk

- The clinical and other symptoms of Covid-19 were no different from other seasonal influenza-like-illnesses. The description of what Covid-19 "was" was reported by doctors as 'different' in different countries and even within countries.
- Covid-19 symptoms are acknowledged to be identical to those associated with colds and flu. This makes each completely indistinguishable from the other based on clinical presentation.

- Despite the similarity of the symptoms of flu with those of SARS-CoV-2 the infection fatality rate for SARS-CoV-2 was said to be different from the flu - its novelty was dependent on its perceived elevated lethality.
- Evidence that SARS-CoV-2 causes a unique condition dubbed spikeopathy, with associated 'blood clots' and unique pulmonary symptoms detectable on CT scans cannot be relied upon. Findings on CT are indistinguishable from those associated with influenza or bacterial pneumonia, except in a small number of cases in the younger age group in New York City during spring 2020 (for which other explanations might better apply).
- Covid-19 was associated with 'blood clots' and 'vascular problems' in 2020, on very weak evidence. Injury and deaths associated with blood clotting were only being widely reported after the vaccines rolled out in 2021 and occurred only in those vaccinated. from 2021 onwards. Vascular injuries blamed on Covid-19 rather than on the vaccines, or on a generic syndrome called 'spikeopathy', which was said to arise from infection by SARS-CoV-2 or the vaccine, are not tenable.
- Similarly, there is no compelling evidence reported linking 'happy hypoxia' and 'dry lung' to SARS-CoV-2 infection.
- From analysis of respiratory deaths data in UK, Australia and the USA there was no significant change in respiratory mortality in 2020 and hence no evidence for a pandemic.
- The pattern of spread of SARS-CoV-2 in spring 2020, and the geographical concentration of the SARS-CoV-2 mortality toll is not what one would expect from a spreading respiratory virus. It is highly localized in specific geographically distant regions and cities. It was a pin-point pandemic.

24.9. Swabs and the 'nasal filter'

- There is no established causal link between a virus or other pathogen discovered in the nasal passages and what may or not be causing respiratory symptoms.
- The inability of swabs to collect causative agents is acknowledged in the medical literature. There is no causal connection between the agent detected in the nose or upper airways and what may be causing symptoms, or lack of them, in the lungs.
- The results of any test are as much determined by the choice of test to apply as by the presence/absence of viruses – 'you will find whatever you want to find'.
- Many people tested will be symptomless, yet the sample taken will contain whatever viruses happen to be around in the air and get trapped in their nose or throat. This is natural - coronaviruses and influenza viruses are trapped by our nasal passages: anyone could just have a few virus particles trapped in their nasal passages, but this does not mean these have made them sick.
- A significant proportion of recently deceased, who have died of other causes, will have detectable levels of influenza and coronaviruses, even though they will not have been diagnosed as infected before death.
- Thus, swabbing as a mechanism of diagnosis is akin to determining the causes of mechanical breakdown in an automobile by inspecting the air filter.

24.10. Bacterial pneumonia

- Conflating pneumonia and Covid-19 repeats an official longstanding tactic of conflating the attribution of influenza and pneumonia. The reduction in the public's perceived threat of flu may have prompted the pharmaceutical industry to attempt a rebranding of the threat along with a new suite of marketable products to respond to that threat.
- The actual burden of risk to hospitalised patients may not have been SARS-CoV-2 (or other viruses) at all but bacterial pneumonia coupled with dystopian treatment protocols, neglect etc.
- High rates of ventilator induced pneumonia were confounded by changes in protocols, delays in admission, and overuse of ventilation etc. and estimates of rates of attribution to SARS-CoV-2 cannot therefore be relied upon.
- Respiratory deaths in hospitals may therefore have been caused by bacterial pneumonia but wrongly attributed to SARS-CoV-2.
- Under modern sanitary conditions large scale pneumonia outbreaks in highly concentrated areas are unlikely to occur naturally. We must look elsewhere for explanations, including the possibility of human agency.
- Given that rates of pneumonia deaths in 2020 were like those seen in previous years, changes in ventilation policy and practices coupled with new PCR testing would be enough to cause the pin-point pandemic effect.
- SARS-CoV-2 might be considered a bystander or decoy virus, and bacterial pneumonia deaths were mistakenly or intentionally used as proof that SARS-CoV-2 was a deadly respiratory pathogen.

24.11. Iatrogenesis

- Many of the elderly and infirm who were said to have died of Covid-19 were instead denied adequate and early antibiotic treatment for what was most probably a bacterial infection leading to pneumonia. The use of ventilators, the inappropriate and unethical use of opioids and social isolation lead to many deaths ascribed to Covid-19. The elderly and vulnerable were being put on an end-of-life pathway, with a huge increase in the use of opioid medication, such as midazolam and fentanyl and the application of do not resuscitate (DNR) orders.
- Incorrect use of ventilators (which were central planks of Western pandemic policy) and the inappropriate use of life-ending drugs and denial of potentially life-saving antibiotics, as well as "softer" issues such as denial of social care, relative visits and the social network which acts as the life-support system for the frail elderly, all contributed to additional mortality.
- The drop in antibiotics correlated with the rise in use of opioids and the change in use of both peak in spring 2020. Antibiotics are essential in a pandemic. Anthony Fauci recommended that stockpiling of antibiotics should also be high priorities for pandemic planning. These stockpiles were either never created or used.
- In the UK and elsewhere a palliative care pathway was introduced for 'end of life' care of Covid-19 patients, and which forbade the use of antibiotics. Where antibiotics were recommended, they were in many cases administered too late,

after bacterial pneumonia had set in. In this way a coordinated policy of euthanasia caused iatrogenic harm and death

- Independent physicians defied government guidance and administered antibiotics and other alternative treatments, such as ivermectin, with some success (though this must be balanced with the beneficial effect of keeping patients away from hospitals).
- Face masking exacerbated the problem, increasing the chance of commensal bacteria and fungi from causing serious lung infections.
- It is the inappropriate use of all these interventions which caused the increased mortality, and not a novel virus.

24.12. Censorship

- Any professionals challenging the 'official' narrative on lockdowns, Covid-19 lethality, or vaccine efficacy were censored, marginalised and ridiculed, called 'covid deniers', 'misinformation spreaders', 'conspiracy theorists', and anti-vaxxers'.
- Medical professionals, journalists and media personalities who refused to remain silent were hounded out of their jobs
- Academics were shunned by their colleagues and students, had their research papers and proposals rejected without proper review, and were disinvited from conferences.
- Dissenters with an online presence were attacked in organised 'twitter storms' demanding they be sacked by their employers (often submitting multiple 'formal' but frivolous complaints) and removed from social media platforms.
- All the major social media platforms censored significant dissenters, in many cases under orders from officials in governments, E.g. the White House. In the case of Facebook, YouTube and twitter/X many accounts were completely removed.
- In the UK, many online attacks on dissenters were organised by an official battalion of the Army called the 77th Brigade.
- Subject Access Information requests made to the Ministry of Defence reveal that Covid-19 dissenters were monitored as a national security threat.

24.13. Vaccine safety and efficacy

- By defining people who tested positive up to 21 days after vaccination as 'unvaccinated' even a 'placebo' vaccine can be shown to be highly effective in the first 3 months of a vaccination programme. It turns out that every major published study showing high vaccine effectiveness applied this 'cheap trick'. Similarly, by treating those who died shortly after vaccination as unvaccinated, the same cheap trick has been used to claim vaccine safety.
- Similarly, the intense scare stories starting in late summer 2021 which claimed that hospitals were being overrun with Covid-19 cases and that almost all of these cases were 'unvaccinated' were based on a mixture of fraudulent data and the miscategorisation of the unvaccinated.

- Concerning safety signals for all the Covid-19 vaccines were evident within weeks of the mass roll-out of the vaccines at the end of 2020. But all attempts to raise public awareness were censored and those raising concerns were subject to vicious coordinated attacks.
- The UK ONS was one of the few national statistics organisations to publish mortality by vaccination status data, but their data were seriously flawed. Not only were they based on a highly biased subset of the population which massively underestimated the proportion of people vaccinated, there was also systemic misclassification and missing vaccinated deaths. Failure to take account of these confounding factors meant that the Covid-19 vaccines were portrayed as having almost miraculous life-preserving properties.
- Data from reporting systems such as VAERS and Yellow Card showed that the level of serious adverse reactions, including deaths, were proportionally orders of magnitude greater than from all previous vaccines dating back 30 years.
- Government bodies including the ONS, UKHSA and MHRA continually produced flawed or misleading data, especially on vaccine safety, but failed to make public corrections when these were pointed out to them. In many cases they simply covered up the errors. The BBC were complicit in promoting government messaging and suppressing any criticism of the same.
- Even using the flawed and biased ONS data, the most recent data on mortality by vaccine status (May 2023) was showing that all-cause mortality was higher in the multiple vaccinated than the unvaccinated in almost every age group. The ONS, and also UKHSA, stopped publishing the data after they ran out of excuses to explain away the adverse data.
- The MHRA has refused to publish the data on vaccine adverse reactions which they collected on 30,000 active participants of the Yellow Card Monitoring Scheme in 2021. This includes crucial information on some 2,000 pregnant women. Yet they, and all arms of the UK Government, declared the vaccines were safe – and strongly recommended – for pregnant and breast-feeding women before any detailed analysis of the data had been conducted.
- The studies claiming the vaccine is safe for pregnant women all suffer from systemic flaws and biases, including especially 'survival bias'
- The Oxford AstraZeneca vaccine proved to be the least safe of the major vaccines used in the UK based on Yellow Card entries. Numerous coroners confirmed deaths of young people as being caused by this vaccine in the UK. It was so widely known to be unsafe that several European countries banned it as early as March 2021 (less than 3 months after its rollout). Although its distribution in the UK was not officially ended until Dec 2023, it was no longer being offered by GPs in the UK as early as May 2021. Yet in June 2021 Dame Sarah Gilbert (who led the AZ vaccine team) was given a standing ovation at Wimbledon.
- The Pfizer RCT (randomized, double-blinded and placebo-controlled trial) of its MRNA vaccine, which claimed to show the vaccine was both safe and "95% effective" was fraudulent in multiple ways. In addition to multiple protocol violations, no safety outcomes were tested in the trial. In fact, there were more

deaths overall in the vaccine arm than the placebo arm, and life changing injuries to several trial participants were ignored.

- An independent analysis of the serious adverse event reports from the ventilators and Moderna RCT trials found the rate of serious adverse events from the vaccines was as high as 1 in 800 doses.
- While it is claimed that 'long covid' affects millions of people, not a single published study had provided any accurate data on the proportion of people suffering from it who have been vaccinated, and the unvaccinated are never reported on separately. We hypothesize that a vastly disproportionate number are simply vaccine injured.

24.14. Recommendations

- The false dichotomy of 'lab leak' versus 'wet market' debate has obscured the other explanation for the pandemic. Prior zoonotic endemicity, coupled with unreliable PCR testing and iatrogenic harm caused the illusion of a pandemic. This explanation needs to be publicly debated, recognised and the reasons for this catastrophe systematically identified and analysed.
- Virological research with the intention of enhancing pathogenicity or transmissibility is unethical and unnecessary and as such should cease.
- The fallacies, dogmas and irrational thinking which underpin virology, vaccinology, epidemiology and much of mainstream medical science have been brutally exposed by the Covid-19 event. If these disciples are to regain public trust they need to engage in root-and-branch scientific and ethical reform.
- The fundamental idea that pandemics are natural rather than man-made events must be challenged. The global pandemic preparedness bureaucracy and the associated enforcement arms of public health must be completely shut down.
- Unethical and immoral pandemic emergency measures that abuse human rights must be banned and these powers placed beyond government use as unconstitutional.
- Vaccine education, trials, research and regulation need wholesale reform, as does the way in which vaccine risks are communicated to the public, and how potential harms and side effects are monitored and reported.
- The choice to take a vaccine, isolate when ill, or take any other treatment for a respiratory (or any other) pathogen should be a matter of personal choice guided by medical advice provided by a physician independent of state, institutional pressure or incentives.
- Freedom of speech must be restored, for scientists and a dissenting public.

References

Chapter 1

[1] https://www.cebm.net/covid-19/global-covid-19-case-fatality-rates/
[2] https://www.bbc.com/future/article/20200401-coronavirus-why-death-and-mortality-rates-differ
[3] https://wherearethenumbers.substack.com/p/coronavirus-country-comparisons-are
[4] https://theconversation.com/coronavirus-country-comparisons-are-pointless-unless-we-account-for-these-biases-in-testing-135464
[5] https://plato.stanford.edu/entries/causal-models/
[6] https://bayesianrisk.blogspot.com/2018/08/second-edition-to-be-published-28.html
[7] https://www.theguardian.com/world/2020/mar/27/coronavirus-test-kits-withdrawn-spain-poor-accuracy-rate
[8] https://7news.com.au/travel/coronavirus/another-country-to-introduce-random-coronavirus-spot-testing-c-770154
[9] https://futurism.com/neoscope/half-coronavirus-carriers-no-symptoms
[10] https://link.springer.com/content/pdf/10.1007/s10608-011-9353-3.pdf
[11] https://doi.org/10.31234/OSF.IO/P39A4
[12] https://arxiv.org/abs/2005.08608
[13] http://doi.org/10.1101/2020.05.04.20090506
[14] https://www.medrxiv.org/content/10.1101/2020.05.06.20092999v1
[15] https://doi.org/10.1101/2020.05.25.20112466
[16] https://arxiv.org/abs/2007.07083
[17] https://www.thelancet.com/journals/laninf/article/PIIS1473-3099(20)30243-7/fulltext
[18] https://www.cnbc.com/2020/03/03/who-says-coronavirus-death-rate-is-3point4percent-globally-higher-than-previously-thought.html
[19] https://www.ons.gov.uk/peoplepopulationandcommunity/birthsdeathsandmarriages/deaths/articles/coronavirusCovid-19relateddeathsbyreligiousgroupenglandandwales/2marchto15may2020
[20] https://blogger.googleusercontent.com/img/b/R29vZ2xl/
[21] https://www.theguardian.com/world/2020/may/07/black-people-four-times-more-likely-to-die-from-covid-19-ons-finds
[22] https://youtu.be/39RZFm4EEzQ
[23] http://causality.cs.ucla.edu/blog/index.php/2020/07/06/race-covid-mortality-and-simpsons-paradox-by-dana-mackenzie/
[24] https://www.medrxiv.org/content/10.1101/2020.06.10.20127621v1
[25] https://probabilityandlaw.blogspot.com/2018/12/book-review-judea-pearl-and-dana.html
[26] http://arxiv.org/abs/2007.07083
[27] https://doi.org/10.1101/2020.07.15.20154286
[28] https://www.qmul.ac.uk/events/digital-library/items/people-and-pandemics--a-better-world.html

Chapter 2

[29] https://youtu.be/jDecehzaVQU
[30] https://coronavirus.data.gov.uk/
[31] https://wherearethenumbers.substack.com/p/uk-plotting-new-covid-cases-per-1000
[32] https://ourworldindata.org/covid-deaths
[33] https://qm-rim.org/wp-content/uploads/2020/09/Neil-et-al-2020-Limits-to-UK-PCR-testing.pdf
[34] https://twitter.com/profnfenton/status/1309813231486218241?s=20
[35] https://www.bmj.com/content/369/bmj.m1808/infographic
[36] https://probabilityandlaw.blogspot.com/2020/07/a-privacy-preserving-bayesian-network.html
[37] https://www.huffingtonpost.co.uk/entry/false-positives-coronavirus_uk_5f686da4c5b6de79b677e909
[38] https://probabilityandlaw.blogspot.com/2020/09/dont-panic-limits-to-what-we-know-about.html
[39] https://theconversation.com/coronavirus-country-comparisons-are-pointless-unless-we-account-for-these-biases-in-testing-135464
[40] https://logicinthetimeofcovid.com/2020/09/07/waiting-for-zero/
[41] https://twitter.com/profnfenton/status/1309813231486218241?s=20
[42] https://wherearethenumbers.substack.com/p/covid19-hospital-admissions-data
[43] https://lockdownsceptics.org/counting-covid-19-cases-is-misleading-everybody/
[44] https://wherearethenumbers.substack.com/p/if-covid-19-is-not-a-high-consequence
[45] https://twitter.com/MartinNeil9/status/1320794985801854976
[46] https://www.gov.uk/government/groups/advisory-committee-on-dangerous-pathogens
[47] https://www.gov.uk/government/news/update-from-sage-delay-phase-modelling
[48] https://twitter.com/MartinNeil9/status/1749163825004253213
[49] https://wherearethenumbers.substack.com/p/time-to-demand-evidence-to-support
[50] https://www.youtube.com/watch?v=adj8MCsZKlg
[51] https://swprs.org/the-trouble-with-pcr-tests/
[52] https://lockdownsceptics.org/how-covid-deaths-are-over-counted/
[53] https://lockdownsceptics.org/lies-damned-lies-and-health-statistics-the-deadly-danger-of-false-positives/
[54] https://spectator.us/covid-19-false-positive-trap-seasonal/
[55] https://twitter.com/ClareCraigPath/status/1312629163036155909?s=20
[56] https://probabilityandlaw.blogspot.com/2021/12/just-discovered-statement-below-on-uk.html
[57] https://www.dailymail.co.uk/health/article-8406621/Coronavirus-tests-return-false-negatives-67-time-theyre-given-four-days-infection.html

Chapter 3

[58] https://covid-dashboard.buckinghamshire.gov.uk/
[59] https://digital.nhs.uk/dashboards/nhs-pathways
[60] https://coronavirus.data.gov.uk/

[61] https://inproportion2.talkigy.com/dashboard/
[62] https://twitter.com/cricketwyvern/status/1338843277232115713?s=20
[63] https://data.london.gov.uk/dataset/coronavirus--covid-19--cases
[64] https://coronavirus.data.gov.uk/details/testing
[65] https://lockdownsceptics.org/pcr-based-covid-testing-has-failed-us/
[66] https://www.england.nhs.uk/coronavirus/publication/pooling-of-asymptomatic-sars-cov-2-covid-19-samples-for-pcr-or-other-testing/
[67] https://www.england.nhs.uk/coronavirus/publication/pooling-of-asymptomatic-sars-cov-2-covid-19-samples-for-pcr-or-other-testing/
[68] https://blogs.bmj.com/bmj/2020/09/30/pooled-testing-for-sars-cov-2-could-provide-the-solution-to-uks-testing-strategy/
[69] https://www.england.nhs.uk/coronavirus/publication/pooling-of-asymptomatic-sars-cov-2-covid-19-samples-for-pcr-or-other-testing/
[70] https://www.england.nhs.uk/coronavirus/publication/pooling-of-asymptomatic-sars-cov-2-covid-19-samples-for-pcr-or-other-testing/
[71] https://probabilityandlaw.blogspot.com/2020/10/why-we-know-so-little-about-covid-19.html
[72] https://academic.oup.com/cid/article/71/16/2073/5828059
[73] https://probabilityandlaw.blogspot.com/2020/12/uk-covid-testing-data-remarkable.html
[74] https://www.eurosurveillance.org/content/10.2807/1560-7917.ES.2020.25.3.2000045
[75] https://covid.joinzoe.com/data
[76] https://www.england.nhs.uk/coronavirus/wp-content/uploads/sites/52/2020/03/guidance-and-sop-covid-19-virus-testing-in-nhs-laboratories-v1.pdf
[77] https://www.cam.ac.uk/coronavirus/stay-safe-cambridge-uni/asymptomatic-covid-19-screening-programme
[78] http://www.doi.org/10.13140/RG.2.2.33939.60968

Chapter 4

[79] https://www.youtube.com/watch?v=p9agUz5cQCk
[80] https://www.independent.co.uk/news/world/americas/nurse-coronavirus-vaccine-tiffany-dover-anti-vaxxers-b1795800.html
[81] https://youtu.be/p9agUz5cQCk
[82] https://podcasts.apple.com/us/podcast/truthers-tiffany-dover-is-dead/id1618512442
[83] https://www.arkmedic.info/p/is-tiffany-dover-responsible-for
[84] https://www.nbcnews.com/tech/misinformation/tiffany-dover-conspiracy-theorists-silence-rcna69401
[85] https://arxiv.org/abs/2102.11612
[86] https://www.bmj.com/content/372/bmj.n208/rr-3
[87] https://www.ons.gov.uk/peoplepopulationandcommunity/healthandsocialcare/conditionsanddiseases/datasets/coronaviruscovid19infectionsurveydata
[88] https://assets.publishing.service.gov.uk/government/uploads/system/uploads/attachment_data/file/959438/Technical_Briefing_VOC_SH_NJL2_SH2.pdf
[89] https://pubmed.ncbi.nlm.nih.gov/31992387/

[90] https://www.who.int/diagnostics_laboratory/eual/200921_final_pqpr_eul_0525_156_00_taqpath_covid19_ce_ivd_rt_pcr_kit.pdf?ua=1#page=77
[91] https://www.who.int/news/item/20-01-2021-who-information-notice-for-ivd-users-2020-05
[92] https://www.ons.gov.uk/peoplepopulationandcommunity/healthandsocialcare/conditionsanddiseases/adhocs/12692covid19infectionsurveyctanalysis
[93] https://arxiv.org/abs/2102.11612
[94] https://amp.theguardian.com/commentisfree/2020/dec/22/new-coronavirus-variant-b117-transmitting?CMP=Share_AndroidApp_Other&__twitter_impression=true
[95] https://doi.org/10.1038/s41564-020-00818-3
[96] Dr John Allen, ONS. Email correspondence to information request from Mr Nicholas Lewis, "Your ad hoc Covid-19 PCR gene detection analysis for the ONS", 22 February 2021.
[97] Zoe (?), ONS. Email correspondence to information request from Mr Nicholas Lewis, ONS, email correspondence to information request from Mr Nicholas Lewis, "ONS ad hoc Covid-19 PCR gene detection analysis", 25 February 2021.
[98] https://www.medrxiv.org/content/10.1101/2020.10.25.20219048v1
[99] https://ons.gov.uk/peoplepopulationandcommunity/healthandsocialcare/conditionsanddiseases/bulletins/coronaviruscovid19infectionsurveypilot/8january2021#the-percentage-of-those-testing-positive-who-are-compatible-for-the-new-uk-variant
[100] https://www.instand-ev.de/System/rv-files/340%20DE%20SARS-CoV-2%20Genom%20April%202020%2020200502j.pdf
[101] https://www.rivm.nl/sites/default/files/2021-02/EQA%2520of%2520Laboratories%2520Performing%2520SARS-CoV-2%2520Diagnostics%2520for%2520the%2520Dutch%2520Population%2520November-2020.pdf
[102] https://wherearethenumbers.substack.com/p/how-wikipedia-defames-and-delegitimizes-anybody-raising-concerns-against-the-who-narrative-on-covid
[103] https://doi.org/10.13140/RG.2.2.33939.60968
[104] https://twitter.com/profnfenton/status/1380468549601398791
[105] https://youtu.be/3qm3zI0j_OA
[106] https://www.medrxiv.org/
[107] https://arxiv.org/
[108] https://www.tandfonline.com/doi/full/10.1080/13669877.2020.1756381
[109] https://twitter.com/ClareCraigPath/status/1380780189941178368
[110] http://www.eecs.qmul.ac.uk/~norman/papers/asymptomatics.pdf
[111] https://www.msn.com/en-us/sports/nfl/nfl-reveals-extensive-restrictions-for-unvaccinated-players-in-training-camp-covid-19-protocols/ar-AAL7siZ
[112] https://youtu.be/39RZFm4EEzQ
[113] https://wherearethenumbers.substack.com/p/paradoxes-in-reporting-of-covid19
[114] http://dx.doi.org/10.13140/RG.2.2.26987.26402
[115] https://wherearethenumbers.substack.com/p/david-fuller-example-of-how-unqualified

[116] https://wherearethenumbers.substack.com/p/how-wikipedia-defames-and-delegitimizes-anybody-raising-concerns-against-the-who-narrative-on-covid

Chapter 5

[117] https://www.thelancet.com/journals/lancet/article/PIIS0140-6736(21)00947-8/fulltext
[118] https://lockdownsceptics.org/2021/05/07/study-claims-pfizer-vaccine-is-95-effective-in-over-65s-but-should-that-be-74/
[119] https://www.fda.gov/media/144245/download
[120] http://dx.doi.org/10.13140/RG.2.2.14176.20483
[121] https://wherearethenumbers.substack.com/p/more-on-the-illusions-of-vaccine-efficacy
[122] https://doi.org/10.1016/S0140-6736(22)00277-X
[123] https://doi.org/10.13140/RG.2.2.30898.07362
[124] http://wherearethenumbers.substack.com/p/the-ons-data-on-vaccine-mortality-is
[125] https://www.washingtoninstitute.org/experts/dr-sharon-alroy-preis
[126] https://www.timesofisrael.com/pfizer-exec-calls-israel-a-sort-of-laboratory-for-covid-vaccines/
[127] https://govextra.gov.il/media/30806/11221-moh-pfizer-collaboration-agreement-redacted.pdf
[128] https://www.frontline.news/post/israel-health-ministry-concealed-manipulated-vaccine-injury-data-say-leaked-documents
[129] https://www.youtube.com/watch?v=8ibKpyKeVEc
[130] https://www.timesofisrael.com/doctors-accused-of-covid-denial-drop-lawsuit-against-top-health-official/
[131] https://twitter.com/profnfenton/status/1612110949279752194
[132] http://wherearethenumbers.substack.com/p/alroy-preis
[133] https://www.spectator.co.uk/article/how-the-lancet-lost-our-trust/
[134] https://wherearethenumbers.substack.com/api/v1/file/ffa5600e-b370-486f-8b58-0abb52eaba3a.pdf
[135] https://wherearethenumbers.substack.com/api/v1/file/96ea7fa2-0ce7-462d-8047-7d2380fc5b4d.pdf
[136] https://dissidentvoice.org/2020/08/lancetgate-why-was-this-monumental-fraud-not-a-huge-scandal/
[137] https://brownstone.org/articles/the-censorship-of-covid-science-three-examples/

Chapter 6

[138] https://www.ons.gov.uk/peoplepopulationandcommunity/birthsdeathsandmarriages/deaths/methodologies/weeklycovid19agestandardisedmortalityratesbyvaccinationstatusenglandmethodology
[139] https://www.ons.gov.uk/file?uri=%2fpeoplepopulationandcommunity%2fbirthsdeathsandmarriages%2fdeaths%2fdatasets%2fdeathsbyvaccinationstatusengland%2fdeathsoccurringbetween2januaryand2july2021/dataset.xlsx

[140] https://www.ons.gov.uk/file?uri=%2fpeoplepopulationandcommunity%2fbirthsdeathsandmarriages%2fdeaths%2fdatasets%2fdeathsbyvaccinationstatusengland%2fdeathsoccurringbetween2januaryand2july2021/dataset.xlsx
[141] https://wherearethenumbers.substack.com/p/all-cause-mortality-rates-in-england
[142] https://www.significancemagazine.com/science/701-misinterpreting-statistical-anomalies-and-risk-assessment-when-analysing-covid-19-deaths-by-ethnicity
[143] https://www.ons.gov.uk/aboutus/transparencyandgovernance/freedomofinformationfoi/deathsintheukfrom1990to2020
[144] http://dx.doi.org/10.13140/RG.2.2.32817.10086
[145] https://youtu.be/DAixfvu6tuY
[146] http://www.eecs.qmul.ac.uk/~norman/papers/inconsistencies_vaccine.pdf
[147] https://wherearethenumbers.substack.com/p/covid-19-claims-and-ludicrous-fact
[148] https://wherearethenumbers.substack.com/p/the-impact-of-misclassifying-deaths-in
[149] https://www.ons.gov.uk/peoplepopulationandcommunity/birthsdeathsandmarriages/deaths/bulletins/deathsinvolvingcovid19byvaccinationstatusengland/deathsoccurringbetween1januaryand31october2021
[150] https://youtu.be/6umArFc-fdc
[151] http://dx.doi.org/10.13140/RG.2.2.14176.20483
[152] https://wherearethenumbers.substack.com/p/update-bmj-rejects-without-review-paper
[153] https://www.researchgate.net/publication/356756711_Latest_statistics_on_England_mortality_data_suggest_systematic_mis-categorisation_of_vaccine_status_and_uncertain_effectiveness_of_Covid-19_vaccination
[154] https://assets.publishing.service.gov.uk/government/uploads/system/uploads/attachment_data/file/1057599/Vaccine_surveillance_report_-_week-8.pdf
[155] https://wherearethenumbers.substack.com/p/debunking-hypothesis-that-healthy
[156] https://www.researchgate.net/publication/357778435_Official_mortality_data_for_England_suggest_systematic_miscategorisation_of_vaccine_status_and_uncertain_effectiveness_of_Covid-19_vaccination
[157] https://coronavirus.data.gov.uk/details/cases
[158] https://coronavirus.data.gov.uk/details/deaths
[159] https://www.england.nhs.uk/statistics/wp-content/uploads/sites/2/2022/04/Publication-definitions-Apr22.pdf
[160] https://www.cdc.gov/mmwr/volumes/70/wr/mm7034e5.htm
[161] http://dx.doi.org/10.13140/RG.2.2.14176.20483
[162] https://www.ons.gov.uk/peoplepopulationandcommunity/birthsdeathsandmarriages/deaths/bulletins/deathsinvolvingcovid19byvaccinationstatusengland/deathsoccurringbetween1januaryand31october2021
[163] https://www.researchgate.net/publication/357778435_Official_mortality_data_for_England_suggest_systematic_miscategorisation_of_vaccine_status_and_uncertain_effectiveness_of_Covid-19_vaccination
[164] https://wherearethenumbers.substack.com/p/why-are-ukhsa-obfuscating-data-on

[165] https://twitter.com/SoutarHamish/status/1499104524023255048?s=20&t=5T-QdKyJz2k03iYCKVSrew
[166] https://youtu.be/IV_9GqTdGF4
[167] https://assets.publishing.service.gov.uk/government/uploads/system/uploads/attachment_data/file/1070356/Vaccine-surveillance-report-week-16.pdf
[168] https://www.instagram.com/p/CcpczmtjY1a/?igshid=YTgzYjQ4ZTY=
[169] https://www.insidethegames.biz/articles/1108104/british-athletes-to-be-fully-vaccinated
[170] https://wherearethenumbers.substack.com/p/censored-youtube-removes-my-video
[171] https://wherearethenumbers.substack.com/p/the-statistical-illusion-of-better-pregnancy-outcomes-for-vaccinated-women
[172] https://www.ncbi.nlm.nih.gov/pmc/articles/PMC9093065/
[173] https://doi.org/10.1126/science.abi9069
[174] http://dx.doi.org/10.13140/RG.2.2.26189.92649
[175] http://dx.doi.org/10.13140/RG.2.2.12472.42248
[176] https://doi.org/10.3389/fped.2021.716898
[177] https://pubmed.ncbi.nlm.nih.gov/33768536/
[178] https://doi.org/10.1038/s41591-021-01627-9
[179] https://investigasi.org/manipulasi-data-ilmiah-untuk-membenarkan-vaksinasi-anak/
[180] https://investigasi.org/tindak-pidana-idai-menyebarkan-berita-bohong-untuk-menciptakan-ketakutan/
[181] https://figshare.com/articles/dataset/English_translation_xlsx/17080991/1
[182] http://www.eecs.qmul.ac.uk/~norman/papers/FrontiersIn_IDAI_study_response.pdf
[183] https://www.thelibertybeacon.com/scientific-journal-censorship-with-dr-robert-malone/

Chapter 7

[184] https://www.bbc.co.uk/mediacentre/2022/unvaccinated-professor-hannah-fry
[185] https://www.normanfenton.com/post/a-critique-of-the-bbc2-documentary-unvaccinated
[186] https://twitter.com/ClareCraigPath/status/1545059907015102464?s=20&t=F3iRtjFPReKsv2S5SsoL6w
[187] https://assets.publishing.service.gov.uk/government/uploads/system/uploads/attachment_data/file/1088929/Weekly_Flu_and_COVID-19_report_w27.pdfhttp://dx.doi.org/10.13140/RG.2.2.28055.09124
[188] http://dx.doi.org/10.13140/RG.2.2.12472.42248
[189] https://probabilityandlaw.blogspot.com/2015/02/the-statistics-of-climate-change.html
[190] https://twitter.com/bbcpress/status/1544970146397229056?s=20&t=U3Gd-DbEjXujsqirn_M8jw
[191] https://www.normanfenton.com/post/bbc-wants-to-understand-why-8-of-the-population-remains-unvaccinated-against-covid

[192] https://www.dailymail.co.uk/health/article-11020717/Did-BBC-team-convince-seven-anti-vaxxers-Covid-jab.html
[193] https://www.pfizer.co.uk/news-and-featured-stories/pfizer%E2%80%99s-vaccine-centre-excellence-launches-university-bristol
[194] https://www.nice.org.uk/Media/Default/Get-involved/Meetings-In-Public/Quality-Standards-Advisory-Committee/QSAC4/DOI-spreadsheet-qsac-4.pdf
[195] https://www.nature.com/articles/s41467-022-30052-w
[196] https://www.frontiersin.org/articles/10.3389/fmed.2022.893292/full
[197] https://www.normanfenton.com/post/bbc-s-independent-vaccine-expert-just-happens-to-be-in-charge-of-pfizer-s-vaccine-centre
[198] https://dailysceptic.org/2022/05/03/looking-into-their-eyes-covid-narrative-dissidents-in-their-own-words/
[199] https://www.dailymail.co.uk/health/article-11020717/Did-BBC-team-convince-seven-anti-vaxxers-Covid-jab.html
[200] https://www.normanfenton.com/post/bbc-wants-to-understand-why-8-of-the-population-remains-unvaccinated-against-covid
[201] https://www.normanfenton.com/post/bbc-s-independent-vaccine-expert-just-happens-to-be-in-charge-of-pfizer-s-vaccine-centre
[202] https://twitter.com/nazarinveronica
[203] https://threadsirish.substack.com/p/prof-hannah-fry-who-presented-bbc
[204] https://twitter.com/vickyborman
[205] https://odysee.com/@MaajidNawaz:d/RadicalEpisode15:b
[206] https://www.normanfenton.com/post/bbc-wants-to-understand-why-8-of-the-population-remains-unvaccinated-against-covid
[207] https://www.icmunlimited.com/our-work/exploring-attitudes-towards-covid-19-vaccinations-for-stv/
[208] https://probabilityandlaw.blogspot.com/2021/10/covid-19-claims-and-ludicrous-fact.html
[209] https://viralimmunologist.substack.com/p/of-29-pregnant-women-that-had-received
[210] https://arkmedic.substack.com/p/the-curious-case-of-the-miscalculated
[211] https://dailysceptic.org/2022/07/21/german-government-acknowledges-covid-vaccines-cause-serious-injury-for-one-in-5000-doses-but-its-own-data-show-the-real-rate-is-one-in-300-doses/
[212] https://www.bbc.co.uk/news/uk-england-tyne-58330796
[213] https://www.bbc.co.uk/news/uk-england-tyne-61885899
[214] https://openvaers.com/
[215] https://probabilityandlaw.blogspot.com/2022/01/no-fancy-statistics-simply-plot-of.html
[216] http://dx.doi.org/10.13140/RG.2.2.28055.09124
[217] https://andrewmadry.substack.com/p/follow-up-to-vaccine-effectiveness
[218] https://iris.ucl.ac.uk/iris/publication/1794138/1
[219] https://www.normanfenton.com/post/a-critique-of-the-bbc2-documentary-unvaccinated
[220] https://youtu.be/ccWOMtmH65U

[221] https://youtu.be/8It4qI9yhzQ
[222] https://rumble.com/v1f7qad-hannah-fry-and-the-bbcs-unvaccinated-exposed-disparities-and-deceptions-par.html
[223] https://off-guardian.org/2022/08/10/the-bbcs-unvaccinated-undisclosed-conflicts-of-interest-part-2/
[224] https://www.bbc.co.uk/contact/sites/default/files/2022-08/18 - 31 July 2022vii.pdf
[225] https://www.normanfenton.com/post/bbc-response-to-my-complain-about-unvaccinated
[226] https://www.normanfenton.com/post/a-critique-of-the-bbc2-documentary-unvaccinated
[227] https://www.normanfenton.com/post/bbc-wants-to-understand-why-8-of-the-population-remains-unvaccinated-against-covid
[228] https://youtu.be/ccWOMtmH65U
[229] https://5fb85da9-953b-4805-9b17-50592f9cfd56.filesusr.com/ugd/d76942_6958df84717c41548cfbc2033097b9f2.pdf
[230] https://5fb85da9-953b-4805-9b17-50592f9cfd56.filesusr.com/ugd/d76942_bec0ea485e9b4af4b18496ca84e37156.pdf
[231] https://d7694293-ffb8-4ed0-a014-3581d49070e4.usrfiles.com/ugd/d76942_523de5e2bd9841fbaf87d988aaacdaee.pdf
[232] https://d7694293-ffb8-4ed0-a014-3581d49070e4.usrfiles.com/ugd/d76942_4572cee2f21d4ceeb43992ba191fd6d9.pdf
[233] https://www.normanfenton.com/post/bbc-response-to-my-follow-up-complaint-about-unvaccinated-documentary
[234] https://d7694293-ffb8-4ed0-a014-3581d49070e4.usrfiles.com/ugd/d76942_acb526c93a584dbc8cc57fb45e93fdab.pdf
[235] https://www.normanfenton.com/post/about-that-ons-estimate-of-only-8-adults-unvaccinated
[236] http://dx.doi.org/10.13140/RG.2.2.12126.92481

Chapter 8

[237] https://www.gov.uk/government/publications/regulatory-approval-of-pfizer-biontech-vaccine-for-covid-19/summary-public-assessment-report-for-pfizerbiontech-covid-19-vaccine
[238] https://www.gov.uk/government/publications/regulatory-approval-of-pfizer-biontech-vaccine-for-covid-19/information-for-healthcare-professionals-on-pfizerbiontech-covid-19-vaccine#pharmacodynamic-properties
[239] https://www.gov.uk/government/publications/covid-19-vaccination-women-of-childbearing-age-currently-pregnant-planning-a-pregnancy-or-breastfeeding/covid-19-vaccination-a-guide-for-women-of-childbearing-age-pregnant-planning-a-pregnancy-or-breastfeeding
[240] https://wherearethenumbers.substack.com/p/a-critique-of-bbc2-documentary

[241] https://www.gov.uk/government/publications/regulatory-approval-of-pfizer-biontech-vaccine-for-covid-19#full-publication-update-history
[242] https://5fb85da9-953b-4805-9b17-50592f9cfd56.filesusr.com/ugd/d76942_524d3ab10f3a474187c6c098fdf7eae1.pdf
[243] https://wherearethenumbers.substack.com/p/uk-government-sneakily-updates-web-page-with-vaccine-report-yet-again
[244] https://www.ons.gov.uk/aboutus/transparencyandgovernance/freedomofinformationfoi/intensivecareuniticuadmissionsofpregnantwomen
[245] https://probabilityandlaw.blogspot.com/2021/09/all-cause-mortality-rates-in-england.html
[246] http://dx.doi.org/10.13140/RG.2.2.28055.09124
[247] https://probabilityandlaw.blogspot.com/2022/07/all-you-need-to-know-to-understand-why.html
[248] http://dx.doi.org/10.13140/RG.2.2.12472.42248
[249] http://dx.doi.org/10.13140/RG.2.2.28055.09124
[250] https://lakaruppropet.se/public-health-agency-reporting-has-distorted-mortality-rates-for-the-unvaccinated-and-vaccinated/
[251] https://arkmedic.substack.com/p/viki-and-the-mutton-crew/comments
[252] https://insulinresistance.org/index.php/jir/article/view/72/228
[253] https://probabilityandlaw.blogspot.com/2022/01/debunking-hypothesis-that-healthy.html
[254] https://wherearethenumbers.substack.com/p/all-you-need-to-know-to-understand-why
[255] https://wherearethenumbers.substack.com/p/more-updates-on-bbc2-documentary-unvaccinated
[256] https://www.researchgate.net/deref/https%3A%2F%2Fassets.publishing.service.gov.uk%2Fgovernment%2Fuploads%2Fsystem%2Fuploads%2Fattachment_data%2Ffile%2F1031157%2FVaccine-surveillance-report-week-44.pdf
[257] https://twitter.com/GidMK/status/1574643817600647168
[258] https://twitter.com/Jikkyleaks/status/1675005406274523137
[259] https://assets.publishing.service.gov.uk/government/uploads/system/uploads/attachment_data/file/1066759/Vaccine-surveillance-report-week-13.pdf
[260] http://dx.doi.org/10.13140/RG.2.2.30898.07362
[261] https://www.ons.gov.uk/peoplepopulationandcommunity/birthsdeathsandmarriages/deaths/datasets/deathsbyvaccinationstatusengland
[262] http://dx.doi.org/10.13140/RG.2.2.28055.09124
[263] http://dx.doi.org/10.13140/RG.2.2.12472.42248
[264] https://code.statisticsauthority.gov.uk/wp-content/uploads/2022/05/Code-of-Practice-for-Statistics-REVISED.pdf
[265] https://d7694293-ffb8-4ed0-a014-3581d49070e4.usrfiles.com/ugd/d76942_bd64e0ebb4754477afd3d9f00bb3dc0f.pdf
[266] https://osr.statisticsauthority.gov.uk/correspondence/ed-humpherson-to-norman-fenton-martin-neil-clare-craig-and-scott-mclachlan-ons-deaths-by-vaccination-status-statistics/

[267] http://wherearethenumbers.substack.com/p/mhra-and-bbc-fail-to-meet-their-own-deadline-for-responding-to-complaints-about-unvaccinated
[268] https://www.thelancet.com/journals/laninf/article/PIIS1473-3099(22)00320-6/fulltext
[269] https://wherearethenumbers.substack.com/p/why-we-cannot-ignore-the-lancet-claim
[270] https://www.astrazeneca.com/media-centre/articles/2021/vaccinating-the-world-op-ed-by-iskra-reic.html
[271] https://doi.org/10.1016/j.amjmed.2022.11.002
[272] https://wherearethenumbers.substack.com/p/a-study-in-stupidity
[273] https://igorchudov.substack.com/p/the-unvaccinated-had-more-car-crashes
[274] https://lawhealthandtech.substack.com/p/we-interrupt-our-regularly-scheduled
[275] https://x.com/ClareCraigPath/status/1602650802186772481
[276] https://youtu.be/LxGSMdE_TN0
[277] http://dx.doi.org/10.13140/RG.2.2.30898.07362
[278] http://dx.doi.org/10.13140/RG.2.2.12126.92481
[279] https://wherearethenumbers.substack.com/p/how-wikipedia-defames-and-delegitimizes
[280] https://open.spotify.com/episode/7uDfZnMddaeZUCSqVHPOBa
[281] https://doi.org/10.1136/bmj.m4037
[282] https://www.ncbi.nlm.nih.gov/pmc/articles/PMC8461570/bin/NEJMoa2110345_appendix.pdf
[283] https://papers.ssrn.com/sol3/papers.cfm?abstract_id=4125239
[284] https://kirschsubstack.com/p/my-latest-all-cause-mortality-survey
[285] https://www.arkmedic.info/p/the-australian-bureau-of-lies-damned
[286] https://doi.org/http:/dx.doi.org/10.13140/RG.2.2.14176.20483
[287] https://doi.org/10.13140/RG.2.2.32817.10086
[288] https://www.ons.gov.uk/peoplepopulationandcommunity/birthsdeathsandmarriages/deaths/datasets/deathsbyvaccinationstatusengland
[289] https://doi.org/10.13140/RG.2.2.12472.42248
[290] https://doi.org/10.13140/RG.2.2.30898.07362
[291] https://twitter.com/TheJikky/status/1601417784587845632
[292] https://doi.org/10.13140/RG.2.2.11570.32962
[293] https://doi.org/10.13140/RG.2.2.12688.28164
[294] https://wherearethenumbers.substack.com/p/the-devils-advocate-an-exploratory
[295] https://www.theepochtimes.com/health/exclusive-cdc-finds-hundreds-of-safety-signals-for-pfizer-and-moderna-covid-19-vaccines_4956733.html
[296] https://childrenshealthdefense.org/defender/cdc-safety-signals-pfizer-moderna-covid-vaccines-et/
[297] https://jackanapes.substack.com/p/cdc-finally-released-its-vaers-safety

Chapter 9

[298] http://pandauncut.substack.com/p/the-lombardy-analysis
[299] https://c2cjournal.ca/2022/03/who-killed-granny-pandemic-death-protocols-in-canadas-long-term-care-facilities/

[300] https://twitter.com/NellyTells/status/1258473555702005760
[301] https://transcriberb.dreamwidth.org/10261.html
[302] https://www.dailymail.co.uk/news/article-8514081/Number-prescriptions-drug-midazolam-doubled-height-pandemic.html
[303] https://twitter.com/Jikkyleaks/status/1624556171964325888
[304] https://www.nice.org.uk/guidance/ng163/resources/covid19-rapid-guideline-managing-symptoms-including-at-the-end-of-life-in-the-community-pdf-66141899069889
[305] http://web.archive.org/web/20200407215603/https:/www.nice.org.uk/guidance/NG163
[306] https://www.bmj.com/content/369/bmj.m1461/rr-1
[307] https://twitter.com/chrislittlewoo8/status/1596913985466486784
[308] https://ugetube.com/watch/a-good-death-jacqui-deevoy-ickonic_mbVzww3HAB6o35v.html
[309] https://open.substack.com/users/66592580-usmortality
[310] https://twitter.com/USMortality/status/1623394604044386309
[311] https://dailysceptic.org/2023/02/17/covid-19-and-excess-deaths-a-defence-of-the-virus-theory/
[312] https://digital.nhs.uk/dashboards/nhs-pathways
[313] https://metatron.substack.com/p/the-fake-pandemic
[314] https://dailysceptic.org/2023/02/17/covid-19-and-excess-deaths-a-defence-of-the-virus-theory/
[315] https://dailysceptic.org/2023/02/24/how-we-know-it-started-in-wuhan/
[316] https://wherearethenumbers.substack.com/p/the-deadly-initial-spring-2020-covid
[317] https://pandauncut.substack.com/p/the-lombardy-analysis
[318] https://woodhouse.substack.com/p/more-data-and-questions-about-spring
[319] https://academic.oup.com/eurpub/article/16/6/583/587693
[320] https://pubmed.ncbi.nlm.nih.gov/36341800/
[321] https://www.nejm.org/doi/full/10.1056/nejmoa032867
[322] https://twitter.com/ClareCraigPath/status/1604954264522358784
[323] https://reaction.life/sage-models-need-a-reality-check/
[324] https://dailysceptic.org/2023/02/23/news-round-up-713/

Chapter 10

[325] https://wherearethenumbers.substack.com/p/more-on-inconsistency-between-official
[326] https://scotland.shinyapps.io/phs-covid-wider-impact/
[327] https://wherearethenumbers.substack.com/p/scottish-cardiac-ambulance-data-shows
[328] https://wherearethenumbers.substack.com/p/the-ons-data-on-vaccine-mortality-is
[329] https://osr.statisticsauthority.gov.uk/correspondence/ed-humpherson-to-norman-fenton-martin-neil-clare-craig-and-scott-mclachlan-ons-deaths-by-vaccination-status-statistics/

[330] https://osr.statisticsauthority.gov.uk/correspondence/ed-humpherson-to-norman-fenton-martin-neil-clare-craig-and-scott-mclachlan-ons-deaths-by-vaccination-status-statistics/
[331] http://wherearethenumbers.substack.com/p/mhra-and-bbc-fail-to-meet-their-own-deadline-for-responding-to-complaints-about-unvaccinated
[332] https://web.archive.org/web/20220707124706/https:/www.bbc.com/mediacentre/2022/unvaccinated-professor-hannah-fry
[333] https://www.bbc.com/mediacentre/2022/unvaccinated-professor-hannah-fry
[334] http://dx.doi.org/10.13140/RG.2.2.28055.09124
[335] http://dx.doi.org/10.13140/RG.2.2.30898.07362
[336] https://wherearethenumbers.substack.com/p/the-impact-of-misclassifying-deaths-in
[337] http://wherearethenumbers.substack.com/p/the-lancet-has-become-a-laughing
[338] https://zenodo.org/record/5243901 .Y8L23BXP0uU
[339] https://www.nejm.org/doi/10.1056/NEJMoa2106599
[340] https://www.ons.gov.uk/peoplepopulationandcommunity/birthsdeathsandmarriages/deaths/datasets/deathsbyvaccinationstatusengland
[341] https://www.dailymail.co.uk/health/article-11775169/Death-rates-NOT-higher-Covid-vaccinated-Brits.html
[342] https://wherearethenumbers.substack.com/p/the-ons-data-on-vaccine-mortality-is
[343] https://youtu.be/DAixfvu6tuY
[344] https://twitter.com/saunasauen/status/1628138191642365958
[345] https://wherearethenumbers.substack.com/p/the-latest-ons-data-on-deaths-by
[346] http://dx.doi.org/10.13140/RG.2.2.30898.07362
[347] https://usmortality.substack.com/p/englands-all-cause-mortality-data
[348] https://igorchudov.substack.com/p/ons-data-25-excess-mortality-among
[349] https://assets.publishing.service.gov.uk/government/uploads/system/uploads/attachment_data/file/1066759/Vaccine-surveillance-report-week-13.pdf
[350] https://metatron.substack.com/p/england-deaths-by-vaccination-status
[351] https://twitter.com/ExcessBurden/status/1628816947788775425
[352] https://drclarecraig.substack.com/p/deaths-among-the-ghost-population
[353] https://boriquagato.substack.com/p/the-new-uk-ons-data-is-out-and-its
[354] https://wherearethenumbers.substack.com/p/postmodern-science-delivers-immortality

Chapter 11

[355] https://www.bbc.com/future/article/20201009-could-social-distancing-make-the-flu-extinct
[356] https://www.eugyppius.com/p/the-mysterious-disappearance-of-influenza
[357] https://app.powerbi.com/view?r=eyJrIjoiZTkyODcyOTEtZjA5YS00ZmI0LWFkZGUtODIxNGI5OTE3YjM0IiwidCI6ImY2MTBjMGI3LWJkMjQtNGIzOS04MTBiLTNkYzI4MGFmYjU5MCIsImMiOjh9
[358] https://wherearethenumbers.substack.com/p/playing-hide-and-seek-with-the-flu
[359] https://wherearethenumbers.substack.com/p/peek-a-boo-flu
[360] https://www.hartgroup.org/the-sars-cov-2-and-influenza-see-saw/

[361] https://blogs.bmj.com/bmj/2021/08/09/the-changing-pattern-of-respiratory-viruses-during-the-covid-19-pandemic-what-does-the-future-hold/
[362] https://www.ncbi.nlm.nih.gov/pmc/articles/PMC8798701/
[363] https://www.ncbi.nlm.nih.gov/pmc/articles/PMC8879759/
[364] https://pubmed.ncbi.nlm.nih.gov/34931581/
[365] https://pubmed.ncbi.nlm.nih.gov/33603116/
[366] https://www.nature.com/articles/s41422-021-00473-1
[367] https://www.ncbi.nlm.nih.gov/pmc/articles/PMC8135706/
[368] https://www.independent.co.uk/news/health/flu-cases-covid-england-phe-latest-b1805124.html
[369] https://wwwnc.cdc.gov/eid/article/28/10/22-0396_article
[370] https://www.nature.com/articles/s41467-021-21361-7
[371] https://pubmed.ncbi.nlm.nih.gov/35262019/
[372] https://onlinelibrary.wiley.com/doi/full/10.1002/jmv.26163
[373] https://wherearethenumbers.substack.com/p/do-not-seek-and-ye-shall-not-find
[374] https://en.wikipedia.org/wiki/Twindemic
[375] https://www.bbc.co.uk/news/world-59656385
[376] https://www.independent.co.uk/news/world/middle-east/covid-variant-symptoms-flurona-flu-b1996224.html
[377] https://www.washingtonpost.com/health/2022/01/05/flurona-coronavirus-flu-symptoms/
[378] https://thedailybeagle.substack.com/p/how-test-kits-are-used-to-perpetuate
[379] https://collateralglobal.org/wp-content/uploads/2022/02/CG-Report-7-PCR-Testing-in-the-UK-During-the-SARS-CoV-2-Pandemic-%E2%80%93-Evidence-From-FOI-Requests.pdf
[380] https://wherearethenumbers.substack.com/p/the-smoking-man-emails
[381] https://www.sciencedirect.com/science/article/pii/S2667038021000065
[382] https://assets.publishing.service.gov.uk/government/uploads/system/uploads/attachment_data/file/897832/Rapid_Assessment_of_GenMark_ePlex_SARS_CoV_2_test_V1.00e.pdf
[383] https://pubmed.ncbi.nlm.nih.gov/33340934/
[384] https://www.health.gov.au/sites/default/files/documents/2020/06/post-market-validation-of-the-beijing-genomics-institute-bgi-sars-cov-2-real-time-pcr-platform.pdf
[385] https://pubmed.ncbi.nlm.nih.gov/32361322/
[386] https://www.ons.gov.uk/aboutus/transparencyandgovernance/freedomofinformationfoi/otherusesandaccuracyofpcrtests
[387] https://mobile.twitter.com/PanData19
[388] https://wherearethenumbers.substack.com/p/on-false-positives-in-covid19-testing
[389] https://www.gov.uk/guidance/high-consequence-infectious-diseases-hcid
[390] http://web.archive.org/web/20200714175623/https://www.cdc.gov/flu/professionals/diagnosis/table-flu-covid19-detection.html
[391] https://syndromictrends.com/
[392] https://seattleflu.org/pathogens
[393] https://www.cdc.gov/flu/about/burden/index.html

[394] https://off-guardian.org/2023/03/30/wuhans-mystery-illness-is-covids-foundational-lie/
[395] https://substack.com/profile/26236720-sl/note/c-17999659

Chapter 12

[396] https://wherearethenumbers.substack.com/p/sensors-set-to-off
[397] http://web.archive.org/web/20200630234109/https://www.cdc.gov/coronavirus/2019-ncov/hcp/broad-based-testing.html
[398] https:/www.cdc.gov/coronavirus/2019-ncov/hcp/testing-overview.html
[399] https://www.cdc.gov/flu/professionals/diagnosis/algorithm-results-not-circulating.htm
[400] https:/www.cdc.gov/coronavirus/2019-ncov/hcp/broad-based-testing.html
[401] https://www.nature.com/articles/ni1343
[402] https://www.ncbi.nlm.nih.gov/pmc/articles/PMC9348440/
[403] https://assets.publishing.service.gov.uk/government/uploads/system/uploads/attachment_data/file/947881/Weekly_Flu_and_COVID-19_report_w52.pdf
[404] https://cdn.who.int/media/docs/default-source/classification/icd/covid-19/guidelines-cause-of-death-covid-19-20200420-en.pdf
[405] https://web.archive.org/web/20210803213630/https:/cambslmc.org/wp-content/uploads/2020/11/COVID.-Verification-and-certification-V7-11-05-2020.pdf
[406] https://www.who.int/teams/global-influenza-programme/influenza-covid19/sentinel-sites-and-specimens
[407] https://wherearethenumbers.substack.com/p/finding-the-flu-is-easy-just-google
[408] https://www.bennettinstitute.cam.ac.uk/blog/pandemic-what-use-google/
[409] https://www.gov.uk/guidance/sources-of-uk-flu-data-influenza-surveillance-in-the-uk
[410] https://trends.google.com/
[411] https://www.who.int/tools/flunet
[412] https://wherearethenumbers.substack.com/p/do-not-seek-and-ye-shall-not-find
[413] https://www.gov.uk/guidance/sources-of-uk-flu-data-influenza-surveillance-in-the-uk
[414] https://fludetector.cs.ucl.ac.uk/
[415] https://www.gov.uk/government/collections/weekly-national-flu-reports
[416] https://flusurvey.net/
[417] http://web.archive.org/web/20210120051145/https:/flusurvey.net/en/results/
[418] http://web.archive.org/web/20201001191550/https:/flusurvey.net/en/results/
[419] http://web.archive.org/web/20210120051145/https:/flusurvey.net/en/results/
[420] http://web.archive.org/web/20211130030556/https:/flusurvey.net/en/results/
[421] https://assets.publishing.service.gov.uk/government/uploads/system/uploads/attachment_data/file/1003027/Weekly_Flu_and_COVID-19_report_w28_v2.pdf
[422] https://assets.publishing.service.gov.uk/government/uploads/system/uploads/attachment_data/file/1050508/Weekly_Flu_and_COVID-19_report_w4.pdf
[423] https://www.gov.uk/guidance/covid-19-and-influenza-point-of-care-testing-results-how-to-report

[424] https://assets.publishing.service.gov.uk/government/uploads/system/uploads/attachment_data/file/942969/Weekly_Flu_and_COVID-19_report_w50_FINAL.PDF
[425] https://wherearethenumbers.substack.com/p/finding-the-flu-is-easy-just-google/comment/16589326
[426] https://www1.racgp.org.au/newsgp/clinical/physical-distancing-and-good-hand-hygiene-australi
[427] https://cdn.who.int/media/docs/default-source/influenza/pcr-wg/report-of-the-11th-meeting-of-the-who-working-group-for-the-molecular-detection-and-subtyping-of-influenza.pdf
[428] https://www.youtube.com/watch?v=oYzdF-VQjvw&t=5s
[429] https://professionals.northwell.edu/sites/northwell.edu/files/2020-03/viral-respiratory-culture-v-vcr-change-3-5-2020pdf.pdf
[430] https://x.com/Wood_House76/status/1635856574374608896
[431] https://www.ons.gov.uk/peoplepopulationandcommunity/birthsdeathsandmarriages/deaths/datasets/weeklyprovisionalfiguresondeathsregisteredinenglandandwales
[432] https://www.ons.gov.uk/file?uri=/peoplepopulationandcommunity/birthsdeathsandmarriages/deaths/datasets/weeklyprovisionalfiguresondeathsregisteredinenglandandwales/2020/publishedweek532020.xlsx
[433] https://www.ons.gov.uk/file?uri=/peoplepopulationandcommunity/birthsdeathsandmarriages/deaths/datasets/weeklyprovisionalfiguresondeathsregisteredinenglandandwales/2021/publishedweek522021.xlsx
[434] https://www.ons.gov.uk/aboutus/transparencyandgovernance/freedomofinformationfoi/deathsfrominfluenzabyagegroupin2020
[435] https://www.ons.gov.uk/peoplepopulationandcommunity/birthsdeathsandmarriages/deaths/datasets/weeklyprovisionalfiguresondeathsregisteredinenglandandwales
[436] https://www.ons.gov.uk/peoplepopulationandcommunity/birthsdeathsandmarriages/deaths/bulletins/deathsregisteredweeklyinenglandandwalesprovisional/latest
[437] https://www.ons.gov.uk/peoplepopulationandcommunity/birthsdeathsandmarriages/deaths/bulletins/deathsinvolvingcovid19englandandwales/deathsoccurringinmarch2020
[438] https://www.ons.gov.uk/peoplepopulationandcommunity/birthsdeathsandmarriages/deaths/bulletins/deathsinvolvingcovid19englandandwales/deathsoccurringinmarch2020/relateddata
[439] https://www.ons.gov.uk/file?uri=/peoplepopulationandcommunity/birthsdeathsandmarriages/deaths/datasets/weeklyprovisionalfiguresondeathsregisteredinenglandandwales/2020/publishedweek532020.xlsx
[440] https://substack.com/@alternativenarrative
[441] https://www.ons.gov.uk/peoplepopulationandcommunity/birthsdeathsandmarriages/deaths/bulletins/deathsregisteredweeklyinenglandandwalesprovisional/weekending29january2021
[442] https://wonder.cdc.gov/

Chapter 13

[443] https://www.bbc.co.uk/news/uk-england-cambridgeshire-59699891

[444] https://wherearethenumbers.substack.com/p/claims-the-unvaccinated-were-at-higher
[445] https://www.bartshealth.nhs.uk/news/almost-90-of-patients-admitted-to-intensive-care-units-in-north-east-london-are-not-fully-vaccinated-11544
[446] https://www.normanfenton.com/post/a-critique-of-the-bbc2-documentary-unvaccinated
[447] https://lawhealthandtech.substack.com/p/who-fact-checks-the-fact-checkers
[448] https://www.ons.gov.uk/peoplepopulationandcommunity/birthsdeathsandmarriages/deaths/datasets/deathsbyvaccinationstatusengland
[449] https://perma.cc/HMV2-Q4V9
[450] https://perma.cc/EVP5-QH63
[451] https://blog.ons.gov.uk/2021/11/19/coronavirus-deaths-understanding-ons-data-on-mortality-and-vaccination-status/
[452] https://www.ons.gov.uk/peoplepopulationandcommunity/birthsdeathsandmarriages/deaths/bulletins/deathsinvolvingcovid19byvaccinationstatusengland/latest
[453] https://www.dailymail.co.uk/health/article-11775169/Death-rates-NOT-higher-Covid-vaccinated-Brits.html

Chapter 14

[454] https://wherearethenumbers.substack.com/p/retrospective-censorship-the-new
[455] https://wherearethenumbers.substack.com/p/the-curious-perfect-p-value-case-study
[456] https://wherearethenumbers.substack.com/p/attempt-to-take-down-paul-mariks
[457] ttps://www.hartgroup.org/
[458] https://pandata.org/
[459] https://www.mdpi.com/2075-471X/11/5/65
[460] https://www.hartgroup.org/bios/
[461] https://web.archive.org/web/20221009064651/ttps://counterdisinformationproject.substack.com/p/the-pandata-file
[462] https://www.mdpi.com/2075-471X/11/5/65
[463] https://counterdisinformationproject.substack.com/p/the-pandata-file
[464] https://www.normanfenton.com/covid-19
[465] https://wherearethenumbers.substack.com/p/the-lancet-heavily-redact-their-response
[466] https://jessicar.substack.com/p/censorship-update-record-keeping
[467] https://www.mdpi.com/1999-4915/13/10/2056
[468] https://arkmedic.substack.com/p/welcome-to-gilead
[469] https://twitter.com/jengleruk/status/1553350526175268864
[470] https://bmcinfectdis.biomedcentral.com/articles/10.1186/s12879-023-07998-3
[471] https://stevekirsch.substack.com/p/mark-skidmores-paper-showing-the
[472] https://stevekirsch.substack.com/p/its-time-we-hold-these-people-accountable
[473] https://odysee.com/@Corona-Ausschuss:3/s155de:c
[474] https://wherearethenumbers.substack.com/p/when-real-misinformation-kills
[475] https://wherearethenumbers.substack.com/p/the-astra-zeneca-vaccine-is-100-effective

[476] https://www.standard.co.uk/news/uk/wimbledon-standing-ovation-oxford-covid-vaccine-sarah-gilbert-b943029.html
[477] https://www.reuters.com/business/healthcare-pharmaceuticals/astrazeneca-withdraws-us-application-covid-vaccine-2022-11-10/
[478] https://nationalpost.com/news/world/u-s-removes-astrazeneca-from-plant-that-ruined-15-million-doses-of-covid-19-vaccine
[479] https://nationalpost.com/news/canada/more-than-half-canadas-astrazeneca-vaccine-came-from-u-s-plant-accused-by-fda-of-quality-control-problems
[480] https://www.newswire.ca/news-releases/statement-from-health-canada-on-astrazeneca-and-janssen-covid-19-vaccines-produced-at-emergent-biosolutions-843630874.html
[481] https://www.nytimes.com/2021/04/23/us/astrazeneca-covid-vaccine-contamination.html
[482] https://nationalpost.com/news/world/johnson-johnson-recorded-contamination-risks-at-baltimore-plant-seven-months-before-vaccine-was-ruined
[483] https://nationalpost.com/news/world/millions-of-astrazeneca-doses-shipped-to-canada-from-u-s-plant-before-complete-inspection
[484] https://www.fiercepharma.com/pharma/emergent-slammed-congressional-report-claiming-contamination-led-millions-discarded-vaccines
[485] https://www.biopharma-reporter.com/Article/2022/06/07/Johnson-Johnson-ending-COVID-19-vaccine-contract-with-Emergent
[486] https://endpts.com/more-than-half-a-billion-covid-vaccine-doses-wasted-after-emergents-baltimore-fiasco/
[487] https://health-infobase.canada.ca/covid-19/vaccine-safety/ a5
[488] https://www.publichealthontario.ca/-/media/documents/ncov/epi/covid-19-aefi-report.pdf
[489] https://www.nytimes.com/topic/company/emergent-biosolutions-inc
[490] https://wherearethenumbers.substack.com/p/manipulating-mortality
[491] https://www.ukcolumn.org/video/uk-column-news-5th-april-2023
[492] https://www.researchprofessionalnews.com/rr-news-uk-politics-2023-3-uk-pays-out-nearly-4m-in-covid-19-vaccine-damages/
[493] https://yellowcard.ukcolumn.org/yellow-card-reports
[494] https://apnews.com/article/fact-check-cdc-covid-vaccine-deaths-910677348223
[495] https://openvaers.com/faq/what-is-underreporting-and-why-it-matters
[496] https://jessicar.substack.com/p/the-under-reporting-factor-in-vaers
[497] https://www.researchgate.net/publication/367030584_Extended_Analysis_of_COVID-19_Vaccine_Death_Reports_from_the_Vaccine_Adverse_Events_Reporting_System_VAERS_Database
[498] https://www.ncbi.nlm.nih.gov/pmc/articles/PMC1495801/pdf/bmjcred00590-0033.pdf
[499] https://wherearethenumbers.substack.com/p/the-devils-advocate-an-exploratory
[500] https://www.gov.uk/government/publications/coronavirus-covid-19-vaccine-adverse-reactions/coronavirus-vaccine-summary-of-yellow-card-reporting--2

[501] https://pharmanewsintel.com/news/european-countries-suspend-use-of-astrazenecas-covid-19-vaccine
[502] https://twitter.com/OpenVAERS/status/1643402285228363778
[503] https://childrenshealthdefense.org/defender/cdc-safety-signals-pfizer-moderna-covid-vaccines-et/
[504] https://pubmed.ncbi.nlm.nih.gov/36055877/
[505] https://www.rasmussenreports.com/public_content/politics/public_surveys/covid_19_virus_deaths_vs_vaccine_deaths
[506] https://valuetainment.com/new-vaccine-analysis-reveals-300000-excess-u-s-deaths-147-billion-in-damage/

Chapter 15

[507] https://wherearethenumbers.substack.com/p/is-vaccine-efficacy-statistical-illusion
[508] https://wherearethenumbers.substack.com/p/more-on-the-illusions-of-vaccine-efficacy
[509] https://youtu.be/6umArFc-fdc
[510] https://youtu.be/hu8akqgPLik
[511] https://wherearethenumbers.substack.com/p/the-illusion-of-vaccine-efficacy
[512] https://www.ons.gov.uk/peoplepopulationandcommunity/birthsdeathsandmarriages/deaths/bulletins/covid19vaccineeffectivenessestimatedusingcensus2021variablesengland/31march2021to20march2022
[513] https://doctorsappeal.com/docs/swedish-public-health-agency-reporting-has-distorted-mortality-rates-for-the-unvaccinated-and-the-vaccinated-2/
[514] https://www.ons.gov.uk/peoplepopulationandcommunity/birthsdeathsandmarriages/deaths/bulletins/covid19vaccineeffectivenessestimatedusingcensus2021variablesengland/31march2021to20march2022
[515] https://jamanetwork.com/journals/jamapediatrics/fullarticle/2805184
[516] https://www.theepochtimes.com/fda-detects-serious-safety-signal-for-covid-19-vaccination-among-kids_5288229.html
[517] https://childrenshealthdefense.org/defender/fda-safety-signal-covid-vaccine-heart-inflammation-kids/
[518] https://www.nature.com/articles/s44161-022-00177-8
[519] https://bestinitiative.org/wp-content/uploads/2022/12/C19-Active-Monitoring-Protocol-Addendum-2022.pdf
[520] https://bestinitiative.org/wp-content/uploads/2022/01/C19-Vax-Safety-AESI-Bkgd-Rate-Protocol-FINAL-2020.pdf
[521] https://coronavirus.data.gov.uk/details/deaths
[522] https://coronavirus.data.gov.uk/details/deaths?areaType=nation&areaName=England
[523] https://wherearethenumbers.substack.com/p/the-uk-governments-flawed-covid-death
[524] https://coronavirus.data.gov.uk/details/deaths?areaType=overview&areaName=United%20Kingdom
[525] http://www.ons.gov.uk/aboutus/transparencyandgovernance/freedomofinformationfoi/covid19deathsandautopsiesfeb2020todec2021

[526] https://wherearethenumbers.substack.com/p/the-very-best-of-cheap-trick
[527] https://www.researchgate.net/publication/357778435_Official_mortality_data_for_England_suggest_systematic_miscategorisation_of_vaccine_status_and_uncertain_effectiveness_of_Covid-19_vaccination
[528] https://wherearethenumbers.substack.com/p/the-dark-horse-podcast-reports-on
[529] https://zenodo.org/records/8120771
[530] https://ia801605.us.archive.org/12/items/b2136140x/b2136140x.pdf
[531] https://www.thelancet.com/journals/lanres/article/PIIS2213-2600(23)00015-2/fulltext
[532] https://www.nejm.org/doi/full/10.1056/NEJMoa2115481
[533] https://bmcinfectdis.biomedcentral.com/articles/10.1186/s12879-022-07814-4
[534] https://jamanetwork.com/journals/jamanetworkopen/article-abstract/2796615
[535] https://www.thelancet.com/journals/laninf/article/PIIS1473-3099(22)00578-3/fulltext
[536] https://academic.oup.com/ofid/article/9/9/ofac449/6693796
[537] https://www.ncbi.nlm.nih.gov/pmc/articles/PMC9319484/
[538] https://www.nejm.org/doi/full/10.1056/nejmoa2101765
[539] https://zenodo.org/record/5243901
[540] https://www.thelancet.com/action/showPdf?pii=S0140-6736%2821%2900947-8
[541] https://wherearethenumbers.substack.com/p/the-lancet-has-become-a-laughing
[542] https://www.ncbi.nlm.nih.gov/pmc/articles/PMC9527398/
[543] https://www.ncbi.nlm.nih.gov/pmc/articles/PMC9244879/
[544] https://www.ncbi.nlm.nih.gov/pmc/articles/PMC8816388/
[545] https://pubmed.ncbi.nlm.nih.gov/34942067/
[546] https://www.ncbi.nlm.nih.gov/pmc/articles/PMC8779277/
[547] https://pubmed.ncbi.nlm.nih.gov/34525277/
[548] https://www.health.nsw.gov.au/Infectious/covid-19/Documents/in-focus/covid-19-vaccination-case-surveillance-051121.pdf
[549] https://www.thelancet.com/journals/lanam/article/PIIS2667-193X(22)00029-1/fulltext
[550] https://doctorsappeal.com/docs/swedish-public-health-agency-reporting-has-distorted-mortality-rates-for-the-unvaccinated-and-the-vaccinated-2/
[551] https://www.cdc.gov/coronavirus/2019-ncov/php/hd-breakthrough.html
[552] https://www.ons.gov.uk/peoplepopulationandcommunity/birthsdeathsandmarriages/deaths/bulletins/covid19vaccineeffectivenessestimatedusingcensus2021variablesengland/31march2021to20march2022
[553] https://www.whatdotheyknow.com/request/809588/response/1937479/attach/html/5/1767 FOI Data classification of those vaccinated within 14 days.pdf.html
[554] https://www.nejm.org/doi/10.1056/NEJMoa2106599
[555] https://www.medrxiv.org/content/10.1101/2023.06.06.23290982v1.full.pdf
[556] https://www.ons.gov.uk/peoplepopulationandcommunity/birthsdeathsandmarriages/deaths/bulletins/covid19vaccineeffectivenessestimatedusingcensus2021variablesengland/31march2021to20march2022
[557] https://pubmed.ncbi.nlm.nih.gov/33956048/
[558] https://www.nejm.org/doi/full/10.1056/NEJMoa2204919

[559] https://www.nejm.org/doi/full/10.1056/NEJMc2306683
[560] https://twitter.com/RetsefL/status/1681907816875925507
[561] https://www.nature.com/articles/s41467-022-33328-3
[562] https://www.ncbi.nlm.nih.gov/pmc/articles/PMC9246705/
[563] https://www.nature.com/articles/s41591-021-01666-2
[564] https://jamanetwork.com/journals/jamanetworkopen/fullarticle/2803959
[565] https://www.nejm.org/doi/full/10.1056/nejmoa2109522
[566] https://apps.who.int/iris/handle/10665/360580
[567] https://www.ncbi.nlm.nih.gov/pmc/articles/PMC9977606/
[568] https://jamanetwork.com/journals/jamaoncology/fullarticle/2807035

Chapter 16

[569] https://uobevents.eventsair.com/haca-2023/
[570] https://www.amazon.co.uk/Bad-Science-Ben-Goldacre/dp/000728487X
[571] https://twitter.com/HACA_Conf/status/1669657718355795968
[572] https://wherearethenumbers.substack.com/t/censorship
[573] https://twitter.com/shellenberger
[574] https://twitter.com/MartinNeil9/status/1671809796905791488
[575] https://twitter.com/Jikkyleaks/status/1658691742915497984
[576] https://www.ageofautism.com/2010/08/whats-behind-ben-goldacre-.html
[577] https://wherearethenumbers.substack.com/api/v1/file/f54b4890-0001-489b-8f73-6a31b14c4812.pdf
[578] https://wherearethenumbers.substack.com/api/v1/file/436477a5-9d39-40db-bd9d-e32330598e69.pdf
[579] https://www.whatdotheyknow.com/request/cancellation_of_presentation_by incoming-2395135
[580] https://wherearethenumbers.substack.com/p/cancelled-by-the-nhs-an-heavily-redacted
[581] https://twitter.com/jontix/status/1671164451658289158
[582] https://wherearethenumbers.substack.com/p/an-update-on-my-nhs-conference-cancellation
[583] https://twitter.com/jontix/status/1391708491761557505
[584] https://youtu.be/lV_C9xkTT-w
[585] https://youtu.be/nLGaINzfEVs
[586] https://doi.org/10.1101/2020.10.22.20217554
[587] https://doi.org/10.1101/2020.10.20.20215814
[588] https://doi.org/10.1101/2020.07.15.20154286
[589] https://doi.org/10.1080/13669877.2020.1778771
[590] https://doi.org/10.1101/2020.05.25.20112466
[591] https://doi.org/10.13140/RG.2.2.33939.60968
[592] https://www.researchgate.net/publication/355437113_Discrepancies_and_inconsistencies_in_UK_Government_datasets_compromise_accuracy_of_mortality_rate_comparisons_between_vaccinated_and_unvaccinated
[593] https://asterisk.dynevor.org/where-do-we-disagree.html
[594] https://sensiblemed.substack.com/p/john-ioannidis-the-pandemic-as-of

[595] https://wherearethenumbers.substack.com/p/the-mhra-is-not-fit-for-purpose
[596] https://www.gov.uk/government/publications/coronavirus-covid-19-vaccine-adverse-reactions/coronavirus-vaccine-summary-of-yellow-card-reporting
[597] https://www.gov.uk/government/publications/report-of-the-commission-on-human-medicines-expert-working-group-on-covid-19-vaccine-safety-surveillance/report-of-the-commission-on-human-medicines-expert-working-group-on-covid-19-vaccine-safety-surveillance
[598] https://wherearethenumbers.substack.com/api/v1/file/bf8785de-4c00-4612-aca8-aa8bc9eb0881.pdf
[599] https://dailysceptic.org/2023/01/03/mhra-caught-hiding-crucial-vaccine-safety-data/
[600] https://dailysceptic.org/2023/01/28/mhra-caught-not-doing-its-promised-vaccine-safety-monitoring-again/
[601] https://wherearethenumbers.substack.com/p/a-week-at-sea-with-dissidents-and
[602] https://twitter.com/julesserkin/status/168815530500378624
[603] https://wherearethenumbers.substack.com/p/when-real-misinformation-kills
[604] https://wherearethenumbers.substack.com/p/the-astra-zeneca-vaccine-is-100-effective
[605] https://wherearethenumbers.substack.com/p/the-scandal-of-the-astrazeneca-vaccine
[606] https://wherearethenumbers.substack.com/p/why-is-the-mhra-hiding-critical-safety
[607] https://www.standard.co.uk/news/uk/wimbledon-standing-ovation-oxford-covid-vaccine-sarah-gilbert-b943029.html

Chapter 17

[608] https://correlation-canada.org/wp-content/uploads/2023/10/2021-10-25-Correlation-Mortality-public-health-disaster-USA.pdf
[609] http://web.archive.org/web/20230331192626/https://jameslyonsweiler.com/2020/09/11/censored-is-cdc-borrowing-pneumonia-deaths-from-flu%E2%80%8B-for-from-covid-19/
[610] https://wherearethenumbers.substack.com/p/whodunnit-abridged
[611] https://www.c-span.org/video/?465845-1/universal-flu-vaccine
[612] https://www.nature.com/articles/s41586-020-2008-3
[613] https://www.sciencedirect.com/science/article/pii/S1076633221002002
[614] https://pubmed.ncbi.nlm.nih.gov/30429395/
[615] https://www.ajronline.org/doi/epdf/10.2214/ajr.160.2.8424326
[616] https://youtu.be/_J60fQr0GWo
[617] https://www.youtube.com/watch?v=gedpJhckEJ4
[618] https://www.nhs.uk/conditions/vaccinations/pneumococcal-vaccination/
[619] https://pubmed.ncbi.nlm.nih.gov/33693636/
[620] https://www.ncbi.nlm.nih.gov/books/NBK526116/ article-27364.s3
[621] https://www.ncbi.nlm.nih.gov/pmc/articles/PMC6810199/
[622] https://www.frontiersin.org/articles/10.3389/fcimb.2023.1161763
[623] https://pubmed.ncbi.nlm.nih.gov/37370910/
[624] https://www.ncbi.nlm.nih.gov/pmc/articles/PMC4299926

[625] https://www.ncbi.nlm.nih.gov/pmc/articles/PMC4299926/ R2
[626] https://www.ncbi.nlm.nih.gov/pmc/articles/PMC7717180/pdf/ciaa1728.pdf
[627] https://pubmed.ncbi.nlm.nih.gov/32711058/
[628] https://pubmed.ncbi.nlm.nih.gov/35100984/
[629] https://nulluslocussinegenio.com/2021/12/22/why-this-new-virus-testing-makes-no-sense/
[630] https://pubmed.ncbi.nlm.nih.gov/34960253/
[631] https://journals.asm.org/doi/10.1128/jcm.00174-22
[632] https://www.sciencedirect.com/science/article/pii/S1438422117304721
[633] https://www.mdpi.com/2076-0817/12/7/932
[634]
[635] https://rebeccacharles.substack.com/p/httpsdeathbyhospitalprotocolcomdanielles
[636] https://pubmed.ncbi.nlm.nih.gov/18710327/
[637] https://pubmed.ncbi.nlm.nih.gov/33693636/
[638] https://www.nature.com/articles/s41598-022-15409-x
[639] https://wherearethenumbers.substack.com/p/whodunnit-abridged
[640] https://t.co/fdWxAcldqe
[641] https://www.nhs.uk/common-health-questions/infections/is-pneumonia-contagious/
[642] https://wherearethenumbers.substack.com/p/do-not-seek-and-ye-shall-not-find
[643] https://www.nejm.org/doi/10.1056/NEJMoa1500245
[644] https://www.nejm.org/doi/10.1056/NEJMoa1405870
[645] https://www.ncbi.nlm.nih.gov/pmc/articles/PMC7436231/
[646] https://pubmed.ncbi.nlm.nih.gov/36560558/

Chapter 18

[647] https://wherearethenumbers.substack.com/p/whodunnit-unabridged
[648] https://www.ronjohnson.senate.gov/covid
[649] https://wherearethenumbers.substack.com/p/how-did-antibiotics-use-change-during
[650] https://wherearethenumbers.substack.com/p/us-covid-19-ventilation-policy-made
[651] https://academic.oup.com/jid/article/198/7/962/2192118
[652] https://www.nice.org.uk/guidance/ng163/resources/covid19-rapid-guideline-managing-symptoms-including-at-the-end-of-life-in-the-community-pdf-66141899069889
[653] http://web.archive.org/web/20200407215603/https:/www.nice.org.uk/guidance/NG163
[654] https://www.gmc-uk.org/ethical-guidance/ethical-guidance-for-doctors/prescribing-and-managing-medicines-and-devices/prescribing-unlicensed-medicines
[655] https://www.bmj.com/content/bmj/369/bmj.m1461.full.pdf
[656] https://www.bmj.com/content/369/bmj.m1461/rr-1
[657] http://web.archive.org/web/20200411192035/https:/www.nice.org.uk/guidance/ng165/chapter/4-Managing-suspected-or-confirmed-pneumonia

[658] https://www.covid19treatmentguidelines.nih.gov/management/clinical-management-of-adults/clinical-management-of-adults-summary/
[659] https://files.covid19treatmentguidelines.nih.gov/guidelines/covid19treatmentguidelines.pdf
[660] https://twitter.com/Jikkyleaks/status/1623147403305193473
[661] https://www.journalofinfection.com/article/S0163-4453(23)00288-8/fulltext
[662] https://openprescribing.net/analyse/org=regional_team&numIds=5.1.5,5.1.2,0501120L0,0501120X0,0501013B0,0501013K0&denom=nothing&selectedTab=chart
[663] https://fmch.bmj.com/content/9/3/e001143.info
[664] https://www.ncbi.nlm.nih.gov/pmc/articles/PMC7799289/
[665] https://www.aerzteblatt.de/nachrichten/132147/Massiver-Einbruch-bei-Antibiotika-Verordnungen-durch-Coronapandemie
[666] https://www.ncbi.nlm.nih.gov/pmc/articles/PMC7833340/
[667] https://www.lifesitenews.com/blogs/romanian-doctor-says-she-cures-100-percent-of-covid-patients/
[668] https://helpstpauls.com/promise/2023/septic-shock-research/
[669] https://onlinelibrary.wiley.com/doi/10.1002/jmv.29507
[670] https://vladimirzelenkomd.com/treatment-protocol/
[671] https://www.amjmed.com/article/S0002-9343(20)30673-2/fulltext
[672] https://www.ncbi.nlm.nih.gov/pmc/articles/PMC8777850/
[673] https://virologyj.biomedcentral.com/articles/10.1186/1743-422X-2-69
[674] https://www.ncbi.nlm.nih.gov/pmc/articles/PMC10125304/
[675] https://pubmed.ncbi.nlm.nih.gov/?term=azithromycin+AND+%22oxidative+stress%22&show_snippets=off&sort=date&size=200
[676] https://europepmc.org/backend/ptpmcrender.fcgi?accid=PMC1889760&blobtype=pdf
[677] https://www.medrxiv.org/content/10.1101/2022.10.11.22280963v1
[678] https://pubmed.ncbi.nlm.nih.gov/360892/
[679] https://off-guardian.org/2020/05/06/covid19-are-ventilators-killing-people/
[680] https://www.ncbi.nlm.nih.gov/pmc/articles/PMC8388913/
[681] https://link.springer.com/article/10.1007/s00134-020-06323-9
[682] https://pubmed.ncbi.nlm.nih.gov/37104035/
[683] https://www.fda.gov/news-events/press-announcements/coronavirus-covid-19-update-fda-takes-action-help-increase-us-supply-ventilators-and-respirators
[684] https://www.ncbi.nlm.nih.gov/pmc/articles/PMC8059113/
[685] https://pubmed.ncbi.nlm.nih.gov/37104035/
[686] https://journals.asm.org/doi/10.1128/jcm.00174-22
[687] https://www.bmj.com/content/368/bmj.m1201
[688] https://archive.is/KX5IQ selection-4609.23-4621.63
[689] https://www.statnews.com/pharmalot/2020/03/31/a-new-covid-19-problem-shortages-of-medicines-needed-for-placing-patients-on-ventilators/
[690] https://whyy.org/articles/philly-area-hospitals-grapple-with-shortage-of-drugs-to-put-patients-on-ventilators/
[691] https://www.ncbi.nlm.nih.gov/pmc/articles/PMC7454318/pdf/zxaa251.pdf

[692] https://substanceabusepolicy.biomedcentral.com/articles/10.1186/s13011-020-00333-y
[693] https://twitter.com/EWoodhouse7/status/1638678544241815558
[694] https://www.reuters.com/article/us-health-coronavirus-ventilators-specia-idUSKCN2251PE
[695] https://www.bmj.com/content/369/bmj.m1828
[696] https://fmch.bmj.com/content/9/3/e001143
[697] https://www.researchgate.net/publication/377266988_Excess_Deaths_in_the_United_Kingdom_Midazolam_and_Euthanasia_in_the_COVID-19_Pandemic
[698] https://globalbiodefense.com/2018/10/31/seizure-drug-approval-expands-countermeasures-for-chemical-weapons-attack/
[699] https://wherearethenumbers.substack.com/p/what-really-caused-the-surge-in-covid
[700] https://pubmed.ncbi.nlm.nih.gov/32711058/
[701] https://academic.oup.com/jid/article/198/7/962/2192118
[702] https://www.ncbi.nlm.nih.gov/pmc/articles/PMC7799289/
[703] https://twitter.com/JavRoJav/status/1625783114541805570
[704] https://www.amnesty.org.uk/press-releases/uk-review-horrifyingly-widespread-use-do-not-resuscitate-orders-care-homes-must
[705] https://www.washingtonpost.com/health/2020/03/25/coronavirus-patients-do-not-resucitate/
[706] https://www.bmj.com/content/369/bmj.m1931
[707] https://biologyphenom.substack.com/
[708] https://open.spotify.com/episode/7edwvm2c6Ieuzun4xtFYCJ
[709] https://twitter.com/elonmusk/status/1242279396226011137
[710] https://twitter.com/ScottWapnerCNBC/status/1242262664732082177
[711] https://www.michaelpsenger.com/p/the-great-covid-ventilator-death
[712] https://pubmed.ncbi.nlm.nih.gov/1757240/
[713] https://pubmed.ncbi.nlm.nih.gov/16215397/
[714] https://web.archive.org/web/20061006144757/http:/www.nyc.gov/html/doh/downloads/pdf/bhpp/bhpp-focus-bio-vent-results.pdf
[715] http://medbox.iiab.me/modules/en-cdc/www.cdc.gov/flu/pandemic-resources/tools/flusurge.htm
[716] https://pubmed.ncbi.nlm.nih.gov/17198049/
[717] https://pubmed.ncbi.nlm.nih.gov/18173862/
[718] https://www.cambridge.org/core/journals/disaster-medicine-and-public-health-preparedness/article/allocating-mechanical-ventilators-during-mass-respiratory-failure-kudos-to-new-york-state-but-more-work-to-be-done/563DFD6CB2109D89FE3A1EF705A63439
[719] https://hartuk.substack.com/p/ethical-boundaries
[720] https://www.health.ny.gov/press/releases/2015/2015-11-25_ventilator_allocation_guidelines.htm
[721] https://www.health.ny.gov/regulations/task_force/reports_publications/docs/ventilator_guidelines.pdf
[722] https://www.michaelpsenger.com/p/the-great-covid-ventilator-death

[723] https://www.researchgate.net/publication/339998871_Handbook_of_COVID-19_Prevention_and_Treatment
[724] https://extranet.who.int/emt/sites/default/files/10-HandbookofCOVID-19PreventionandTreatment.pdf

Chapter 19

[725] https://dailysceptic.org/2023/08/30/the-scandalous-eu-contract-with-pfizer-biontech-has-been-online-for-two-years-why-has-nobody-seen-it/
[726] https://wherearethenumbers.substack.com/p/still-unknown-safety-efficacy-in-pfizer-contracts-slovenia
[727] https://d7694293-ffb8-4ed0-a014-3581d49070e4.usrfiles.com/ugd/d76942_5af19ff7389d405585ae0c9db50eb306.pdf
[728] https://www.gov.uk/government/publications/regulatory-approval-of-pfizer-biontech-vaccine-for-covid-19/conditions-of-authorisation-for-pfizerbiontech-covid-19-vaccine
[729] https://wherearethenumbers.substack.com/p/informed-consent-statement-on-covid
[730] https://scholar.google.co.uk/citations?user=wKIBcKEAAAAJ&hl=en&oi=ao
[731] https://wherearethenumbers.substack.com/p/an-explosive-discussion-with-ex-cdc
[732] https://wherearethenumbers.substack.com/p/whodunnit-unabridged
[733] https://twitter.com/Jockthedog2/status/1333502166829502465
[734] https://pubmed.ncbi.nlm.nih.gov/17238820/
[735] https://pubmed.ncbi.nlm.nih.gov/32015508/
[736] https://en.wikipedia.org/wiki/Bronchoalveolar_lavage
[737] https://www.nejm.org/doi/10.1056/NEJMoa1500245
[738] https://www.nejm.org/doi/10.1056/NEJMoa1405870
[739] https://pubmed.ncbi.nlm.nih.gov/32015508/
[740] https://wmcresearch.org/
[741] https://en.wikipedia.org/wiki/Tokyo_subway_sarin_attack
[742] https://www.cell.com/cell-host-microbe/fulltext/S1931-3128(22)00572-8
[743] https://threadreaderapp.com/thread/1712237556752859452

Chapter 20

[744] https://pubmed.ncbi.nlm.nih.gov/18710327/
[745] https://wherearethenumbers.substack.com/t/flu
[746] https://wherearethenumbers.substack.com/p/a-closer-look-at-spikeopathy-as-the
[747] https://wherearethenumbers.substack.com/p/our-response-to-dr-pierre-kory
[748] https://www.hsgac.senate.gov/hearings/covid-19-how-new-information-should-drive-policy/
[749] https://covid19criticalcare.com/
[750] https://covid19criticalcare.com/wp-content/uploads/2023/11/Understanding-Remdesivir.pdf
[751] https://www.nejm.org/doi/10.1056/NEJMoa2002032?url_ver=Z39.88-2003&rfr_id=ori:rid:crossref.org&rfr_dat=cr_pub%20%200pubmed
[752] https://www.ncbi.nlm.nih.gov/pmc/articles/PMC4367726/

[753] https://pubmed.ncbi.nlm.nih.gov/32963028/
[754] https://pubmed.ncbi.nlm.nih.gov/32017662/
[755] https://www.sciencedirect.com/science/article/pii/S1076633221002002
[756] https://link.springer.com/article/10.1007/s00330-020-06920-8
[757] https://pubmed.ncbi.nlm.nih.gov/32291197/
[758] https://www.ajronline.org/doi/10.2214/AJR.20.23214
[759] https://www.ncbi.nlm.nih.gov/pmc/articles/PMC8814899/
[760] https://www.bmj.com/content/370/bmj.m2426
[761] https://www.sciencedirect.com/science/article/pii/S0049384820301201
[762] https://pubmed.ncbi.nlm.nih.gov/32314058/
[763] https://erj.ersjournals.com/content/erj/18/1/196.full.pdf
[764] https://respiratory-research.biomedcentral.com/articles/10.1186/s12931-020-01462-5
[765] https://pubmed.ncbi.nlm.nih.gov/37788896/
[766] https://pubmed.ncbi.nlm.nih.gov/35490510/
[767] https://pubmed.ncbi.nlm.nih.gov/36902815/
[768] https://www.atsjournals.org/doi/full/10.1164/rccm.201501-0017OC
[769] https://europepmc.org/article/med/18571356
[770] https://pubs.rsna.org/doi/full/10.1148/radiol.2020201365
[771] https://pubmed.ncbi.nlm.nih.gov/32963028/
[772] https://www.sciencedirect.com/science/article/pii/S1076633221002002
[773] https://pubmed.ncbi.nlm.nih.gov/32314058/
[774] https:/www.nejm.org/doi/10.1056/NEJMoa1405870
[775] https://www.nejm.org/doi/10.1056/NEJMoa1500245
[776] https://nakedemperor.substack.com/p/47-of-deceased-persons-had-a-respiratory
[777] https://wwwnc.cdc.gov/eid/article/24/7/18-0162_article
[778] https://pubmed.ncbi.nlm.nih.gov/33487401/
[779] https://www.nejm.org/doi/full/10.1056/NEJMoa1911614
[780] https://www.nejm.org/doi/full/10.1056/NEJMe1912032
[781] https:/academic.oup.com/pmj/article/96/1132/61/6971614
[782] https://en.wikipedia.org/wiki/DRASTIC
[783] https://www.researchgate.net/publication/359231017_Is_SARS-CoV-2_the_causative_agent_of_EVALI_cases_prior_to_the_Covid-19_pandemic/stats
[784] https://twitter.com/RemnantMd/status/1503834564925575174
[785] https://eu.usatoday.com/story/opinion/2020/07/01/slow-covid-19-more-americans-need-wear-n-95-masks-indoors-column/3278779001/
[786] https://pierrekorymedicalmusings.com/p/debate-was-covid-19-a-pandemic-caused
[787] https://www.ncbi.nlm.nih.gov/pmc/articles/PMC7498137/
[788] https://my.clevelandclinic.org/health/diagnostics/22327-differential-diagnosis
[789] https://www.sgu.edu/news-and-events/intensivist-dr-house-grooms-aspiring-doctors-for-future-success/
[790] https://journal.chestnet.org/article/S0012-3692(21)00218-X/fulltext

Chapter 21

[791] https://wherearethenumbers.substack.com/p/does-unacceptably-high-cross-reactivity

[792] https://anandamide.substack.com/p/the-smoking-gun

[793] https://twitter.com/Jikkyleaks/status/1756079847066267861

[794] https://wherearethenumbers.substack.com/t/pcr-testing

[795] https://wherearethenumbers.substack.com/p/the-smoking-man-emails

[796] https://www.eurosurveillanceandtent/10.2807/1560-7917.ES.2020.25.3.2000045

[797] https://www.ncbi.nlm.nih.gov/pmc/articles/PMC7364759/

[798] https://www.instand-ev.de/System/rv-files/340%20DE%20SARS-CoV-2%20Genom%20April%202020%2020200502j.pdf

[799] https://wherearethenumbers.substack.com/p/uk-lighthouse-laboratories-testing-for

[800] https://www.health.gov.au/sites/default/files/documents/2020/06/post-market-validation-of-the-beijing-genomics-institute-bgi-sars-cov-2-real-time-pcr-platform.pdf

[801] https://www.health.gov.au/sites/default/files/documents/2020/06/post-market-validation-of-the-beijing-genomics-institute-bgi-sars-cov-2-real-time-pcr-platform.pdf

[802] https://wherearethenumbers.substack.com/p/peek-a-boo-flu

[803] https://wherearethenumbers.substack.com/cp/136588888

[804] https://diagnostics.roche.com/us/en/products/lab/cobas-sars-cov-2-and-influenza-a-b-v2-test-5800-6800-8800-pid00000617.html

[805] https://wherearethenumbers.substack.com/p/sensors-set-to-off

[806] https://www.ncbi.nlm.nih.gov/pmc/articles/PMC7355678/

[807] https://www.ncbi.nlm.nih.gov/pmc/articles/PMC7392437/

[808] https://www.sciencedirect.com/science/article/pii/S1386653215001675

[809] https://www.ndr.de/nachrichten/info/16-Coronavirus-Update-Wir-brauchen-Abkuerzungen-bei-der-Impfstoffzulassung,podcastcoronavirus140.html#wodarg

[810] https://pubmed.ncbi.nlm.nih.gov/18382647/

[811] https://www.nytimes.com/2007/01/22/health/22whoop.html

[812] https://wherearethenumbers.substack.com/p/did-operation-moonshot-inadvertently

[813] https://www.arkmedic.info/p/there-was-no-virus

[814] https://wherearethenumbers.substack.com/p/does-unacceptably-high-cross-reactivity

[815] https://wherearethenumbers.substack.com/p/smashing-1-in-3-people-with-covid-19

[816] https://www.nejm.org/doi/10.1056/NEJMoa1500245

[817] https://www.nejm.org/doi/10.1056/NEJMoa1405870

[818] https://www.youtube.com/watch?v=4qopWRosPDA&t=122s

[819] https://wherearethenumbers.substack.com/p/does-unacceptably-high-cross-reactivity

[820] https://wherearethenumbers.substack.com/cp/136588888

[821] https://professionals.northwell.edu/sites/northwell.edu/files/2020-03/viral-respiratory-culture-v-vcr-change-3-5-2020pdf.pdf

[822] https://wherearethenumbers.substack.com/p/on-false-positives-in-covid19-testing
[823] https://www.health.gov.au/sites/default/files/documents/2022/10/aisr-fortnightly-report-no-17-16-november-to-29-november-2020.pdf
[824] https://www.abs.gov.au/statistics/health/causes-death/causes-death-australia/2020 data-downloads
[825] https://wherearethenumbers.substack.com/p/do-not-seek-and-ye-shall-not-find
[826] https://wherearethenumbers.substack.com/p/finding-the-flu-is-easy-just-google
[827] https://www.randox.com/coronavirus-randox-test/
[828] https://wherearethenumbers.substack.com/p/was-declaring-pcr-positives-using
[829] https://wherearethenumbers.substack.com/p/uk-lighthouse-laboratories-testing-for
[830] https://wherearethenumbers.substack.com/p/was-declaring-pcr-positives-using

Chapter 22

[831] https://wherearethenumbers.substack.com/p/virus-origins-and-gain-claim-of-function
[832] https://www.umassmed.edu/globalassets/ambros-lab/meetings/rna-biology-club-2019_20/masters-and-perlman-2013-in-fields-virology_1.pdf
[833] https://www.amazon.co.uk/Fields-Virology-Emerging-Howley-Knipe/dp/1975112547
[834] https://www.frontiersin.org/journals/microbiology/articles/10.3389/fmicb.2021.649314/full
[835] https://www.ncbi.nlm.nih.gov/pmc/articles/PMC1866027/
[836] https://www.pennmedicine.org/news/news-releases/2019/may/how-do-you-find-a-virus-thats-completely-unknown-study-says-look-to-the-genome
[837] https://www.ncbi.nlm.nih.gov/pmc/articles/PMC7104603/
[838] https://en.wikipedia.org/wiki/2015_Middle_East_respiratory_syndrome_outbreak_in_South_Korea
[839] https://en.wikipedia.org/wiki/2018_Middle_East_respiratory_syndrome_outbreak
[840] https://pubmed.ncbi.nlm.nih.gov/24920393/
[841] https://pubmed.ncbi.nlm.nih.gov/34325501/
[842] https://www.ncbi.nlm.nih.gov/pmc/articles/PMC8127614/
[843] https://wherearethenumbers.substack.com/p/how-did-antibiotics-use-change-during
[844] https://royalsocietypublishing.org/doi/pdf/10.1098/rstb.2004.1490
[845] https://en.wikipedia.org/wiki/SARS
[846] https://wherearethenumbers.substack.com/p/a-closer-look-at-spikeopathy-as-the
[847] https://en.wikipedia.org/wiki/MERS
[848] https://www.who.int/health-topics/severe-acute-respiratory-syndrome
[849] https://web.archive.org/web/20200511191228/https:/www.cdc.gov/sars/surveillance/absence.html
[850] https://www.statnews.com/2024/04/05/bird-flu-ron-fouchier-h5n1-risk-to-people/
[851] https://sanityunleashed.substack.com/p/sars-cov-2-whats-in-a-name-everything
[852] https://www.biorxiv.org/content/10.1101/2020.02.07.937862v1.full
[853] https://journals.asm.org/doi/10.1128/jvi.07173-11
[854] https://www.nature.com/articles/s41564-020-0695-z author-information

[855] https://www.who.int/emergencies/diseases/novel-coronavirus-2019
[856] https://apps.who.int/iris/handle/10665/163636
[857] https://en.wikipedia.org/wiki/Liger
[858] https://link.springer.com/chapter/10.1007/978-3-7091-6607-9_1
[859] https://www.nature.com/articles/s41392-020-0184-0
[860] https://wmcresearch.substack.com/p/the-purpose-of-the-furin-cleavage
[861] https://web.archive.org/web/20220722052227/http:/adeno-news.com/2022/07/18/fragility-of-the-spike-protein-against-antibodies-raise-questions-about-the-origin-of-the-sars-cov-2-furin-cleacage-site/
[862] https://www.frontiersin.org/journals/microbiology/articles/10.3389/fmicb.2021.649314/full
[863] https://www.frontiersin.org/articles/10.3389/fviro.2022.834808/full
[864] https://www.frontiersin.org/articles/10.3389/fviro.2022.914888/full
[865] https://journals.physiology.org/doi/pdf/10.1152/physiolgenomics.00087.2020
[866] https://www.biorxiv.org/content/10.1101/2020.01.30.927871v1.full
[867] https://pubmed.ncbi.nlm.nih.gov/10649986/
[868] https://usrtk.org/wp-content/uploads/2024/01/USGS-DEFUSE-2021-006245-Combined-Records_Redacted.pdf
[869] https://merylnass.substack.com/p/a-new-study-reports-309-lab-acquired
[870] https://www.biorxiv.org/content/10.1101/2022.10.18.512756v1.full.pdf
[871] https://www.ncbi.nlm.nih.gov/pmc/articles/PMC9937728/
[872] https://thebulletin.org/2022/06/gain-of-function-research-cant-deliver-pandemic-predictions-are-there-alternatives/
[873] https://www.frontiersin.org/articles/10.3389/fpubh.2014.00077/full
[874] https://pubmed.ncbi.nlm.nih.gov/24186378/
[875] https://twitter.com/DKlemitz/status/1766157759257690357
[876] https://www.thelancet.com/journals/lanmic/article/PIIS2666-5247%2824%2900025-9/fulltext
[877] https://www.frontiersin.org/journals/public-health/articles/10.3389/fpubh.2014.00077/full
[878] https://www.ncbi.nlm.nih.gov/pmc/articles/PMC3388103/
[879] https://www.ncbi.nlm.nih.gov/pmc/articles/PMC4003409/
[880] https://pubmed.ncbi.nlm.nih.gov/24696487/
[881] https://www.cell.com/cell-host-microbe/fulltext/S1931-3128(22)00572-8
[882] https://www.ncbi.nlm.nih.gov/pmc/articles/PMC3840482/
[883] https://www.nature.com/articles/s41586-021-03237-4.pdf
[884] https://www.nature.com/articles/s41564-021-00908-w
[885] https://www.ncbi.nlm.nih.gov/pmc/articles/PMC7878750/
[886] https://pubmed.ncbi.nlm.nih.gov/38324940/
[887] https://www.ncbi.nlm.nih.gov/pmc/articles/PMC4465284/
[888] https://wherearethenumbers.substack.com/p/a-closer-look-at-spikeopathy-as-the
[889] https://www.science.org/doi/10.1126/science.abe5901
[890] https://pubmed.ncbi.nlm.nih.gov/32724171/
[891] https://www.annualreviews.org/content/journals/10.1146/annurev-virology-093022-013037

[892] https://www.nature.com/articles/s41579-023-00878-2
[893] https://www.nature.com/articles/s41598-023-39232-0
[894] https://academic.oup.com/mbe/article/38/8/3046/6257226
[895] https://dailysceptic.org/2022/12/30/the-evidence-covid-19-was-spreading-silently-around-the-world-in-late-2019
[896] https://www.medrxiv.org/content/10.1101/2020.06.13.20129627v1
[897] https://journals.asm.org/doi/full/10.1128/aem.02750-20
[898] https://anthonycolpo.substack.com/p/peer-reviewed-fact-what-they-are
[899] https://www.biorxiv.org/content/10.1101/2022.10.18.512756v1.full.pdf
[900] https://journals.asm.org/doi/10.1128/jvi.00385-06
[901] https://pubmed.ncbi.nlm.nih.gov/19036930/
[902] https://www.nature.com/articles/s41598-018-28900-1
[903] https://www.scientificamerican.com/article/u-s-lifts-moratorium-on-funding-controversial-high-risk-virus-research/
[904] https://pubmed.ncbi.nlm.nih.gov/35881005/
[905] https://correlation-canada.org/no-plague-mass-homicide-2020/
[906] https://sanityunleashed.substack.com/p/two-articles-which-destroy-the-pandemic
[907] https://medium.com/@JohnPospichal/questions-for-lockdown-apologists-32a9bbf2e247
[908] https://sanityunleashed.substack.com/p/austrian-officials-must-have-known
[909] https://gigaohmbiological.com/
[910] https://x.com/heliodown/status/1681670067027623941
[911] https://sanityunleashed.substack.com/p/did-the-nocebo-effect-play-a-huge

Chapter 23

[912] https://www.conservativewoman.co.uk/faked-figures-that-drove-the-worlds-reaction-to-covid/
[913] https://wherearethenumbers.substack.com/p/exaggerated-estimates-from-epidemiological
[914] https://pandauncut.substack.com/p/the-dashboard-that-ruled-the-world
[915] https://threadreaderapp.com/thread/1333502166829502465.html
[916] https://ourworldindata.org/explorers/coronavirus-data-explorer
[917] https://justin-hart.medium.com/almost-all-the-covid-19-dashboard-dates-you-see-are-wrong-5e2e9f809c63
[918] https://www.nytimes.com/2021/05/14/learning/the-math-of-ending-the-pandemic-exponential-growth-and-decay.html
[919] https://justin-hart.medium.com/the-coronavirus-dashboards-will-doom-us-all-7dbbaf419d6f
[920] https://web.archive.org/web/20200407061231/https:/www.imperial.ac.uk/mrc-global-infectious-disease-analysis/covid-19/report-9-impact-of-npis-on-covid-19/
[921] https://www.eurosurveillance.org/content/10.2807/1560-7917.ES.2020.25.4.2000058
[922] https://www.nejm.org/doi/full/10.1056/NEJMOa2001316
[923] https://principia-scientific.com/the-false-premise-of-covid-19/

[924] https://www.researchgate.net/profile/Nicholas-Juleff/publication/51106448_Relationship_Between_Clinical_Signs_and_Transmission_of_an_Infectious_Disease_and_the_Implications_for_Control/links/0c96051791435e1c63000000/Relationship-Between-Clinical-Signs-and-Transmission-of-an-Infectious-Disease-and-the-Implications-for-Control.pdf
[925] https://citeseerx.ist.psu.edu/document?repid=rep1&type=pdf&doi=dd89599a7e8ce402fb6e91e111457b2b72692706
[926] https://www.academia.edu/download/87206658/Ferguson-Estimating-the-human-health-risk-from-possible-BSE-infection-of-the-British-sheep-flock.pdf
[927] https://www.nationalreview.com/corner/professor-lockdown-modeler-resigns-in-disgrace/
[928] https://www.bbc.com/news/science-environment-13299666
[929] https://www.telegraph.co.uk/news/2020/03/28/neil-ferguson-scientist-convinced-boris-johnson-uk-coronavirus-lockdown-criticised/
[930] https://www.theguardian.com/world/2022/feb/26/patrick-vallance-chris-whitty-best-bits-covid
[931] https://committees.parliament.uk/writtenevidence/13847/default/
[932] https://www.researchgate.net/publication/365202828_What_the_ONS_Mortality_Covid-19_Surveillance_Data_can_tell_us_about_Vaccine_Safety_and_Efficacy
[933] https://www.normanfenton.com/post/the-ons-data-on-vaccine-mortality-is-not-fit-for-purpose
[934] https://coronavirus.data.gov.uk/details/deaths
[935] https://www.ons.gov.uk/peoplepopulationandcommunity/healthandsocialcare/conditionsanddiseases/articles/coronaviruscovid192020incharts/2020-12-18
[936] https://www.gov.uk/government/publications/covid-19-reported-sars-cov-2-deaths-in-england/covid-19-confirmed-deaths-in-england-to-31-december-2020-report
[937] https://www.timesofisrael.com/the-end-of-exponential-growth-the-decline-in-the-spread-of-coronavirus/
[938] https://www.spectator.co.uk/article/why-can-t-neil-ferguson-s-imperial-model-be-replicated-
[939] https://pubmed.ncbi.nlm.nih.gov/32512579/
[940] https://player.odycdn.com/v6/streams/e1d999dc0aec0ad991e16269e984cf234acbc78d/859e6c.mp4
[941] https://data.spectator.co.uk/sage
[942] https://heatherrenkel.github.io/
[943] https://medium.com/wintoncentre/how-much-normal-risk-does-covid-represent-4539118e1196
[944] https://sanityunleashed.substack.com/p/another-virus-challenge-trial-spectacularly
[945] https://www.thelancet.com/journals/lanmic/article/PIIS2666-5247%2824%2900025-9/fulltext
[946] https://pubmed.ncbi.nlm.nih.gov/30770534/
[947] https://pubmed.ncbi.nlm.nih.gov/25416753/
[948] https://www.ncbi.nlm.nih.gov/pmc/articles/PMC7947934/pdf/BLT.20.265892.pdf/

[949] https://wherearethenumbers.substack.com/p/updating-our-own-priors-to-accommodate
[950] http://dx.doi.org/10.13140/RG.2.2.28055.09124
[951] https://wherearethenumbers.substack.com/p/can-our-detractors-decide-if-vaccinees-are-especially-healthy-or-especially-unhealthy
[952] https://x.com/ClareCraigPath/status/1793622868565299341
[953] http://dx.doi.org/10.13140/RG.2.2.12472.42248
[954] https://wherearethenumbers.substack.com/p/the-very-best-of-cheap-trick

Index

Academic hypocrisy, 8, 183, 185, 390
Age Standardised Mortality Rate (ASMR), 140, 141, 339
All-cause mortality, 71-73, 79, 89, 94, 106, 112-114, 140-141, 143, 181, 267, 357
Alroy-Preis, Sharon, 61-62, 66
Antibiotics, 130, 231, 234, 238, 243-255, 268-275, 289, 313, 314, 349, 355, 356, 381, 387
Antibodies, 13, 14, 123, 270, 271, 317, 327, 329, 332, 388
Arteta, Mikel, 1
arXiv, 50, 100, 111, 112, 221, 222, 223
Asymptomatics, 14-15, 22, 35-36, 41, 42-43, 51, 197, 268, 294, 299, 304-305, 314, 319, 342, 350, 353, 361, 362
Bacterial pneumonia, 114, 231-242, 243-255, 268, 273-292, 314, 325, 349, 354, 355, 356
Bayes Theorem (Network), 2, 4, 7, 10, 17, 18, 40, 86, 117, 162, 213, 214, 221, 222, 299, 300
BBC Unvaccinated documentary, 89-102, 176
Bergamo, Italy, 126, 127, 128, 233, 234, 331, 335, 353
BioFire, 151, 153, 154, 155, 240, 300
Blood clots, 200, 354
Causal Model, 2, 3, 7, 13, 14, 86
CDC (Center for Disease Control), 83, 115-118, 153, 158-161, 170, 173, 194, 207, 241, 257, 268-272
Censorship, 5, 103, 111, 125, 136, 183, 185, 213, 214, 351, 356, 363, 365, 375, 379
Cheap Trick, 195, 202, 335, 345, 356
Climate change, 218, 347
Conspiracy theorist, 45, 46, 93, 186, 356
Contact Tracing, 7, 39, 122, 221
Coronaviruses, 37, 47, 129-131, 149-155, 236, 242, 269, 270, 278, 295, 301, 303, 311-319, 323-325, 327, 328, 329, 331, 332, 350, 352, 354
Covid-19
  Cases data, 1, 10, 11, 12, 15, 16, 22, 26, 28, 52, 59, 82, 124, 154, 206, 237, 239, 240, 244, 279, 283, 340, 349, 350, 356
  Country comparisons, 1-3
  deaths data, 6, 7, 71-89, 106, 108, 112, 114, 121, 139-143, 193, 223, 237, 250, 251, 254, 275, 307, 323, 344
  High Consequence Infectious Disease, 18, 19, 153, 347
  Hospitalisations, 10-16, 21, 27, 30-34, 82, 93-94, 123, 138-139, 175-180, 182, 192, 202, 205, 208, 219, 234, 238, 265, 266, 294, 304, 349, 350
  Infection fatality rate, 4, 5, 87, 128, 138, 155, 248, 250, 267, 332, 340, 342, 343, 348, 354, 356
  Infection prevalence rate, 4, 5, 11, 16
  Religion impact, 6, 7
  Risk factors, 3, 4, 7, 19, 221, 248
  Symptoms, 1, 17, 29, 82, 130, 137, 276, 289, 305, 353
  Testing, *see PCR Testing*
  Waves, 9-10, 119, 353
Craig, Clare, 14, 20, 26, 34, 83, 89, 108, 111, 129, 141, 143, 345
CT Scans, 262, 274, 275, 276, 277, 278, 279, 280, 281, 282, 284, 287, 354
DNR (Do not resuscitate), 121, 130, 255, 349, 355
Dover, Tiffany, 45, 46
Emergent Biosolutions, 186, 188
Engler, Jonathan, 34, 36, 119, 124, 343
Epidemiology, 22, 91, 98, 101, 313, 330, 335, 358
European Medicines Agency (EMA), 187, 266
Fact checkers, iv, 104, 180, 181, 190
False positives, *see PCR testing*
Fauci, Anthony, 176, 232, 239, 243, 253, 254, 268, 272, 273, 322, 355
Flawed studies, 87-88, 101, 109-110, 111, 136, 202-211
Flu (influenza), 145-173, 231-236, 239, 240, 273-274, 278-279, 282-283, 299-307, 351-355,

Surveillance, 162-173
Vanishing flu, 145-156
Frontiers, 87-88
Fry, Hannah, 89, 90, 92, 93, 94, 135
Gain of function, 271, 311-333
Gilbert, Sarah, 186, 229, 357
Grainger, Cheryl, 223, 224, 225, 228
Guetzkow, Josh, 116, 142, 199
Happy hypoxia, 274, 275, 276, 277, 278, 280, 282, 284, 288, 354
Healthy vaccinee effect (HVE), 79, 80, 81, 106, 109, 135, 141, 197, 344, 345
Hurricane Katrina, 259
Iatrogenesis, 119, 120, 122, 123, 333, 343, 349, 355, 356, 358
Influenza, *see Flu*
Informed consent, v, 261, 265
Intensive Care Units (ICUs), 93, 101, 105, 123, 176, 210, 238, 248-254, 274-276, 280, 287, 292
Jikkyleaks, 107, 120, 245, 368, 370, 379, 382, 386
Johnson, Boris, 1, 261
Jones, Will, 58, 122, 125
Kenny, Laura, 85
Kirsch, Steve, 112, 185
Kory, Pierre, 88, 273, 274, 276, 277, 282, 286, 287, 288, 289, 290, 291
Lockdowns, 1, 3, 7-9, 18-25, 29-33, 94, 122-123, 128, 306, 330, 338-340, 342, 347, 351
London, 7, 21, 26, 30, 31, 33, 34, 35, 91, 95, 176, 353
Malone, Robert, xv, 88
Masks, iii, ii, ix, 86, 87, 156, 158, 235, 242, 267, 286, 289, 351, 385
McCullough, Peter, xv, 184
McLachlan, Scott, 13, 16, 21, 34, 55, 108, 199, 222, 223
Medicines and Healthcare products Regulatory Agency (MHRA), 98-101, 223-227, 228, 265, 266, 357
medRxiv, 100, 223
MERS, 257, 278, 279, 295, 302, 312, 313, 314, 317, 325, 329, 387
Midazolam. *See Opiods*
Miscategorisation, 61, 78, 79, 81, 84, 142, 202, 203, 206, 209, 345, 356, 364, 378
Misinformation, 64, 66, 67, 68, 69, 93, 101, 125, 184, 185, 186, 190, 220, 346, 356, 361, 375, 380
New York City (NYC), 126-128, 238-241, 253-259, 272, 285, 287-288, 335, 353, 354
NFL Covid-19 protocols, 1
NHS (National Health Service), 7, 13, 20, 24, 30, 35, 37, 38, 39, 80, 82, 96, 103, 104, 105, 106, 124, 166, 175, 176, 177, 178, 213, 214, 215, 216, 217, 218, 219, 220, 261, 262, 263, 264, 305, 306, 308, 309, 344, 353
NICE (National Institute for Health and Care Excellence), 91, 120, 121, 243, 244
NIMS (National Immunisation Management System), 76, 83, 106, 142, 176, 177, 345
NOMIS mortality statistics, 166, 172, 173
NPI (Non pharmaceutical intervention), 122, 170, 269
ONS (Office for National Statistics), 6, 23-25, 41-48, 71-73, 76-84, 89, 92, 95-98, 100-101, 104-111, 134-135, 139-144, 152, 166, 170-173, 180-182, 195-198, 207, 208, 335, 339, 344-345
Opioids, 120, 121, 243, 253, 349, 355
Fentanyl 253
Midazolam, 120, 121, 244, 245, 253, 254, 259, 355, 370, 383
PANDATA, 152, 183
Pandemic, 7-8, 143-155, 170-173, 256,-260, 273, 293-294, 321, 322, 323, 325, 326, 327, 329, 330,
Pinpoint pandemic, 241
PCR testing, 13-14, 17, 22, 23, 27, 34-36, 41-42, 46-48, 58- 60, 82-83, 151-155-161, 24-242, 263-264, 269, 270, 279, 293-309, 349-350
Confirmatory testing, 32, 36, 38-40, 42, 46, 48, 152, 158, 299
Cross Reactivity, 47, 151, 293, 294, 295, 296, 297, 299, 302, 303
False positives, 2, 3, 9, 10, 12-14, 15, 17, 22, 23, 26-39, 42, 47, 51, 149-163, 190, 191, 236, 294-307, 350
Positivity rate, 31, 32, 35, 40, 240, 296

Personal stories, 45-46, 85, 104, 185, 189-190, 213-220, 228-229, 256, 261-264, 270, 272, 287-289
Pieniazek, Norman, 241, 268-272
Pneumonia, *see Bacterial pneumonia*
Pregnancy, 84-86, 91, 95-96, 97-98, 103-105, 184, 209-210, 223-228, 268, 357
Raine, June, 224, 228
Rose, Jessica, 184
SAGE group, 18, 19, 20, 23, 25, 163, 340, 342, 347, 351
SARS, 257, 311-318
Schwab, Klaus, 7
Smally, Joel, 34, 122, 142, 207
Spikeopathy, 273, 274, 283, 287, 303, 314, 354, 384, 387, 388
Statistical illusion, 73, 76, 77, 84, 138
Stillbirths, 84, 85
Survivor bias, 85, 86, 138, 218
The Great Reset, 7, 219
The Lancet, 57-69, 109-110,
The Times, 48, 49, 62, 116, 150, 151, 185, 187, 188, 198, 302, 336, 340
Twindemic, 150, 372
UK lighthouse laboratories, 46, 47, 48, 308
UK Statistics Regulator, 61, 134
UKHSA (UK Health Security Agency), 83-85, 89, 96, 98, 101, 106, 107, 142, 153, 166-168, 179, 207, 266, 339, 352, 357
Unhealthy Vaccinee effect, 107, 345
Unvaccinated
  Definition, 59, 60, 83, 197
  Proportions, 96, 108, 112, 139
Vaccinated
  Definition, 93, 137, 195, 197
Vaccines, 203, 204, 205, 270
  AstraZeneca, 49, 110, 185, 186, 187, 188, 189, 193, 194, 209, 228, 229, 357
  Efficacy, 54, 73, 76, 77, 83, 84, 89, 93, 94, 96, 105, 109, 114, 135, 136, 137, 140, 181, 195, 196, 198, 203, 211, 266, 356
  Moderna, 83, 115, 116, 118, 136, 188, 189, 193, 194, 209, 224, 227, 267, 270, 358
  Pfizer, 45, 57-69, 90-95, 104, 113, 115-118, 136, 188-189, 209
  Placebo, 59, 60, 74, 76, 77, 94, 113, 138, 195, 196, 197, 198, 205, 345, 356, 357
  Rollout, i, 29, 46, 78, 79, 81, 138, 170, 266, 344, 357
  Safety, 77, 89, 101, 103, 104, 105, 108, 114, 115, 134, 135, 139, 140, 144, 214, 223, 267, 356, 357
VAERS (Vaccine Adverse Event Reporting System), ii, 54, 55, 56, 94, 115, 189, 190, 191, 192, 193, 194, 267, 357, 376
VALI (Vaping Acquired Lung Injury), 284, 285, 286, 290
Ventilators, 122, 149, 238, 240-245, 248-253, 256-260, 3553
Veronica, Nazarin, 91
Viruses and virus origins, 131, 256, 270, 311, 312, 316, 317, 319, 320, 325, 327, 329, 330, 333, 348, 387, 388
Wikipedia, 49, 50, 112, 313, 314
WONDER mortality statistics, 172, 173, 353
World Economic Forum (WEF), 7, 110, 347
Wuhan, 125-126, 232-234, 256, 269, 272, 276, 319-320, 327-333, 348, 353
Yellow Card, 189-193, 224-228, 266-267, 357

Made in United States
North Haven, CT
19 September 2026

18841672R00232